Salivary Diagnostics

$165.00

Salivary Diagnostics

250201

Edited by

David T. Wong
DMD, DMSc

WILEY-BLACKWELL

A John Wiley & Sons, Ltd., Publication

Blackwell Munksgaard, formerly an imprint of Blackwell Publishing was acquired by John Wiley & Sons in February 2007. Blackwell's publishing program has been merged with Wiley's global Scientific, Technical, and Medical business to form Wiley-Blackwell.

Editorial Office
2121 State Avenue, Ames, Iowa 50014-8300, USA

For details of our global editorial offices, for customer services and for information about how to apply for permission to reuse the copyright material in this book please see our website at www.wiley.com/wiley-blackwell.

Library of Congress Cataloging-in-Publication Data

Salivary diagnostics / edited by David T. Wong.
    p. ; cm.
Includes bibliographical references and index.
ISBN 978-0-8138-1333-2 (alk. paper)
1. Saliva–Examination.   2. Mouth–Diseases–Diagnosis.   I. Wong, David, 1954–
[DNLM: 1. Saliva–physiology.   2. Biological Markers.   3. Communicable Diseases–diagnosis.
4. Mouth Diseases–diagnosis. QY 125 S1678 2008]
RB52.5.S25   2008
616.3′16075–dc22   2008025004

A catalogue record for this book is available from the U.S. Library of Congress.

Set in 10/12pt Palatino by Aptara® Inc., New Delhi, India
Printed in Singapore by Fabulous Printers Pte Ltd

1   2008

Contents

Contributors

Arie van Nieuw Amerongen, PhD
Professor, Department of Oral Biochemistry, ACTA, Medical Faculty, Vrije Universiteit, Van der Boechorststraat 7, 1081 BT Amsterdam, the Netherlands

Jack Ballantyne, PhD
University of Central Florida, 4000 Central Florida, Orlando, FL 32816

Bruce J. Baum, DMD, PhD
National Institute of Dental and Craniofacial Research, 9402 Balfour Drive, Bethesda, MD 20814

R. Michael Buch, PhD
GlaxoSmithKline (GSK), Parsippany, NJ 07054

Joseph A. Califano, MD
Professor, Johns Hopkins Medical Center, Baltimore, MD 21287

Paul L.A.M. Corstjens, PhD
Assistant Professor, Department of Molecular Cell Biology, Leiden University Medical Center, 2300 RC Leiden, the Netherlands

Ana P. Cotrim, DDS, PhD
Gene Transfer Section, Gene Therapy and Therapeutics Branch, National Institute of Dental and Craniofacial Research, National Institutes of Health, Department of Health and Human Services, Bethesda, MD 20892

James J. Crall, DDS, ScD
Professor and Chair, Section of Pediatric Dentistry Director, MCHB National Oral Health Policy Center, UCLA School of Dentistry, CHS 23-020A, 10833 Le Conte Avenue, Los Angeles, CA 90095

Paul C. Denny, PhD
Professor, Division of Diagnostic Sciences, School of Dentistry, University of
Southern California, Los Angeles, CA 90089

Patricia A. Denny, MA
Division of Diagnostic Sciences, School of Dentistry, University of Southern
California, Los Angeles, CA 90089

Meghan Dubois, BS
Research Fellow, Michigan Center for Oral Health Research, University of
Michigan Clinical Center, 24 Frank Lloyd Wright Dr, Lobby M, Box 422,
Ann Arbor, MI 48106

Susan J. Fisher, PhD
Department of Cell and Tissue Biology, University of California at San
Francisco, 513 Parnassus Avenue, San Francisco, CA 94143

Christine K. Fortunato, BS
Department of Human Development and Family Studies, Pennsylvania State
University, University Park, PA 16803

Philip C. Fox, DDS
Visiting Scientist, Department of Oral Medicine, Carolinas Medical Center,
Charlotte, NC, and, President, PC Fox Consulting, LLCVia Monterione, 29,
06038 Spello (PG), Italy

Uttam Garg, PhD
Professor, University of Missouri Kansas City School of Medicine, Director,
Clinical Chemistry and Toxicology Laboratories, Department of Pathology
and Laboratory Medicine, Children's Mercy Hospitals and Clinics, Kansas
City, MO 64108

William V. Giannobile, DDS, DMedSc
Najjar Professor of Dentistry and Director, Michigan Center for Oral Health
Research, University of Michigan Clinical Center, Professor of Biomedical
Engineering, 24 Frank Lloyd Wright Dr, Lobby M, Box 422, Ann Arbor, MI
48106

Corinne M. Goldsmith, BS
Gene Transfer Section, Gene Therapy and Therapeutics Branch, National
Institute of Dental and Craniofacial Research, National Institutes of Health,
Department of Health and Human Services, Bethesda, MD 20892

Douglas A. Granger, PhD
Pennsylvania State University, University Park, PA 16802

Markus Hardt, PhD
Department of Cell and Tissue Biology, University of California at San
Francisco, 513 Parnassus Avenue, San Francisco, CA 94143

Leah C. Hibel, BS
Department of Biobehavioral Health, Pennsylvania State University, University Park, PA 16802

Matthew P. Hoffman, BDS, PhD
Matrix and Morphogenesis Unit, CDBRB, National Institutes of Health/NIDCR, 30 Convent Dr MSC 4370, Bethesda, MD 20892

Shen Hu, PhD
Associate Professor, Division of Oral Biology, UCLA School of Dentistry, 10833 Le Conte Avenue, Los Angeles, CA 90095

Zhanzhi Hu, PhD
Postdoctoral Research Fellow, Division of Oral Biology, UCLA School of Dentistry, Los Angeles, CA

Jane Juusola, PhD
Educational Programs Coordinator, Molecular Diagnostics Laboratory, Department of Pathology, Virginia Commonwealth University Medical Center, Richmond, VA 23298

Cees G.M. Kallenberg, MD
University Medical Center Groningen, Hanzeplein 1, PO Box 30 001, 9700 RB, Groninger, the Netherlands

Janet S. Kinney, RDH, MS
Assistant Professor, Michigan Center for Oral Health Research, University of Michigan Clinical Center, 24 Frank Lloyd Wright Dr, Lobby M, Box 422, Ann Arbor, MI 48106

Sarah M. Knox, PhD
Visiting Fellow, Matrix and Morphogenesis Unit, LCDB, NIDCR, NIH, 30 Convent Dr, Bethesda, MD 20892

Sreenivas Koka, DDS, MS, PhD
Professor, Mayo Clinic School of Medicine, Rochester, MN 55905

Eleni Kousvelari, DDS, DSc
Sandia National Laboratories, 1515 Eubank Boulevard, SE 5800, Albuquerque, NM 87185-1413

Karl E. Krueger, PhD
Program Director, Cancer Biomarkers Research Group, Division of Cancer Prevention, National Cancer Institute, 6130 Executive Plaza North, Suite 3136, Rockville, MD 20852

Joseph A. Loo, PhD
Professor, UCLA, Department of Biochemistry, 402 Boyer Hall, Los Angeles, CA 90095

Daniel Malamud, PhD
Professor, New York University College of Dentistry, New York, NY 10010

Irwin D. Mandel, DDS
Cedar Grove, NJ

Milton V. Marshall, PhD, DABT
Baylor College of Medicine, Department of Radiology, Division of Molecular Imaging, One Baylor Plaza MS, BCM 360, Houston, TX 77030

John T. McDevitt, PhD
Professor, Department of Chemistry and Biochemistry, Center for Nano and Molecular Science and Technology, Texas Materials Institute, University of Texas at Austin, 1 University Station A5300 Austin, TX 78712

Jiska Marianne Meijer, MD
Department of Oral and Maxillofacial Surgery, University Medical Center Groningen, 9700 RB Groningen, the Netherlands

James E. Melvin, DDS, PhD
Director, Center for Oral Biology, Professor of Pharmacology and Physiology, Aab Institute for Biomedical Sciences, University of Rochester, Medical Center Box 611, 601 Elmwood Avenue, Rochester, NY 14642

Fumi Mineshiba, DDS, PhD
Gene Transfer Section, Gene Therapy and Therapeutics Branch, National Institute of Dental and Craniofacial Research, National Institutes of Health, Department of Health and Human Services, Bethesda, MD 20892

Suhail K. Mithani, MD
Johns Hopkins Medical Center, Baltimore, MD 21287

Thiago Morelli, DDS
Research Fellow, Michigan Center for Oral Health Research, University of Michigan Clinical Center, 24 Frank Lloyd Wright Dr, Lobby M, Box 422, Ann Arbor, MI 48106

R. Sam Niedbala, PhD
Lehigh University, 6 East Parker Avenue, Bethelehem, PA 18015

Frank G. Oppenheim, DDS, PhD
Professor and Chair, BU Goldman School Of Graduate Dentistry, W-201, Boston, MA 02118

D. Stott Parker, PhD
Professor, Department of Computer Science, University of California at Los Angeles, Box 951596, 3532H BH, Los Angeles, CA 90095

Lance Presley, PhD, DABFT
Quest Diagnostics, Lenexa, KS 66219

Senrong Qi, DDS, PhD
Gene Transfer Section, Gene Therapy and Therapeutics Branch, National Institute of Dental and Craniofacial Research, National Institutes of Health, Department of Health and Human Services, Bethesda, MD 20892

Renli Qiao, MD, PhD
Associate Professor of Clinical Medicine, Pulmonary and Critical Care Medicine, Keck School of Medicine, University of Southern California, 2011 Zonal Avenue, HMR911, Los Angeles, CA 90033

Gabor Z. Racz, PhD
Gene Transfer Section, Gene Therapy and Therapeutics Branch, National Institute of Dental and Craniofacial Research, National Institutes of Health, Department of Health and Human Services, Bethesda, MD 20892

Christoph A. Ramseier, DMD
School of Dental Medicine, Department of Periodontology, University of Berne, Freiburgstrasse 7, 3012 Bern, Switzerland

Lindsay Rayburn, BS
Research Specialist, Michigan Center for Oral Health Research, University of Michigan Clinical Center, 24 Frank Lloyd Wright Dr, Lobby M, Box 422, Ann Arbor, MI 48106

Nelson L. Rhodus, DMD, MPH, FACD
Professor and Director, Division of Oral Medicine, School of Dentistry, Adjunct Professor, Department of Otolaryngology, School of Medicine, Academy of Distinguished Teachers, Diplomate, American Board of Oral Medicine, University of Minnesota, 7536 Moos HST; 515 Delaware St SE, Minneapolis, MN 55455

Victor G. Romanenko, PhD
Research Assistant Professor, University of Rochester Medical Center, 601 Elmwood Avenue, Rochester, NY 14642

Yuval Samuni, DMD, PhD
Gene Transfer Section, Gene Therapy and Therapeutics Branch, National Institute of Dental and Craniofacial Research, National Institutes of Health, Department of Health and Human Services, Bethesda, MD 20892

Jonathan A. Ship, DDS, PhD
New York University College of Dentistry, Professor, Division of David B
Kriser Dental Center, Department of Clinical Research Center, Weissman, 421
First Ave, 233 W, New York, NY 10010, NYU Mail Code: 9447

Chakwan Siew, PhD
American Dental Association, 211 East Chicago Avenue, Chicago, IL 60611

Stuart R. Smith, BDS, PhD
GlaxoSmithKline (GSK), Weybridge, Surrey, United Kingdom KT130DE

Sudhir Srivastava, PhD, MPH, MS
Program Director, EDRN, National Cancer Institute, 6130 Executive
Boulevard, EPN 330F, Bethesda, MD 20892

Takayuki Sugito, DDS, PhD
Gene Transfer Section, Gene Therapy and Therapeutics Branch, National
Institute of Dental and Craniofacial Research, National Institutes of Health,
Department of Health and Human Services, Bethesda, MD 20892

Lawrence A. Tabak, DDS, PhD
Director, National Institute of Dental and Craniofacial Research, 30 Convent
Drive, Bethesda, MD 20892

Shawn Than, MS
University of California at Los Angeles, School of Dentistry, 10833 Le Conte
Avenue, 73-017 CHS, Los Angeles, CA 90095

Michael D. Turner, DDS, MD
Assistant Professor, New York University College of Dentistry, New York, NY
10010

Enno C.I. Veerman, PhD
Professor, Academic Centre for Dentistry Amsterdam (ACTA), van der
Boechorststraat 7, 1081 BT Amsterdam, the Netherlands

Arjan Vissink, DMD, MD, PhD
Professor, Department of Oral and Maxillofacial Surgery, University Medical
Center Groningen, Groningen, the Netherlands

Antonis Voutetakis, MD, PhD
Gene Transfer Section, Gene Therapy and Therapeutics Branch, National
Institute of Dental and Craniofacial Research, National Institutes of Health,
Department of Health and Human Services, Bethesda, MD 20892

David R. Walt, PhD
Robinson Professor of Chemistry, Tufts University, Department of Chemistry,
62 Talbot Avenue, Medford, MA 02155

Andy Wolff, DMD
Saliwell Ltd Medical Systems, Hatamar St, Harutzim 60917, Israel

David T. Wong, DMD, DMSc
University of California at Los Angeles, Professor and Associate Dean of
Research, School of Dentistry, Director, Dental Research Institute, 10833 Le
Conte Avenue, 73-017 CHS, Los Angeles, CA 90095

Weihong Yan, PhD
Keck Bioinformatics User Center, Department of Chemistry and
Biochemistry, UCLA, 607 Charles E. Young Drive East, Los Angeles, CA 90095

John R. Yates, PhD
Professor, Scripps Research Institute, 10550, North Torrey Pines Rd, SR11,
Department Cell Biology, La Jolla, CA 92037

Weixia Yu, PhD
University of California at Los Angeles, School of Dentistry, 10833 Le Conte
Avenue, 73-017 CHS, Los Angeles, CA 90095

Changyu Zheng, MD, PhD
Gene Transfer Section, Gene Therapy and Therapeutics Branch, National
Institute of Dental and Craniofacial Research, National Institutes of Health,
Department of Health and Human Services, Bethesda, MD 20892

Bernhard G. Zimmermann, PhD
Assistant Researcher, Division of Oral Biology, UCLA School of Dentistry, Los
Angeles, CA 90095

Foreword

"...there is no disease that I spit on more than treachery."
Aeschylus (525-456 BC)

Saliva is one of those things you love or hate. Although historically scorned in literature, viewed by many cultures as the ultimate insult and clinically "damned," investigators, clinicians, and our patients are increasingly turning to saliva as a safe and "non-invasive" indicator of health and disease. Many biomarkers may be measured using oral fluids. This opens up the extraordinary opportunity of enhancing research conducted in the field or expanding the versatility of point-of-care diagnostics by using saliva as the diagnostic fluid.

Behavioral research that seeks to correlate physiological with psychological status has been revolutionized by the availability of assays that accurately measure such hormones as cortisol in saliva. Reaction (and sometimes aversion) to a needle stick for collection of blood has a far greater chance of disturbing the subject than does the collection of oral fluid. Accurate and rapid diagnostic tests that can be performed in the privacy of one's home or in a community or field setting are proving crucial to controlling a number of diseases and conditions. For example, such tests for sexually transmitted diseases can yield diagnosis in the early stages of the infection resulting in a decreased transmission from asymptomatic patients. Infectious diseases kill approximately 15 million persons worldwide each year. Saliva-based point-of-care diagnostic tests, which dispense with the need for a phlebotomist, have the potential to overcome some of the limitations and challenges of the modest medical infrastructures found in the developing world.

Continued advances in biomedical engineering coupled to enhance understanding of the salivary proteome will make it possible to one day implant biosensors directly in the mouth. These in-dwelling "labs on a chip" will help catalyze a shift from our current practice of disease detection to a health surveillance through detection and measurement of multiple, relevant biomarkers in saliva. With the advances of this technology comes the additional significant obligation to ensure the privacy of patients. While saliva collection is facile and anatomically non-invasive, oral fluids have sufficient quantities of DNA to decode genotypes. Thus, one must be equally discreet with saliva and blood samples.

The numerous contributors to this volume are experts in their respective areas and provide the historical background as well as the status of current research. They see salivary diagnosis developing into a new "industry;" they deal with its utilization in dentists' and physicians' offices and explore reimbursement mechanisms for the services. The projection into the future also considers testing at home and concerns regarding the commercial market.

Salivary Diagnostics provides insight into an area that will increasingly involve many disciplines.

Lawrence A. Tabak, DDS, PhD
Irwin D. Mandel, DDS

Preface

This book is dedicated to the visionaries who planted and nurtured the seeds for saliva diagnostics to flourish and bear harvest.

The publication of "Salivary Diagnostics" marks a defining moment. Revolutionary genome-wide research tools have spawned remarkable advances in human genomics, proteomics, and metabolomics. These interrelated developments, largely driven by the Human Genome Project, ushered a new dawn on the ancient study of saliva. We have learned that human saliva contains a repertoire of proteins, glycoproteins, lipids, metabolites, RNA and genomic information, in addition to the 700 microbial species and is endowed with many of the same diagnostic analytes inherent in other bodily fluids such as blood, cerebral spinal fluid, and urine.

The National Institute of Dental and Craniofacial Research charged into the inclement waters of risky science and planted its flag on the *terra incognita* of saliva omics. The completion of the human salivary proteome project is a landmark accomplishment marking the discovery of the first diagnostic alphabet in saliva. Now, the race is on for a self-contained diagnostic chip that can provide clinical information to a physician or dentist at point-of-care before a patient leaves the clinician's office during a regular visit.

From the adventurer's past, saliva diagnostics emerges into the clockmaker's present. Now is the time for us to exchange adventurer's leather jacket for a clockmaker's loupe. We are in the critical phase where the scientific foundations of saliva for clinical disease detection must be established beyond any doubt. Only on the broadest foundation of absolute scientific integrity can we build the highest edifice of saliva diagnostics in the shortest possible time.

And the future? With the potential to revolutionize delivery of diagnostic services both on the personal and public health levels, the future of saliva diagnostics is enormous.

David T. Wong, DMD, DMSc

Acknowledgment

I am thankful to Tanya Lazzar, the project manager; Carol Field, the task master; Shelby Hayes and Sophia Joyce at Wiley-Blackwell for their skills and professionalism in putting the book together.

To Alik Segal, who patiently assisted me in the editorial tasks of this book. And to my wife, Sharon, who supports me unconditionally.

Part I

Background and Foundation

Salivary gland development and regeneration

Sarah M. Knox and Matthew P. Hoffman

INTRODUCTION

The formation of salivary glands throughout embryogenesis is exquisitely or-chestrated so that at birth the organ system is primed and ready to produce sali-vary secretions under the control of autonomic innervation. An appreciation for the developmental mechanisms that give rise to this complex and highly regulated system is an important foundation to understanding the physiology and biochemistry of postnatal saliva production, which is the fluid required for salivary diagnostics. In this chapter, we compare what is known about human salivary gland development with mouse submandibular gland development and highlight human genetic conditions that provide profound insight into gland development. We have also included a section on potential strategies for salivary gland regeneration.

SALIVARY GLAND DEVELOPMENT

The salivary organ system is composed of three pairs of major glands: the sub-mandibular (SMG), parotid, and sublingual (SLG), which together produce more than 90% of saliva, as well as numerous minor glands lining the oral cavity. The major salivary glands share homologous mechanisms of branch-ing morphogenesis during organogenesis to produce an intricate branched structure of ducts with terminal buds that differentiate into acinar structures. They are also well supplied by the vascular system, which develops alongside, and is intimately associated with the branching epithelial structures. Little is known about vascular development in the salivary gland; salivary secretion is accompanied by increased blood flow to the glands, and an extensive cap-illary network is found around the striated duct where ion exchange occurs. The salivary glands are innervated by the parasympathetic and sympathetic branches of the autonomic nervous system, which are essential for postnatal saliva secretion and will be the focus of a section below. Human salivary glands are composed of different types of acinar cells that produce distinct types of saliva: parotid acinar cells are serous and secrete a watery serous saliva; SMG acinar cells are approximately 80% serous and also contain mucous secretory units capped by seromucous demilunes, producing a seromucous saliva; SLG acinar cells are mixed secretory units but are mainly composed of mucous cells and produce a mucous saliva. The reader is directed to a textbook for a comprehensive histological description of cell types within the glands.[1]

The development of human and mouse salivary glands is similar in many aspects, and to highlight this point, we will compare human and mouse development in this chapter. There have been a few histological reports documenting human salivary gland development[2–4] that basically corroborate the early histological descriptions by Thoma in 1919, shown in Figure 1.1.[5] The parotid gland is derived from the oral ectoderm, and the mesenchyme is neural crest-derived ectomesenchyme. However, the origin of the SMG and SLG epithelium has not been clearly defined. Humans with mutations in the ectodysplasin A (*EDA*) gene develop hypohidrotic ectodermal dysplasia (HED), characterized by defects in teeth, hair, sweat glands, and salivary glands, and mice lacking the EDA receptor (*Edar*) have SMG aplasia or hypoplasia (recently reviewed in reference 6). Mice lacking p63, an ectodermal marker, have no salivary glands,[7] suggesting that the origins of the SMG and SLG are ectodermal.

Human salivary gland development begins with the thickening of the oral epithelium to form a placode at a specific site in the oral cavity. Figure 1.1 shows the parotid placode forming in the lateral border of the buccal sulcus of a human embryo. Factors that define the site of placode initiation of human and mouse salivary glands are not known. However, a recent review of salivary gland development in *Drosophila* describes how global patterning genes, such as the homeotic gene *scr*, define the site of salivary gland initiation, whereas other genes repress gland initiation in the anterior–posterior and dorsal–ventral axes.[8] Experimental evidence from *Drosophila* provides a paradigm for how gland initiation is likely to occur in humans and mice, and the reader is referred to Denny et al.[9] for discussion.

The next stage in development is the expansion and invagination of the placode as an epithelial bud into a condensing mesenchyme at around 6–8 weeks in humans (Fig. 1.2) and embryonic day 12 (E12) in mice.[4,5] The condensing mesenchyme provides growth factors and extracellular matrix that play an instructive role in branching morphogenesis of the mouse salivary gland (reviewed in references 6 and 10). The human SMG epithelium then undergoes successive rounds of branching morphogenesis, which involves cleft formation, end bud expansion, and duct elongation, finally appearing as solid end buds and cords of epithelial cells (Fig. 1.3) at 10 weeks,[2,5] similar to an E14 mouse SMG (Fig. 1.2). By 14 weeks, functional differentiation of the gland has started with branches and terminal buds forming lumens to establish presumptive ducts and acini.

Branching morphogenesis continues until approximately 12 weeks where lumenization of ducts and polarization of the end bud epithelium begins, similar to E15 in the mouse. However, from approximately 12 to 28 weeks, cellular differentiation begins with polarization of the end buds and lumenization of the ducts with secretory material appearing in the lumens of the ducts and end buds, similar to E17 in the mouse SMG (Fig. 1.2). Also, during mouse SMG development, the gene expression of secretory products, such as parotid secretory protein (PSP) and submandibular gland protein C (SMGc), is barely detectable

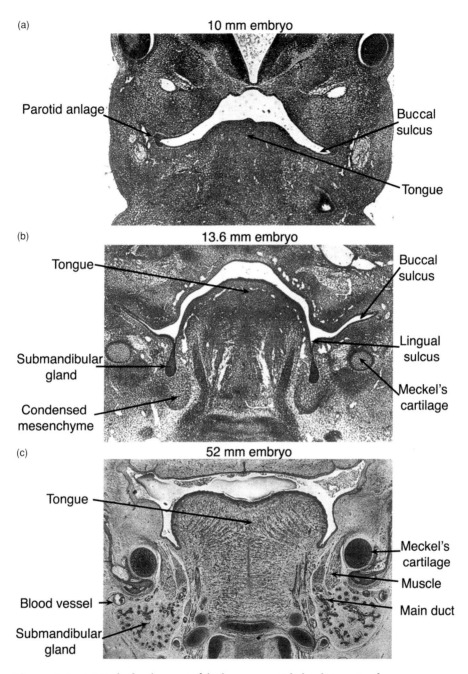

Figure 1.1 (a) Early development of the human parotid gland. A section from an approximately 6–8-week-old human embryo shows the thickening of the parotid placode, which forms in the major groove of the buccal sulcus. (b) Development of the human SMG. At approximately 6–8 weeks, but later than that in part (a), the SMG rudiment extends into a condensed mesenchyme capsule that provides growth factors and matrix, which stimulate branching morphogenesis. (c) At 10 weeks, the SMG has undergone extensive branching within the mesenchymal capsule. The main duct is visible, and lumens can be seen in some minor ducts. (All figures from Reference 5.)

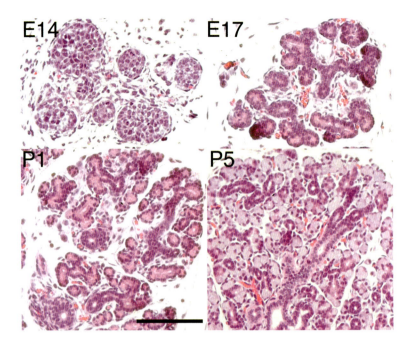

Figure 1.2 Development of the mouse SMG. At E14, the branched epithelium consists of solid end buds and ducts. By E17, functional differentiation has begun with lumen formation and end bud polarization. At P1, the acinar cells are differentiated, but connective tissue remains around the parenchyma. By P5, the functioning acini have continued to enlarge, and ductal differentiation is apparent. Bar = 200 μm.

by real-time polymerase chain reaction (PCR) at E15, but increase at E17 and after birth at postnatal day 1 (P1) (Fig. 1.3). By 13–16 weeks in human SMGs, cells adjacent to lumens show the presence of desmosomes and numerous microvilli projecting into the intercellular space. The cytoplasm of some cells contained serous, but not mucous, granules, and the luminal contents were strongly positive for glycosaminoglycans.[11] The epithelium is surrounded by a well-developed basal lamina and contains a few elongated cells that appear similar to myoepithelial cells. By 16 weeks, both striated ducts and intercalated ducts are distinguishable. From 20 to 24 weeks, acinar cells begin to predominate; in rodents (E18), granular convoluted tubules (GCTs) appear. By 28 weeks there is a marked increase in the amount of acini (and GCT cells in rodents),

Figure 1.3 Differential gene expression of secretory products highlights the development of secretory function during mouse SMG development. FGF2 expression is increased during branching morphogenesis, whereas PSP and SMGc expression begins after E15 when functional differentiation begins. During postnatal development, EGF and NGF expression dramatically increases after puberty. Gene expression, normalized to the housekeeping gene 29S, was measured by real-time PCR, over a developmental time course from E12 to adult (Adt).

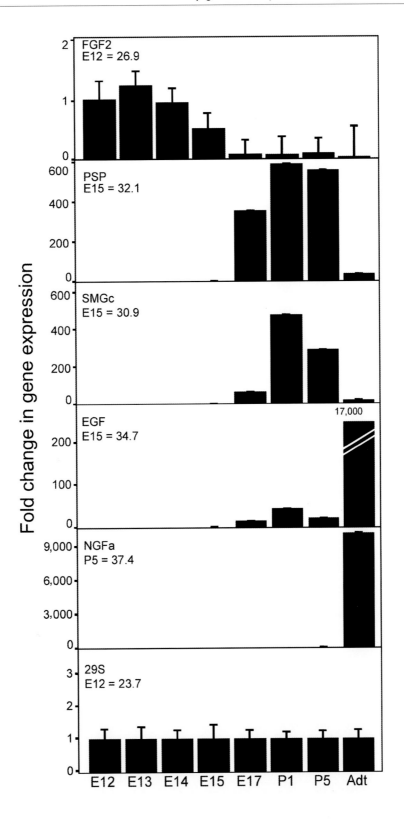

although less secretory products are apparent.[2] At birth, only serous cells are present, with connective tissue spaces between the acini, similar to P1 of mouse SMG development (Fig. 1.2). In humans, prenatal growth and differentiation continue after 28 weeks such that the glands are capable of secreting saliva in response to parasympathetic stimulation at P1. In comparison, postnatal mouse SMG development, particularly the differentiation of the GCTs by puberty, is evidenced by expression of GCT secretory gene products such as EGF, which is weakly expressed from E17 and at birth but dramatically increases after puberty, and NGF, which is barely detectable at P5 but also dramatically increases with postnatal ductal differentiation (Fig. 1.3).

DEVELOPMENT OF THE AUTONOMIC INNERVATION OF SALIVARY GLANDS

Innervation of salivary glands by the parasympathetic and sympathetic branches of the autonomic nervous system is essential for secretion and tissue homeostasis because denervation results in loss of saliva production and atrophy of the tissue. For a comprehensive review of salivary gland innervation, the reader is directed to Proctor and Carpenter (2007).[12] Embryonic innervation of the human salivary glands has been described from histological sections,[4] but most experimental investigations have used rodent SMGs.

There are important differences between sympathetic and parasympathetic nerve development in salivary glands. First, sympathetic innervation is postnatal, around P3–P5. In contrast, parasympathetic innervation develops at the same time as the gland and requires an interaction with the salivary epithelium.[13] Second, the sympathetic efferent nerves, which release norepinephrine, arise from the superior cervical ganglion located away from the gland in the thoracic spinal cord. However, the parasympathetic nerves secrete acetylcholine and extend either from the otic ganglion, which innervates the parotid, or from the submandibular ganglion, which innervates both the SMG and SLG. The submandibular ganglion lies within the SMG, whereas the otic ganglion is separate from the parotid. Interestingly, branching morphogenesis of the parotid gland does not begin until otic neurons reach the initial epithelial bud. Most of what is known about embryonic development of the glandular parasympathetic ganglions is derived from early studies on mouse SMG development.[14,15]

HUMAN GENETIC CONDITIONS AFFECTING SALIVARY GLAND DEVELOPMENT

There are a few human genetic conditions that affect salivary gland development leading to aplasia or hypoplasia. However, two of the most informative are due to mutations in genes that affect fibroblast growth factor (FGF) receptor signaling. Mutations in FGF10, resulting in haploinsufficiency, have been linked to aplasia of lacrimal and salivary glands (ALSGs) syndrome (OMIM

180920),[16] an autosomal dominant anomaly with aplasia or hypoplasia of the lacrimal and salivary systems. Importantly, mice also missing one copy of FGF10 or its receptor, FGFR2b, have severe salivary gland hypoplasia. Additionally, lacrimoauriculodentodigital (LADD) syndrome is an autosomal dominant disorder characterized by aplasia or hypoplasia of the lacrimal and salivary systems as well as abnormalities of the face, ears, eyes, mouth, teeth, digits, and genitourinary system. LADD syndrome occurs as a result of mutations in fibroblast growth factor receptors 2 and 3 (FGFR2, FGFR3), as well as in FGF10.[17,18] ALSG and LADD syndrome are thought to be allelic disorders with variable expressivity, possibly due to different types of FGF10 mutations.[18]

Other genetic diseases showing salivary gland phenotypes include mutations in EDA and its receptor, EDAR, which result in HED, characterized by abnormal ectodermal organs such as hair, teeth, sweat glands, and salivary glands. Similar phenotypes occur in *Tabby* (Eda^{Ta}) and *Downless* ($Edar^{dl}$) mutant mice.[19] Eda^{Ta} SMGs are hypoplastic, while $Edar^{dl}$ SMGs are dysplastic. Eda/Edar signaling is essential for branching morphogenesis, lumen formation, and differentiation, but not for initial gland formation.[20]

MODEL SYSTEMS TO STUDY SALIVARY GLAND DEVELOPMENT

As described earlier, there are many similarities in the development of the mouse SMG compared to human salivary glands, both in the histological development and also in the development of the secretory function of the gland. A major advantage of using mouse SMG to model human gland development is the ability to experimentally manipulate the mouse genome. Ex vivo mouse SMG organ culture allows the investigation of branching morphogenesis in a complex system that contains mesenchyme, epithelium, parasympathetic neurons, and endothelial cells forming the developing vasculature (Fig. 1.4). E12 SMGs, beginning with a single epithelial bud in a condensed mesenchyme, display reproducible branching morphogenesis in serum-free culture and appear similar to SMGs in vivo. SMG organ culture has been used extensively to explore the molecular mechanisms of epithelium–mesenchyme interactions, and a broad range of molecules have been identified that regulate epithelial branching, including constituents of the extracellular matrix, cell adhesion receptors, proteases, and growth factors. The reader is referred to recent detailed reviews on mouse SMG branching morphogenesis.[6,10]

THE GOAL OF FUNCTIONAL SALIVARY GLAND REGENERATION

An irreversible loss of salivary gland function often occurs in humans after removal of salivary tumors, after therapeutic radiation of head and neck tumors, as a result of Sjögren's syndrome, and in certain rare genetic syndromes affecting FGF signaling. The loss of salivary gland function impairs the oral health of

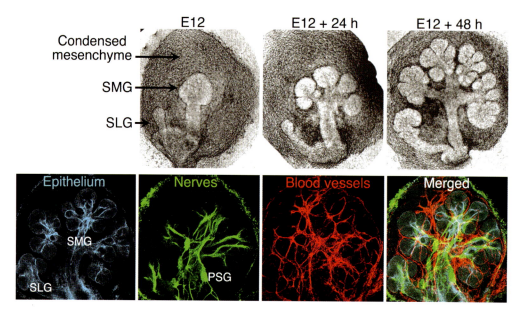

Figure 1.4 Ex vivo organ culture of E12 mouse SMGs for 48 h in serum-free media recapitulates the development of the gland in vivo. A single epithelial bud undergoes branching morphogenesis. The lower panel highlights the cellular complexity of the SMG. The epithelium (blue, laminin α1) is surrounded by nerves (green, β3-tubulin) that extend from the parasympathetic submandibular ganglion at the base of the primary duct. The mesenchyme contains a large network of blood vessels (red, PECAM). The image is a projection of a confocal stack.

these patients and significantly affects their quality of life. Currently, patients are treated with parasympathetic mimetics such as pilocarpine, which rely on some gland function. Patients with some remaining salivary tissue could benefit from genetic reengineering to restore tissue function or from a regenerative approach to repair the gland. Patients with little or no functional gland tissue may need regenerative therapy or replacement with artificial salivary glands.[21]

Animal models used to investigate and develop techniques for functional regeneration of salivary glands include rodents, minipigs, and primates. Rat models have been used to investigate the effects of irradiation,[22] denervation, and ductal ligation,[12] and intraductal adenovirus injection for gene therapy.[23] Minipigs are a large animal model whose SMGs resemble the human gland and are useful for studying changes after gland irradiation[24] and for preclinical applications of gene transfer to salivary glands.[25]

Genetic reengineering

Most research to date has focused on the reengineering and replacement of salivary glands. Reengineering of salivary glands is based on inductive gene transfer technology using recombinant viruses. A number of genes have been delivered successfully to nonhuman salivary glands in vivo, including human aquaporin 1 (*Aqp1*)[26] and aquaporin 5 (*Aqp5*).[27] Aquaporins are water channels located in acinar cells that facilitate the movement of water across the plasma bilayer. Aqp1 has been shown to be acutely downregulated after radiation therapy. Gene transfer of Aqp1 using adeno-associated virus into salivary glands partially transformed ductal cells into functional secretory cells in rats and minipigs.[25,28] Aqp1 gene therapy on irradiated human patients using adeno-associated virus is currently in clinical trials. This topic is elaborated in Chapter 27.

Regenerate and repair

The use of stem cells to regenerate tissue is increasingly being utilized in many organ systems. Recently, Lombaert and coworkers[29] used GFP-labeled bone marrow stem cells (BMSCs) to regenerate irradiated mouse SMGs. They measured an increase in salivary secretion after mobilization of BMSCs in the irradiated tissue. However, the stem cells were not part of the epithelial compartment of the gland, but were exerting their effect from the mesenchyme.[29] Potentially, the effect may be mediated by repopulation of the vasculature or nerves to increase blood supply or innervation, as a reduction in either of these structures leads to gland atrophy.[12]

Replace

Patients who have lost parenchyma because of disease, radiation therapy, or surgery are not candidates for gene transfer or regenerative/repair strategies, and total organ replacement is required. Organ replacement is hampered by the cellular complexity of the salivary gland and the necessity to regenerate functional secretory epithelium, nerves, blood vessels, and stromal tissue in an encapsulated organ space. Engineering of an "artificial" salivary gland may involve the use of synthetic or ECM-derived 3D scaffolds onto which cells are seeded to form a polarized secretory epithelium.[26,30]

In conclusion, understanding how salivary glands develop may facilitate gland regeneration and/or tissue-engineering approaches to restore secretory function in adult glands. Fundamental scientific knowledge provides a foundation for therapeutic interventions and will benefit from the translational and clinical utilities of saliva and its analytes, the thematic topic of this book.

Acknowledgments

The authors thank Harry Grant, Vaishali Patel, and Ivan Rebustini for critical reading of the manuscript. This work was supported by the Intramural Research Program of the National Institute for Dental and Craniofacial Research at the National Institutes of Health.

REFERENCES

1. Ten Cate AR. *Oral Histology: Development, Structure, and Function*, 5th edn. St. Louis: Mosby; 1998.
2. el-Mohandes EA, Botros KG, Bondok AA. Prenatal development of the human submandibular gland. Acta Anat (Basel) 1987;130(3):213–18.

3. Guizetti B, Radlanski RJ. Development of the submandibular gland and its closer neighboring structures in human embryos and fetuses of 19–67 mm CRL. Ann Anat 1996;178(6):509–14.

4. Merida-Velasco JA, Sanchez-Montesinos I, Espin-Ferra J, Garcia-Garcia JD, Garcia-Gomez S, Roldan-Schilling V. Development of the human submandibular salivary gland. J Dent Res 1993;72(8):1227–32.

5. Thoma KH. A contribution to the knowledge of the development of the submaxillary and sublingual salivary glands in human embryos. J Dent Res 1919;1:95–143.

6. Tucker AS. Salivary gland development. Semin Cell Dev Biol 2007;18(2):237–44.

7. Yang A, Schweitzer R, Sun D, et al. p63 is essential for regenerative proliferation in limb, craniofacial and epithelial development. Nature 1999;398(6729):714–18.

8. Kerman BE, Cheshire AM, Andrew DJ. From fate to function: the *Drosophila* trachea and salivary gland as models for tubulogenesis. Differentiation 2006;74(7):326–48.

9. Denny PC, Ball WD, Redman RS. Salivary glands: a paradigm for diversity of gland development. Crit Rev Oral Biol Med 1997;8(1):51–75.

10. Patel VN, Rebustini IT, Hoffman MP. Salivary gland branching morphogenesis. Differentiation 2006;74(7):349–64.

11. Gibson MH. The prenatal human submandibular gland: a histological, histochemical and ultrastructural study. Anat Anz 1983;153(1):91–105.

12. Proctor GB, Carpenter GH. Regulation of salivary gland function by autonomic nerves. Auton Neurosci 2007;133(1):3–18.

13. Coughlin MD. Target organ stimulation of parasympathetic nerve growth in the developing mouse submandibular gland. Dev Biol 1975;43(1):140–58.

14. Coughlin MD. Early development of parasympathetic nerves in the mouse submandibular gland. Dev Biol 1975;43(1):123–39.

15. Nishi R. Ability of developing epithelia to attract neurite outgrowth in culture is not correlated with the appearance of laminin. J Neurosci Res 1988;21(2–4):307–14.

16. Entesarian M, Matsson H, Klar J, et al. Mutations in the gene encoding fibroblast growth factor 10 are associated with aplasia of lacrimal and salivary glands. Nat Genet 2005;37:125–7.

17. Rohmann E, Brunner HG, Kayserili H, et al. Mutations in different components of FGF signaling in LADD syndrome. Nat Genet 2006;38(4):414–17.

18. Milunsky JM, Zhao G, Maher TA, Colby R, Everman DB. LADD syndrome is caused FGF10 mutations. Clin Genet 2006;69(4):349–54.

19. Thesleff I, Mikkola ML. Death receptor signaling giving life to ectodermal organs. Sci STKE 2002;2002(131):PE22.

20. Jaskoll T, Zhou YM, Trump G, Melnick M. Ectodysplasin receptor-mediated signaling is essential for embryonic submandibular salivary gland development. Anat Rec A Discov Mol Cell Evol Biol 2003;271(2):322–31.

21. Baum BJ. Prospects for re-engineering salivary glands. Adv Dent Res 2000;14:84–8.

22. Vissink A, s-Gravenmade EJ, Ligeon EE, Konings WT. A functional and chemical study of radiation effects on rat parotid and submandibular/sublingual glands. Radiat Res 1990;124(3):259–65.

23. Mastrangeli A, O'Connell B, Aladib W, Fox PC, Baum BJ, Crystal RG. Direct in vivo adenovirus-mediated gene transfer to salivary glands. Am J Physiol 1994;266(6, Pt 1):G1146–55.

24. Radfar L, Sirois DA. Structural and functional injury in minipig salivary glands following fractionated exposure to 70 Gy of ionizing radiation: an animal model for human radiation-induced salivary gland injury. Oral Surg Oral Med Oral Pathol Oral Radiol Endod 2003;96(3):267–74.

25. Shan Z, Li J, Zheng C, et al. Increased fluid secretion after adenoviral-mediated transfer of the human aquaporin-1 cDNA to irradiated miniature pig parotid glands. Mol Ther 2005;11(3):444–51.

26. Tran SD, Sugito T, Dipasquale G, et al. Re-engineering primary epithelial cells from rhesus monkey parotid glands for use in developing an artificial salivary gland. Tissue Eng 2006;12(10):2939–48.

27. Delporte C, Baum BJ. Preclinical and biological studies using recombinant adenoviruses encoding aquaporins 1 and 5. Eur J Morphol 1998;36 (Suppl):118–22.

28. Zheng C, Hoque AT, Braddon VR, Baum BJ, O'Connell BC. Evaluation of salivary gland acinar and ductal cell-specific promoters in vivo with recombinant adenoviral vectors. Hum Gene Ther 2001;12(18):2215–23.

29. Lombaert IM, Wierenga PK, Kok T, Kampinga HH, deHaan G, Coppes RP. Mobilization of bone marrow stem cells by granulocyte colony-stimulating factor ameliorates radiation-induced damage to salivary glands. Clin Cancer Res 2006;12(6):1804–12.

30. Sun T, Zhu J, Yang X, Wang S. Growth of miniature pig parotid cells on biomaterials in vitro. Arch Oral Biol 2006;51(5):351–8.

Salivary gland physiology relevant to diagnostics

Victor G. Romanenko and James E. Melvin

INTRODUCTION

Oral fluid, also known as "whole" or "total" saliva, is typically collected by having the subject drool into a cup, with or without stimulation (see Chapter 3). Oral fluid is composed primarily of saliva secreted by the three major paired glands—parotid, submandibular, and sublingual—and numerous minor glands located throughout the oral cavity. Whole saliva also contains gingival crevicular fluid, sloughed oral epithelial cells, nasopharyngeal discharge, food debris, and bacteria and their products. Despite this "contamination," the flow rate and composition of oral fluid overwhelmingly reflects secretions from the major salivary glands. Ductal saliva can be collected using gland-specific devices to restrict analysis to the output from an individual gland, and thereby eliminate nonsaliva constituents (see Chapter 4). The analysis of oral fluid is proving to be an invaluable diagnostic tool because (i) saliva sampling is a noninvasive, fast, and inexpensive process; (ii) saliva flow rate and ionic composition are easy to measure by straightforward methods; and importantly (iii) recent advances in understanding the salivation mechanism should help to confirm the molecular basis of many disorders and thus provide critical information for developing more specific and efficient treatment modalities.

Fluid and electrolyte secretion by salivary glands is considered to be a two-step process (Fig. 2.1). Initially, the acinus, also known as a secretory end piece, secretes a plasmalike primary saliva. This process is driven by transepithelial Cl^- movement.[1-3] The acinar tight junctions provide a cation-selective pathway for Na^+ flux down its electrical gradient into the acinar lumen. The resultant osmotic gradient for NaCl causes water movement, via water channels and across tight junctions, to produce an isotonic, plasmalike primary fluid. Secondarily, the ion composition of the primary fluid is modified in the salivary ducts by the action of absorption and secretion pathways. While there is a general consensus regarding the secretion mechanism as well as the molecular identity of the key participants in the production of the primary saliva, the ductal transport machinery that modifies the ionic composition of saliva is less well understood.

Fluid secretion by the major salivary glands is largely initiated in response to stimulation of muscarinic receptors on the cell surface of acinar cells when

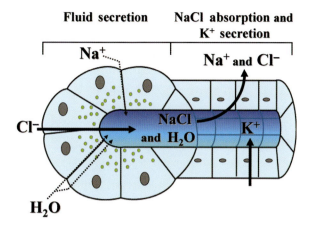

Figure 2.1 Secretion model. Fluid secretion is a two-step process. Transepithelial Cl⁻ move-ment drives the fluid and electrolyte secretion process in acinar cells. The accumulation of Cl⁻ in the acinar lumen is neutralized by Na⁺ movement across tight junctions and water fol-lows osmotically. As the primary saliva transits through the ductal network, much of the NaCl secreted by the acinar cells is reabsorbed while K⁺ is secreted.

the neurotransmitter acetylcholine is released by parasympathetic nerve ter-minals (Fig. 2.2). Association of acetylcholine with its receptor is coupled to the activation of G proteins, and consequently, an elevation of intracel-lular $[Ca^{2+}]$ through a phospholipase C (PLC)/inositol trisphosphate (IP_3)-dependent pathway. In turn, this increase in intracellular $[Ca^{2+}]$ triggers the opening of apical Cl⁻ channels. The extent of the outwardly directed electro-chemical gradient for Cl⁻ defines the magnitude of intracellular Cl⁻ efflux across the apical membrane of acinar cells. Na⁺ and then water follow Cl⁻ into the acinar lumen. Thus, for sustained secretion, as during a meal, the intra-cellular Cl⁻ must remain concentrated above its electrochemical gradient. The driving force for Cl⁻ uptake is provided by the Na⁺, K⁺-ATPase that extrudes intracellular Na⁺ in exchange for the accumulation of K⁺ in the cytosol. Us-ing the resultant large inward-directed Na⁺ gradient, Cl⁻ uptake is primarily achieved by the electroneutral basolateral Na⁺–K⁺–2Cl⁻ cotransporter. A sec-ondary Na⁺-driven Cl⁻ uptake pathway, provided by the concerted activity of Cl⁻/HCO_3^- and Na⁺/H⁺ exchangers, is also generally found in salivary gland acinar cells. In this latter process, extracellular NaCl is exchanged for intracellular HCO_3^- and protons generated from water and CO_2 in a reaction catalyzed by carbonic anhydrases. Importantly, K⁺ efflux via Ca^{2+}-activated K⁺ channels in the basolateral membrane counteracts the depolarizing activity of the apical Cl⁻ channels. Simultaneous activation of the Ca^{2+}-activated K⁺ and Cl⁻ channels produces a lumen-negative, transepithelial electrical poten-tial difference. Therefore, the cooperative activities of these ion transporters and channels result in net trans-acinar Cl⁻ flux.

The salivary gland duct system modifies the concentration of electrolytes in the final secreted fluid. The epithelial cells of the salivary duct mainly reabsorb Na⁺ and Cl⁻ and secrete K⁺ (and also HCO_3^-, depending on the

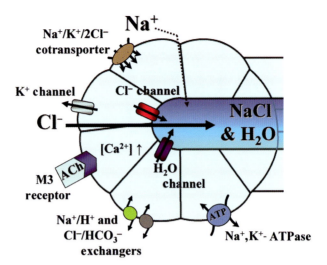

Figure 2.2 Fluid secretion mechanism. Basolateral Na^+, K^+-ATPase produces the driving force for Cl^--secreting acinar cells by concentrating Cl^- above its electrochemical equilibrium via the electroneutral Na^+–K^+–$2Cl^-$ cotransporter and paired Na^+/H^+ and Cl^-/HCO_3^- exchangers. Secretion is activated once acetylcholine (ACh) binds the M3 muscarinic receptor to mobilize intracellular Ca^{2+}. K^+ and Cl^- exit acinar cells when the K^+ and Cl^- channels open in response to this increase in the intracellular $[Ca^{2+}]$. Apical water channels allow water to follow Na^+ and Cl^- into the acinar lumen. Note that acinar cells are homogeneous; therefore, the different transport elements are spread out for clarity, but all occur in each cell.

gland type and species). Salivary gland ducts absorb little water, except at very slow flow rates. Because NaCl absorption is almost always greater than K^+ secretion, the resulting saliva is hypotonic, generally less than 200 mOsm. The transepithelial flux of Na^+ and Cl^- is supported by distinct transport pathways in the apical and basolateral membranes of the duct cells. The main route for Cl^- absorption is most likely through the apical cystic fibrosis transmembrane conductance regulator (CFTR) Cl^- channel, although Ca^{2+}-activated Cl^- channel (CLCA) and/or CLC-2 Cl^- channels may also play a role. In some salivary glands, the concerted activity of apical Na^+/H^+ and Cl^-/HCO_3^- exchangers is also thought to provide an alternative route for Cl^- reabsorption.

Like Cl^- uptake, absorption of Na^+ across the apical membrane of duct cells is mediated through channels and/or carrier-mediated pathways (Fig. 2.3). Two carriers have been proposed to mediate Na^+ uptake, a Na^+/HCO_3^- cotransporter, which can be electrogenic or electroneutral, and Na^+/H^+ exchangers. Nevertheless, the main Na^+ absorption mechanism is most likely an amiloride-sensitive Na^+ channel. Na^+ entry is thus driven by a combination of the Na^+ concentration gradient, the membrane potential and, in the case of the carrier-mediated transporters, by the pH gradient (proton equivalents). Extrusion of intracellular Na^+ across the basolateral membrane is carried out

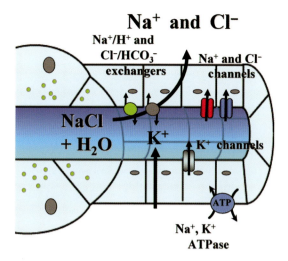

Figure 2.3 NaCl absorption and K^+ secretion. Duct cells reabsorb the NaCl secreted by the acinar cells while K^+ is secreted. The mechanisms involved in these processes are cell and gland type dependent, as well as species specific. In general, Na^+ and Cl^- channels and paired Na^+/H^+ and Cl^-/HCO_3^- exchangers located in the apical membrane reabsorb NaCl. Na^+ efflux across the basolateral membrane occurs by the Na^+, K^+-ATPase. K^+ secretion is mediated by an apical K^+ channel. Because the ducts are relatively impermeable to water, the final saliva is typically hypotonic.

by the Na^+, K^+-ATPase, but the high expression of Na^+/H^+ exchangers in the basolateral membrane of the ducts suggest that Na^+/H^+ exchange may also play a role.[4] In exchange for Na^+ extrusion, the Na^+, K^+-ATPase drives interstitial K^+ into the cytosol of duct cells. Intracellular K^+ is then secreted into the duct lumen and/or released back into the interstitial space via apical and basolateral K^+ channels, respectively. Electrogenic K^+ efflux via channels hyperpolarizes the membrane and provides an additional driving force for Na^+ absorption through apical Na^+ channels (and electrogenic carriers), as well as for Cl^- efflux across the basolateral membrane. However, the negative membrane potential also opposes Cl^- absorption through the apical Cl^- channels. It has been proposed that the spatially isolated apical Cl^- absorption and basolateral efflux of intracellular Cl^- are temporally segregated processes.[5] The Cl^- absorption phase is coordinated with the membrane depolarization activity of Na^+ channels. Na^+ influx occurs through these channels sufficiently to depolarize the cell membrane to allow the Cl^- concentration to increase. In contrast, during the Cl^- secretion phase, K^+ channels open and hyperpolarize the cell enough to drive basolateral Cl^- efflux via an electrogenic pathway. Because one of the major K^+ channels in duct cells is activated by an increase in the intracellular $[Ca^{2+}]$ (see below), this hypothesis is consistent with the oscillatory Ca^{2+} signaling observed in stimulated human duct cells.[6] That is, K^+ secretion by ductal cells appears to be regulated by the maxi-K channel, a voltage- and Ca^{2+}-activated K^+ channel.[7,8]

MOLECULAR IDENTITY OF THE FLUID SECRETION MECHANISM

Over the past decade, the molecular identities of many of the ion and water transporters involved in the fluid secretion process have been established in nonprimate animal models, and then confirmed, by taking advantage of knock-out mice where null mutations in individual genes have been introduced by homologous recombination (Table 2.1). Although further studies are required, a significant effort has recently been made to validate the key players in the fluid secretion mechanism of the human parotid gland.[9] Such information may prove critical in the development of therapies that directly target different forms of salivary gland dysfunction (see Chapter 5).

Chloride channels

While the properties of several different types of Cl^- channels have been characterized in salivary acinar cells, the Ca^{2+}-activated Cl^- channel is the key anion channel necessary for secretion. The molecular identity of this latter channel remains unknown. Among the proposed Ca^{2+}-activated Cl^- channel, candidates in salivary acinar cells are members of the Bestrophin, CLCA, and Tweety gene families. The Bestrophin family of proteins is composed of four members (BEST1-4). It has been recently demonstrated that the translation products of mouse Best2 are capable of forming functional Cl^- channels that are sensitive to physiologically relevant concentrations of Ca^{2+}.[40] Inhibition (knockdown) of Best1 and Best2 expression with siRNA significantly suppressed Ca^{2+}-activated Cl^- currents in airway and colonic epithelial cells.[41–43] Moreover, members of the BEST family have been shown to be expressed in human and mouse salivary glands.[9,44] Mutations in the BEST1 gene (*VMD2*) are associated with vitelliform macular dystrophy in humans.[19] The effects of ablation of BEST function on saliva production have not yet been investigated in either humans or mice.

Several members of the CLCA family also mediate Ca^{2+}-activated Cl^- currents in heterologous expression systems, albeit in response to very high Ca^{2+} concentration.[45,46] Expression of several CLCA isoforms was detected in human and mouse salivary glands.[9,47] Interestingly, the low Ca^{2+} sensitivity of CLCA was markedly increased when mCLCA1 was coexpressed with the β1-subunit of the calcium- and voltage-activated $K_{Ca}1.1$ potassium channel,[48] which coincidentally is endogenously present with CLCA1 in salivary glands. Ishibashi and colleagues suppressed CLCA function in the rat submandibular glands using an siRNA approach. Knockdown of the Cl^- channel resulted in saliva with high Cl^- levels indicating that CLCA may play an important role in Cl^- reabsorption by rat salivary ducts.[20] While an association has not been reported for mutations in *CLCA* genes with human disease, a potential role of CLCA2 in cancer metastasis has been noted.[49]

Some members of the tweety (tty) family of proteins originally cloned in *Drosophila melanogaster* have also been demonstrated to form functional Ca^{2+}-activated Cl^- channels.[50] Nevertheless, the role of the tweety channel family in

Table 2.1 Effects of functional ablation.

Function	Gene	Saliva (mouse)	Other dysfunctions in mice	Human dysfunctions
$K_{Ca}1.1$	Kcnma1	Low K^+, high Cl^-, Na^+, osm.[7]	Bladder overactivity,[10] erectile dysfunction,[11] cerebellar dysfunction,[12] progressive deafness[13]	Autism and mental retardation[14]
$K_{Ca}3.1$	Kcnn4	No effect[15]	Impaired cell volume regulation in T lymphocytes and RBCs[15]	Diamond–Blackfan anemia[16] (?)
Kir1.1	Kcnj1	Unk?	Phenotype of Bartter syndrome[17]	Type II Bartter syndrome[18]
BEST	Vmd2	Unk?	Unk?	Vitelliform macular dystrophy[19]
CLCA	Clca	High Cl^- (rat knockdown)[20]	Unk?	Unk?
Tweety	Tty	Unk?	Unk?	Unk?
CFTR	Cftr	High Cl^-, K^+ (rat knockdown)[20]	Cystic fibrosis[21]	Cystic fibrosis, high Cl^-, K^+, and osm. of saliva[22]
CLC-2	Clcn2	No effect[23]	Blind, male infertility[23,24]	Unk?
ENaC	Scnn1	Unk?	Lethal[25]	Systemic pseudohypoaldosteronism type I (PHAI),[26] Liddle's syndrome[27]
NKCC1	Slc2a2	Hyposalivation[28]	Deafness,[29] male infertility,[30] low blood pressure[31]	Unk?
AE2	Slc4a2	Unk?	Male infertility,[32] edentulous and achlorhydria[33]	Unk?
NHE1	Slc9a1	Hyposalivation,[4] defective pH regulation[34,35]	Ataxia and seizures[36]	Unk?
AQP5	Aqp5	Hyposalivation[37,38]	Lung alveolar water permeability deficit[39]	Unk?

Note: The functional and gene names are provided in columns 1 and 2, respectively. The effect of gene ablation on salivary glands is given in column 3 and systemic effects in column 4. Human diseases associated with individual genes are shown in column 5. Unk?, unknown.

animal physiology, and specifically in salivary glands, is unclear. However, expression of a human homologue termed TTYH2 is typically upregulated in renal cell carcinoma, suggesting that it may play a role in kidney tumorigenesis.[51]

Much of the anion conductance in salivary duct cells is supported by CFTR channels. Mutations in this cAMP-activated Cl^- channel cause cystic fibrosis, the most common inherited disease of Caucasians. Cystic fibrosis primarily affects the secretory function of the lungs, gastrointestinal tract, liver, and pancreas. Expression of CFTR channels has been detected both in human and mouse salivary glands.[9] Suppression of CFTR expression by siRNA in rat submandibular glands resulted in high levels of Cl^- in secreted saliva.[20] Accordingly, both parotid and submandibular glands of *Cftr*-null mice produce saliva with a high Cl^- content and elevated $[Na^+]$ (Nakamoto and Melvin, unpublished observations). Although muscarinic receptor stimulation is required for robust fluid secretion, it is noteworthy that when salivary glands are stimulated with a β-adrenergic agonist, saliva secretion nearly disappeared in *Cftr*-null mice, indicating that the CFTR channel may also be important in fluid secretion by acinar cells.[21] In humans, more than a thousand different CFTR mutations have been linked to cystic fibrosis, the severity of the disease depending on the type of mutation. Like sweat glands, a significantly higher salivary $[Cl^-]$ and saliva osmolarity have been found in humans with cystic fibrosis.[22]

Potassium channels

The molecular identities of two Ca^{2+}-gated K^+ channels—$K_{Ca}1.1$ and $K_{Ca}3.1$—were recently determined in mouse salivary glands. $K_{Ca}1.1$ channels are expressed in both acinar and duct cells, whereas $K_{Ca}3.1$ channels appear to be only in acinar cells.[7,8,15,52] The functional and molecular properties of these two channels were also characterized in human parotid acinar cells.[9] $K_{Ca}3.1$ channels were found to be involved in cell volume regulation in lymphocytes and red blood cells,[15] whereas $K_{Ca}1.1$ channels were required for salivary acinar cells to recover from a hypotonic challenge.[7] Simultaneous loss of both $K_{Ca}1.1$ and $K_{Ca}3.1$ channels was required to strongly suppress saliva production, suggesting that these channels functionally compensate for each other in mice. Ablation of $K_{Ca}1.1$, but not $K_{Ca}3.1$ channels, results in a substantial decrease in K^+ secretion and in a significant increase in the $[Na^+]$ of secreted saliva, consistent with a functional link between K^+ secretion and Na^+ absorption.[7,8] A null mutation of the *$K_{Ca}3.1$* channel gene did not produce significant effects on saliva flow or ion composition in mice.[15] In humans, a functional defect of the $K_{Ca}1.1$ channel is associated with autistic disorder,[14] and deletion of *$K_{Ca}3.1$* channel gene is associated with Diamond–Blackfan anemia.[16] The molecular identity of K^+ channel(s) in duct cells is not clear. Both ROMK1-type (likely Kir1.1) and Ca^{2+}-activated (likely $K_{Ca}1.1$) channels have been detected in the human submandibular gland ductal cell line.[53] In human parotid salivary glands, Kir1.1 mRNA expression was detected.[9] Nevertheless, the low $[K^+]$ secreted in the saliva from *$K_{Ca}1.1$* null mice is consistent with these channels being the major K^+ secretion pathway of salivary ducts.[7,9] Indeed, impaired function of Kir1.1 channel results in type II Bartter syndrome in humans,[18] but no salivary gland defect has been reported in these individuals.

Sodium channels

The amiloride-sensitive epithelial Na^+ channel (ENaC) is almost certainly the most important Na^+ absorption mechanism in salivary duct cells. The ENaC channel consists of three subunits (α, β, and γ), and all these subunits are expressed in both human and mouse salivary glands.[9] Null mutations in any of these subunits lead to prenatal lethality in mice.[25] In humans, *ENaC* gene mutations are associated with systemic pseudohypoaldosteronism type I (PHAI)[26] and Liddle's syndrome.[27]

Sodium-dependent chloride uptake mechanisms

As described earlier, there are two distinct Na^+-dependent Cl^- uptake pathways in salivary gland acinar cells: the Na^+–K^+–$2Cl^-$ cotransporter and the paired Cl^-/HCO_3^- and Na^+/H^+ exchangers. Disruption of the Na^+–K^+–$2Cl^-$ cotransporter gene *Nkcc1* dramatically reduces the amount of fluid produced by mouse salivary glands,[28] inhibits intestinal Na^+ absorption, and appears to be important for the maintenance of normal blood pressure.[31,54,55] *Nkcc1*-null mice are congenitally deaf.[29]

The residual saliva produced by *Nkcc1*-null mice is generated by the paired Cl^-/HCO_3^- and Na^+/H^+ exchangers. The NHE1 isoform is the dominant Na^+/H^+ exchanger in salivary gland acinar cells and is a major regulator of intracellular pH in many tissues. Knockout of the *Nhe1* gene reduces saliva production by about 30%,[4] and the ability to recover from an acid load is essentially eliminated in the acinar cells from these mice.[34,35] Mice lacking Nhe1 exhibit ataxia and a unique epilepsy phenotype.[36] AE2 appears to be the dominant Cl^-/HCO_3^- exchanger isoform in most salivary acinar cells. Mice lacking Ae2 expression were edentulous and display severe growth retardation.[33] Unfortunately, most $Ae2^{-/-}$ mice die before weaning, excluding studies to examine adult salivary gland function. The Ae2 gene drives alternative transcription, which results in several Ae2 variants. Targeted disruption of specific Ae2 variants expressed in the testes results in male, but not female, infertility.[32]

Water channels

Evidence for 5 of the 13 members of the aquaporin (*AQP*), or water channel, gene family has been described in salivary glands. Of these, only the AQP5 water channel appears to play a major role in salivation. A null mutation in the *Aqp5* gene dramatically inhibits in vivo saliva production by about 60%,[37,38] whereas disruption of *Aqp1*, *Aqp3*, or *Aqp4* did not. Moreover, mice lacking Aqp5 exhibit a dramatic decrease in the water permeability of acinar cells,[37] consistent with Aqp5's role in secretion. There is no evidence that mutations in *AQP5* lead to salivary gland dysfunction in humans.

PROTEOMIC ANALYSIS OF THE SECRETION MECHANISM

In addition to ions and water, saliva contains a complex mixture of more than a thousand proteins derived from several sources (see Chapters 11 and 22). The majority of high-abundance proteins such as amylase, cystatins, and gustin are synthesized and secreted by acinar cells, while others, like the kallikreins and growth factors, are excreted by the duct cells of the salivary glands. These proteins are segregated into granules and then secreted primarily in response to stimulation via regulated pathways, but are also released via constitutive pathway(s). Mass spectrometry analysis has recently revealed that in addition to the dozens of major secretory proteins, more than a thousand less abundant proteins are also found in saliva.[56,57] Some of these proteins are excreted using the same secretion pathways as major proteins, that is, discharge into the ductal lumen upon fusion of secretory granules to the apical membrane. However, hundreds of proteins found in saliva are also present in blood plasma, suggesting that plasma proteins make their way into saliva.[56] The blood plasma proteins released into saliva are not likely to be secreted by granules. Because this latter study collected ductal saliva from individual glands of healthy individuals, the detection of plasma proteins in saliva does not represent contamination by gingival crevicular fluid, food debris, or bacteria. Consequently, because the salivary gland acinar complexes are "leaky" epithelia, many of these proteins must enter saliva by diffusion across tight junction complexes. Regardless of the mechanism for the secretion of plasma proteins in ductal saliva, the results of this study suggest that saliva is an easily accessible source for monitoring numerous proteins that originate in blood. Thus, in some cases these proteins may serve as disease biomarkers.

It was surprising to find that a large number of the low-abundant proteins excreted in saliva are the same plasma membrane-associated ion transport proteins described earlier.[56] The simplest explanation for the appearance of these membrane-associated proteins in ductal saliva is that some salivary gland cells normally slough off. This may be true to a limited extent, but it also appears likely that many of these proteins are released with exosomes. Exosomes are the internal vesicles of multivesicular bodies found in nearly all cells. Plasma membrane-associated proteins found in exosomes display a unique orientation. Endosomes, which retrieve proteins from the plasma membrane, fuse with the outer membrane of multivesicular bodies, followed by invagination to form exosomes that are "cytoplasmic-side inward." The function of exosomes is not clear, but in some cell types they may provide for intercell communication, such as antigen presentation by cells of the immune system, or as a route for protein elimination, for example, the excretion of the transferrin receptor by red blood cells during maturation. Valadi et al.[58] also provide convincing evidence that exosomes can mediate the transfer of mRNAs between cells. The delivered mRNAs are subsequently translated into proteins, confirming that the mRNAs remain functionally intact. It will be interesting to determine if exosomes are the source of the mRNAs found in saliva (see Chapter 12).

Thus, it is theoretically possible that plasma membrane-associated proteins enter saliva when exosomes are released into saliva after multivesicular bodies fuse with the apical plasma membrane of acinar and/or duct cells. Proteins isolated from urine.[59] and from saliva.[56] contain representative exosomal proteins formed by other types of cells, suggesting that exosomes are excreted by these organs. Urinary plasma membrane protein biomarkers have been proposed for use in clinical diagnostics, for example, aquaporin-2 for diabetes insipidus and carbonic anhydrase II for one form of autosomal recessive metabolic acidosis. Proteins derived from genes associated with renal as well as systemic diseases have been found in urine exosomes. The fact that many of the transporter and channel proteins expressed in salivary glands are secreted, and saliva can be collected in large quantities, suggests that saliva may substitute for blood as a source of biomarkers in some diseases associated with defective ion and water transport. Moreover, the multiple pathways for excretion of proteins and mRNAs in saliva demonstrate the potential use of saliva biomarkers in disease diagnostics in general.

REFERENCES

1. Cook DI, Van Lennep EW, Roberts ML, Young JA. Secretion by the major salivary glands. In: Johnson LR, ed., *Physiology of the Gastrointestinal Tract*, 3rd edn. New York: Raven Press; 1994:1061–1117.
2. Melvin JE, Yule D, Shuttleworth T, Begenisich T. Regulation of fluid and electrolyte secretion in salivary gland acinar cells. Annu Rev Physiol 2005;67:445–69.
3. Nauntofte B. Regulation of electrolyte and fluid secretion in salivary acinar cells. Am J Physiol 1992;263:G823–37.
4. Park K, Evans RL, Watson GE, et al. Defective fluid secretion and NaCl absorption in the parotid glands of Na^+/H^+ exchanger-deficient mice. J Biol Chem 2001;276:27042–50.
5. Kasai H and Augustine GJ. Cytosolic Ca^{2+} gradients triggering unidirectional fluid secretion from exocrine pancreas. Nature 1990;348:735–8.
6. Tojyo Y, Tanimura A, Nezu A, Morita T. Possible mechanisms regulating ATP- and thimerosal-induced Ca^{2+} oscillations in the HSY salivary duct cell line. Biochim Biophys Acta 2001;1539:114–21.
7. Romanenko V, Nakamoto T, Srivastava A, Melvin JE, Begenisich T. Molecular identification and physiological roles of parotid acinar cell maxi-K channels. J Biol Chem 2006;281:27964–72.
8. Romanenko VG, Nakamoto T, Srivastava A, Begenisich T, Melvin JE. Regulation of membrane potential and fluid secretion by Ca^{2+}-activated K channels in mouse submandibular glands. J Physiol 2007;581:801–17.
9. Nakamoto T, Srivastava A, Romanenko VG, et al. Functional and molecular characterization of the fluid secretion mechanism in human parotid acinar cells. Am J Physiol Regul Integr Comp Physiol 2007;292:R2380–90.
10. Thorneloe KS, Meredith AL, Knorn AM, Aldrich RW, Nelson MT. Urodynamic properties and neurotransmitter dependence of urinary bladder contractility in the BK channel deletion model of overactive bladder. Am J Physiol Renal Physiol 2005;289:F604–10.
11. Werner ME, Zvara P, Meredith AL, Aldrich RW, Nelson MT. Erectile dysfunction in mice lacking the large-conductance calcium-activated potassium (BK) channel. J Physiol 2005;567:545–56.
12. Sausbier M, Hu H, Arntz C, et al. Cerebellar ataxia and Purkinje cell dysfunction caused by Ca^{2+}-activated K^+ channel deficiency. Proc Natl Acad Sci U S A 2004;101:9474–8.
13. Ruttiger L, Sausbier M, Zimmermann U, et al. Deletion of the Ca^{2+}-activated potassium (BK) alpha-subunit but not the BKbeta1-subunit leads to progressive hearing loss. Proc Natl Acad Sci USA 2004;101:12922–7.

14. Laumonnier F, Roger S, Guerin P, et al. Association of a functional deficit of the BKCa channel, a synaptic regulator of neuronal excitability, with autism and mental retardation. Am J Psychiatry 2006;163:1622–9.
15. Begenisich T, Nakamoto T, Ovitt CE, et al. Physiological roles of the intermediate conductance, Ca^{2+}-activated potassium channel Kcnn4. J Biol Chem 2004;279:47681–7.
16. Ghanshani S, Coleman M, Gustavsson P, et al. Human calcium-activated potassium channel gene KCNN4 maps to chromosome 19q13.2 in the region deleted in diamond-blackfan anemia. Genomics 1998;51:160–161.
17. Lorenz JN, Baird NR, Judd LM, et al. Impaired renal NaCl absorption in mice lacking the ROMK potassium channel, a model for type II Bartter's syndrome. J Biol Chem 2002;277:37871–80.
18. Bhandari S. The pathophysiological and molecular basis of Bartter's and Gitelman's syndromes. Postgrad Med J 1999;75:391–6.
19. White K, Marquardt A, Weber BH. VMD2 mutations in vitelliform macular dystrophy (Best disease) and other maculopathies. Hum Mutat 2000;15:301–8.
20. Ishibashi K, Yamazaki J, Okamura K, Teng Y, Kitamura K, Abe K. Roles of CLCA and CFTR in electrolyte re-absorption from rat saliva. J Dent Res 2006;85:1101–5.
21. Best JA, Quinton PM. Salivary secretion assay for drug efficacy for cystic fibrosis in mice. Exp Physiol 2005;90:189–93.
22. Aps JK, Delanghe J, Martens LC. Salivary electrolyte concentrations are associated with cystic fibrosis transmembrane regulator genotypes. Clin Chem Lab Med 2002;40:345–50.
23. Nehrke K, Arreola J, Nguyen HV, et al. Loss of hyperpolarization-activated Cl^- current in salivary acinar cells from Clcn2 knockout mice. J Biol Chem 2002;277:23604–11.
24. Bosl MR, Stein V, Hubner C, et al. Male germ cells and photoreceptors, both dependent on close cell-cell interactions, degenerate upon ClC-2 Cl^- channel disruption. Embo J 2001;20:1289–99.
25. Hummler E and Beermann F. Scnn1 sodium channel gene family in genetically engineered mice. J Am Soc Nephrol 2000;11 Suppl 16:S129–34.
26. Thomas CP, Zhou J, Liu KZ, Mick VE, MacLaughlin E, Knowles M. Systemic pseudohypoaldosteronism from deletion of the promoter region of the human Beta epithelial Na^+ channel subunit. Am J Respir Cell Mol Biol 2002;27:314–19.
27. Knight KK, Olson DR, Zhou R, Snyder PM. Liddle's syndrome mutations increase Na^+ transport through dual effects on epithelial Na^+ channel surface expression and proteolytic cleavage. Proc Natl Acad Sci USA 2006;103:2805–18.
28. Evans RL, Park K, Turner RJ, et al. Severe impairment of salivation in $Na^+/K^+/2Cl^-$ cotransporter (NKCC1)-deficient mice. J Biol Chem 2000;275:26720–26.
29. Flagella M, Clarke LL, Miller ML, et al. Mice lacking the basolateral Na-K-2Cl cotransporter have impaired epithelial chloride secretion and are profoundly deaf. J Biol Chem 1999;274:26946–55.

30. Pace AJ, Lee E, Athirakul K, Coffman TM, O'Brien DA, Koller BH. Failure of spermatogenesis in mouse lines deficient in the Na^+-K^+-$2Cl^-$ cotransporter. J Clin Invest 2000;105:441–50.

31. Meyer JW, Flagella M, Sutliff RL, et al. Decreased blood pressure and vascular smooth muscle tone in mice lacking basolateral Na^+-K^+-$2Cl^-$ cotransporter. Am J Physiol Heart Circ Physiol 2002;283:H1846–55.

32. Medina JF, Recalde S, Prieto J, et al. Anion exchanger 2 is essential for spermiogenesis in mice. Proc Natl Acad Sci USA 2003;100:15847–52.

33. Gawenis LR, Ledoussal C, Judd LM, et al. Mice with a targeted disruption of the AE2 Cl^-/HCO_3^- exchanger are achlorhydric. J Biol Chem 2004;279:30531–9.

34. Evans RL, Bell SM, Schultheis PJ, Shull GE, Melvin JE. Targeted disruption of the Nhe1 gene prevents muscarinic agonist-induced up-regulation of Na^+/H^+ exchange in mouse parotid acinar cells. J Biol Chem 1999;274:29025–30.

35. Nguyen HV, Stuart-Tilley A, Alper SL, Melvin JE. Cl^-/HCO_3^- exchange is acetazolamide sensitive and activated by a muscarinic receptor-induced $[Ca^{2+}]$ (i) increase in salivary acinar cells. Am J Physiol Gastrointest Liver Physiol 2004;286:G312–20.

36. Bell SM, Schreiner CM, Schultheis PJ, et al. Targeted disruption of the murine Nhe1 locus induces ataxia, growth retardation, and seizures. Am J Physiol 1999;276:C788–95.

37. Krane CM, Melvin JE, Nguyen HV, et al. Salivary acinar cells from aquaporin 5-deficient mice have decreased membrane water permeability and altered cell volume regulation. J Biol Chem 2001;276:23413–20.

38. Ma T, Song Y, Gillespie A, Carlson EJ, Epstein CJ, Verkman AS. Defective secretion of saliva in transgenic mice lacking aquaporin-5 water channels. J Biol Chem 1999;274:20071–4.

39. Ma T, Fukuda N, Song Y, Matthay MA, Verkman AS. Lung fluid transport in aquaporin-5 knockout mice. J Clin Invest 2000;105:93–100.

40. Qu Z, Fischmeister R, Hartzell C. Mouse bestrophin-2 is a bona fide Cl^- channel: identification of a residue important in anion binding and conduction. J Gen Physiol 2004;123:327–40.

41. Barro Soria R, Spitzner M, Schreiber R, Kunzelmann K. Bestrophin 1 enables Ca^{2+} activated Cl^- conductance in epithelia. J Biol Chem 2006;281:17460–67.

42. Chien LT, Zhang ZR, Hartzell HC. Single Cl^- channels activated by Ca^{2+} in *Drosophila* S2 cells are mediated by bestrophins. J Gen Physiol 2006;128:247–59.

43. Duta V, Szkotak AJ, Nahirney D, Duszyk M. The role of bestrophin in airway epithelial ion transport. FEBS Lett 2004;577:551–4.

44. Kunzelmann K, Milenkovic VM, Spitzner M, Soria RB, Schreiber R. Calcium-dependent chloride conductance in epithelia: is there a contribution by Bestrophin? Pflugers Arch 2007;454:879–89.

45. Eggermont J. Calcium-activated chloride channels: (un)known, (un)loved? Proc Am Thorac Soc 2004;1:22–7.

46. Fuller CM, Ji HL, Tousson A, Elble RC, Pauli BU, Benos DJ. Ca^{2+}-activated Cl^- channels: a newly emerging anion transport family. Pflugers Arch 2001;443 (Suppl 1):S107–10.
47. Loewen ME and Forsyth GW. Structure and function of CLCA proteins. Physiol Rev 2005;85:1061–92.
48. Greenwood IA, Miller LJ, Ohya S, Horowitz B. The large conductance potassium channel beta-subunit can interact with and modulate the functional properties of a calcium-activated chloride channel, CLCA1. J Biol Chem 2002;277:22119–22.
49. Abdel-Ghany M, Cheng HC, Elble RC, Pauli BU. The breast cancer beta 4 integrin and endothelial human CLCA2 mediate lung metastasis. J Biol Chem 2001;276:25438–46.
50. Suzuki M. The *Drosophila* tweety family: molecular candidates for large-conductance Ca^{2+}-activated Cl^- channels. Exp Physiol 2006;91:141–7.
51. Rae FK, Hooper JD, Eyre HJ, Sutherland GR, Nicol DL, Clements JA. TTYH2, a human homologue of the *Drosophila melanogaster* gene tweety, is located on 17q24 and upregulated in renal cell carcinoma. Genomics 2001;77:200–207.
52. Nehrke K, Quinn CC, Begenisich T. Molecular identification of Ca^{2+}-activated K^+ channels in parotid acinar cells. Am J Physiol Cell Physiol 2003;284:C535–46.
53. Liu X, Singh BB, Ambudkar IS. ATP-dependent activation of K(Ca) and ROMK-type K(ATP) channels in human submandibular gland ductal cells. J Biol Chem 1999;274:25121–9.
54. Gawenis LR, Hut H, Bot AG, Shull GE, de Jonge HR, Stien X, Miller ML, Clarke LL. Electroneutral sodium absorption and electrogenic anion secretion across murine small intestine are regulated in parallel. Am J Physiol Gastrointest Liver Physiol 2004;287:G1140–49.
55. Oppermann M, Hansen PB, Castrop H, Schnermann JB. Vasodilatation of afferent arterioles and paradoxical increase of renal vascular resistance by furosemide in mice. Am J Physiol Renal Physiol 2007;293:F279–87.
56. Denny P, Hagen FK, Hardt M, et al. The proteomics of human parotid and submandibular/sublingual gland salivas collected as the ductal secretions. J Proteome Res 2008;7:1994–2006.
57. Guo T, Rudnick PA, Wang W, Lee CS, Devoe DL, Balgley BM. Characterization of the human salivary proteome by capillary isoelectric focusing/nanoreversed-phase liquid chromatography coupled with ESI-tandem MS. J Proteome Res 2006;5:1469–78.
58. Valadi H, Ekstrom K, Bossios A, Sjostrand M, Lee JJ, Lotvall JO. Exosome-mediated transfer of mRNAs and microRNAs is a novel mechanism of genetic exchange between cells. Nat Cell Biol, 2007;9:654–9.
59. Pisitkun T, Shen RF, Knepper MA. Identification and proteomic profiling of exosomes in human urine. Proc Natl Acad Sci U S A 2004;101:13368–73.

Saliva: Properties and functions 3

Arie van Nieuw Amerongen, Enno C.I. Veerman,
and Arjan Vissink

INTRODUCTION

Oral fluid (whole saliva) is for the larger part produced and secreted by the various salivary glands, such as the submandibular, sublingual, and parotid glands. In addition, it contains serum components that enter the oral cavity via damaged oral mucosa or the periodontium (crevicular fluid).[1] The secretion of a specific gland type of saliva has a characteristic protein composition.[2] For example, sublingual saliva is very rich in mucins and contains little amylase, while parotid saliva, which is the main source of salivary amylase and basic proline-rich proteins, does not contain mucin. During the day the contribution of the individual salivary glands can vary considerably, depending on applied stimuli, which results in changes in fluid secretion and salivary protein composition.

Saliva has several types of functions that are of profound importance for the oral health.[3] In the absence of saliva, not only teeth will rapidly decay, but also the oral mucosa will become vulnerable to bacterial, viral, and fungal infections.[4] Thus, patients with chronic dry mouth are prone to develop rampant caries, because of the diminished protection by saliva, are highly susceptible for development of oral infections, again as a result of the diminished protection of, in particular, the protein composition of saliva, and are more vulnerable for dental wear, due to the combined processes of attrition, abrasion, and erosion (Fig. 3.1).

Saliva protects the oral tissues in various ways (Fig. 3.2). Upon stimulation, the cleansing action of the continuous flow of watery saliva clears the mouth from bacteria and food particles. Buffering ions, particularly bicarbonate, aid in acid neutralization, in this way protecting dental enamel against demineralization. Furthermore, saliva forms a lubricating protein film on the dental enamel, denoted pellicle, which prevents direct access of acids to the dental surface, and thus protects the enamel surface against erosion.[5] Moreover, because of its lubricating properties, saliva reduces friction between tissue surfaces and diminishes mechanical wear.

The digestive functions of saliva include the moistening of food and aiding in the formation of a food bolus, thus facilitating swallowing and assisting in taste

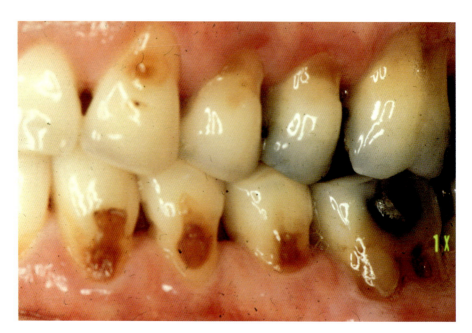

Figure 3.1   Dental decay, both dental caries and dental wear and erosion, easily occurs in patients with Sjögren's syndrome. This occurs both due to the loss of protection by saliva and the use of sweet and acidic foods to relieve the dry mouth feeling.

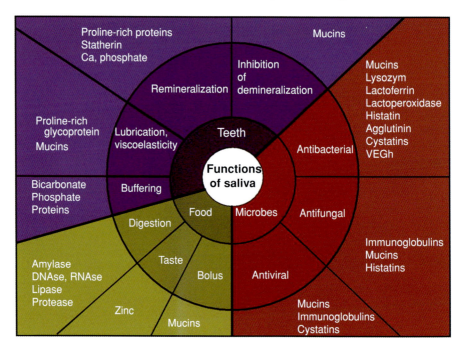

Figure 3.2   Overview of the relationship between the various functions of saliva and the salivary constituents involved. A number of salivary proteins participate in more than one function.

perception. Saliva contains amylase, an enzyme that breaks down starch into soluble maltose and dextrin fragments, and in this way initiates the digestion of food. Also, the digestion of fat is initiated in saliva due to the presence of salivary lipase.

SALIVA—A MIXED SECRETION

Whole saliva is, for the large part, composed of secretions coming from three pairs of major salivary glands (parotid, submandibular, and sublingual) and numerous minor ones (labial, buccal, lingual, palatal).[2] Each type of gland secretes a fluid with a characteristic protein composition. Thus, whole saliva is a mixed secretion. Upon mechanical or gustatory (taste) stimulation, the parotid gland is triggered to secrete a watery fluid that is rich in bicarbonate. The main protein constituents of parotid saliva are amylase (20%), phosphoproteins, such as statherin (7%), and proline-rich proteins (60%). Phosphoproteins and proline-rich proteins are major constituents of the protein pellicle on dental surfaces and also play a role in keeping saliva supersaturated in calcium. So, parotid saliva is important for rinsing, neutralization of acids, and pellicle formation.

At rest, mainly submandibular and sublingual glands are active. Together with the numerous minor salivary glands, they are the main source of the salivary mucins, MUC5B and MUC7.[6–8] The main function of MUC5B, a large gel-forming molecule, is to protect both hard and soft oral tissues against chemical, physical, and microbial damage.[9,10] MUC5B is the backbone of the slime layers that cover oral surfaces, acting as a diffusion barrier impeding the entry of noxious agents, including protons. Furthermore, this layer helps in reducing the friction between antagonistic teeth, and in this way diminishes dental wear. The role of MUC5B can only partially be replaced by the artificial constituents added to saliva substitutes, such as carboxymethylcellulose, mucins from animal sources, and organic gums such as xanthan gum.[11,12] MUC5B can bind to only a limited number of oral bacteria, particularly to *Helicobacter pylori*, *Haemophilus parainfluenza*, and *Candida albicans*.[13,14] In addition, MUC5B can also bind to HIV-1.[15] The low-molecular-weight mucin MUC7 has broad-spectrum bacteria-binding properties and as such plays an important role in the oral clearance of bacteria. In addition to bacteria, a number of viruses, including HIV, are encapsulated and inactivated by MUC7. On the other hand, as a constituent of the dental pellicle, MUC7 may support the adhesion of oral bacteria such as *Streptococcus mutans* and as such enhance their colonization on the dental surface. Without mucins, the oral mucosa and the dental surface become highly vulnerable to infection, inflammation, and mechanical wear (see Figs. 3.1 and 3.3).[16]

Altogether, the saliva quality and quantity, together with diet and oral hygiene, determine the caries risk of an individual. In the absence of saliva, for example, after nearly complete destruction of the salivary glands by radiotherapeutic treatment of head and neck cancer, it is extremely difficult to maintain the oral tissues healthy.

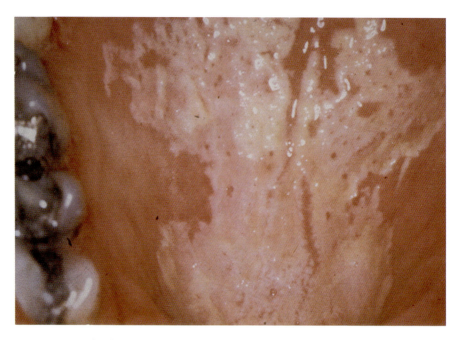

Figure 3.3   Palatal candidiasis in a patient with hyposalivation and a decreased antimicrobial protection.

CONSEQUENCES OF HYPOSALIVATION AND DRY MOUTH

Xerostomia is defined as the subjective feeling of a dry mouth.[17] Hyposalivation, on the other hand, is a decrease in salivary flow, which can be objectively assessed by measuring the amount of saliva secreted per minute. These two conditions are not necessarily congruent, so a patient with a completely normal saliva secretion can complain about a dry mouth, while people with an objective decrease in salivary flow may have no complaints at all.[4]

Hyposalivation results in drying up of the oral epithelium tissues causing pain in the tongue epithelium with fissures (Fig. 3.4). In the majority of the patients, a dry mouth is caused by the use of xerogenic medication, for example, β-blockers, sedatives, and antipsychotic medication, which blocks the neurotransmission to the salivary gland. This blockage can be overcome by mechanical or gustatory triggers. A second, much smaller group of patients suffering from hyposalivation consists of individuals with an autoimmune disease, in particular the Sjögren's syndrome. In the first stage of this disease process, the reduction in salivary flow can be overcome by mechanical or gustatory stimulants, but this secretory ability will decline gradually when the disease progresses.[18] Nevertheless, stimulation of saliva secretion can give relief, even at later stages of the disease. In less than 1% of patients, the shortage of saliva is caused by radiotherapy in the head/neck region. Conventional radiotherapy of a tumor in the oral cavity or oropharynx often results in a complete,

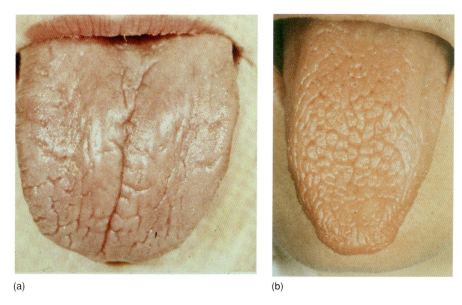

(a)   (b)

Figure 3.4 Two tongues of patients with the Sjögren's syndrome showing dry epithelium with fissures caused by severe hyposalivation.

irreversible destruction of the major salivary glands, and thus leads to severe hyposalivation. In these cases stimulation of the salivary glands is no longer a feasible option, and one has to resort to palliative treatment using artificial saliva and hydrating gels.[4,19] Newer schedules of radiotherapy (3D conformal radiotherapy and intensity-modified radiotherapy) have been shown to result in less involvement of the salivary glands in the treatment portals (at least a lower overall dose to the gland tissue) and thus to less hyposalivation.

THE EFFECT OF AGING ON SALIVA

Hyposalivation increases with age.[20] Whereas in the whole population, 6–10% suffers from dry mouth, this percentage increases to 25% for people >50-year old and even to 40% for those >80-year old. In the majority of the cases, this age-related increase is caused by increased use of medications in the elderly population, such as β-blockers, antihypertensives, sedatives, tranquillizers, and antipsychotics.[21] In general, neuropharmaceuticals, acting on specific neurotransmitter receptors, have no absolute specificity for their target organ, for example, antihypertensives will also block neuroreceptors present on the salivary glands. As a rule of thumb, it can be said that when the daily number of different medicines is >4, hyposalivation and xerostomia are likely to occur.[22] Pharmaceutical inhibition can be overcome by application of gustatory and mechanical stimuli, for example, by chewing gum. Histochemical studies revealed that with increasing age the amount of secretory tissue in the salivary gland decreased, but apparently this did not lead to an appreciable loss of secretory performance.

PROTECTIVE SYSTEMS IN SALIVA

In saliva a number of antimicrobial proteins and peptides are present, which together keep the oral microflora under control.[23,24] When due to a diminished salivary flow the salivary defense is compromised, a shift in the composition of the oral microflora can occur toward more virulent gram-negative species. Furthermore, carriers of the opportunistic pathogen, *C. albicans*, may develop oral candidiasis within a few days after the onset of hyposalivation, because of uncontrolled outgrowth of the fungus (Figs. 3.1 and 3.3). Because the clearance of sugar is diminished, an increase in the number of *S. mutans* has also been reported.

Mucosal tissues, which are vulnerable to infection, are covered by a mucous slimy layer, which protects the underlying epithelia against mechanical, chemical, and microbial injury. A decrease in the mucin content of saliva, for example, due to a surgical removal of mucous glands, will therefore result in increased susceptibility for infections, inflammation, and tissue damage (Fig. 3.3). This phenomenon has, for example, been observed in drooling children in whom the sublingual glands had been removed and the Wharton's ducts had been redirected toward the oropharynx.

The mineral of dental enamel, calcium hydroxyapatite, is composed mainly of calcium and phosphate. Both are constituents of saliva, which normally bathes the dental surfaces. In addition, protection is afforded by a pellicle consisting of salivary proteins, which covers the dental surfaces. The enamel pellicle consists of calcium-binding phosphoproteins present in saliva. Important constituents of older pellicles are, in addition, salivary mucins that protect the dental enamel against acidic attacks.[5] Salivary proteins not only protect the dental surface, but also perform the function of increasing the local concentration of calcium and phosphate on the mineral surface, which then become available for tooth remineralization.[16]

The enamel and dentin mineral is a basic salt, hydroxyapatite, which at neutral pH value is insoluble in saliva. However, when the pH of the plaque fluid, which is directly in contact with the dental surface, becomes low, because of lactic acid produced by bacteria or dietary acids, hydroxyapatite crystals will dissolve. A high concentration of buffering ions, mainly sodium bicarbonate, will bring back the pH to neutral values, and in this way protects against demineralization. Under normal conditions the pH of unstimulated saliva is about neutral (mean value pH 6.8), and upon stimulation the concentration of bicarbonate increases, resulting in a higher pH (mean value 7.4). Individuals having an intrinsically low salivary pH, for example, pH 6.2, will thus be prone to develop dental caries or erosion, depending on their dietary and oral hygiene habits. In sum, a high salivary flow rate contributes to a healthy oral condition: the rinsing action promotes the removal of food remnants and also accelerates the neutralization and dilution of acid (see Fig. 3.2). Furthermore, under these conditions the output of antimicrobial proteins will be higher, resulting in a more effective bacterial clearing. So, stimulation of the salivary flow, either by (dental safe) gustatory or masticatory stimuli, has beneficial effects for the oral health (Nieuw Amerongen *et al.*, 2004).[25] But the opposite is also true: a reduced salivary flow rate will increase the susceptibility for tooth decay and oral infection and inflammation (Figs 3.1, 3.3, and 3.4).

ANTIMICROBIAL MECHANISM IN SALIVA

Besides affording direct protection against tooth decay, described earlier, saliva also actively lowers the microbial burden in the mouth through various antimicrobial components, including bacteria-agglutinating factors and bactericidal components. An example of an agglutinating factor in saliva is sIgA, the main secretory protein that represents the adaptive immunity in saliva. After secretion, sIgA binds selectively to antigens, a characteristic feature of immunoglobulins. This binding prevents antigens, such as microbes and viruses, from attaching to mucosal and dental surfaces. Binding can be prevented, for example, by agglutination of microbes, by hampering their motility through interference with the action of flagella, and by blocking interactions between microbial receptors and their ligands on epithelial cells. The cells responsible for local IgA production originate from the various lymphoid structures surrounding the mucosa, such as the tonsils and the Peyer's patches, collectively referred to as the mucosa-associated lymphoid tissue. After activation they migrate to exocrine glands, including the salivary glands, where they reside in the interstitium as IgA-producing plasma cells. They produce a polymeric form of IgA, which after uptake by glandular acinar cells, becomes secreted into saliva as sIgA. The other main agglutinating factors in saliva are the low-molecular-weight mucin MUC7, secreted by the serous cells of the sublingual and submandibular glands, and salivary agglutinin gp340, which is secreted by the parotid glands, and the submandibular glands.[26–28] Like sIgA, these proteins interfere in the soluble phase with the binding of microbes to oral surfaces. At variance with IgA, however, MUC7 and gp340 have a broad specificity, binding a variety of bacterial species and viruses. In addition to these bacteria-agglutinating factors, saliva harbors a multitude of proteins that inactivate or kill bacteria. These include lysozyme, which acts on gram-positive bacteria, lactoperoxidase, lactoferrin, and antimicrobial peptides, such as histatins and the cathelicidin LL-37.[24,25,29]

CONCLUDING REMARKS

- Saliva is a mixed fluid continuously changing in composition and rheological properties varying from thin watery to slimy and sticky.
- The main functions of saliva are related to maintaining all oral tissues lifelong healthy.
- A great number of salivary (glycol)proteins have antimicrobial properties preventing oral infections and inflammations.

- In addition, a number of salivary proteins form a pellicle on the tooth surface protecting the dental enamel against dental wear, both physical wear (attrition and abrasion) and chemical wear (dental erosion).
- The viscoelastic properties of the salivary mucins, combined with their resistance to proteolytic degradation, make these molecules the most important constituents of saliva.
- Patients with hyposalivation are vulnerable to all types of oral diseases, both to infection and inflammation of the mucosa and epithelium and to dental wear.
- Saliva of healthy elderly people is sufficient in volume and has adequate protecting properties. If they have dry mouth complaints, this is caused largely as side effects by the medications used or as a consequence of a systemic disease.

REFERENCES

1. Schenkels LCPM, Veerman ECI, Nieuw Amerongen AV. Biochemical composition of human saliva in relation to other mucosal fluids. Crit Rev Oral Biol Med 1995;6:161–75.
2. Veerman ECI, van den Keijbus PAM, Vissink A, Nieuw Amerongen AV. Human glandular salivas: their separate collection and analysis. Eur J Oral Sci 1996;104:346–52.
3. Mandel ID. The role of saliva in maintaining oral homeostasis. J Am Dental Ass 1989;119:298–304.
4. Vissink A, Schaub RMH, van Rijn LJ, 's Gravenmade EJ, Panders AK, Vermey A. The efficacy of mucin-containing artificial saliva in alleviating symptoms of xerostomia. Gerodontology 1987;6:95–101.
5. Nieuw Amerongen AV, Oderkerk CH, Driessen AA. Role of mucins from human whole saliva in the protection of tooth enamel against demineralization *in vitro*. Caries Res 1987;21:297–309.
6. Nieuw Amerongen AV, Bolscher JGM, Veerman ECI. Salivary mucins: protective functions in relation to their diversity. Glycobiology 1995;5:733–40.
7. Nieuw Amerongen AV, Bolscher JGM, Bloemena E, Veerman ECI. Sulfomucins in the human body. Biol Chem 1998;379:1–18.
8. Thornton DJ, Khan N, Mehrotra R, et al. Salivary mucin MG1 is comprised almost entirely of different glycosylated forms of the MUC5B gene product. Glycobiology 1999;9:293–302.
9. Bolscher JGM, Veerman ECI, Nieuw Amerongen AV, Tulp A, Verwoerd D. Distinct populations of high-M_r mucins secreted by different human salivary glands discriminated by density-gradient electrophoresis. Biochem J 1995;309:801–906.
10. Veerman ECI, Bolscher JGM, Appelmelk BJ, Bloemena E, van den Berg TK, Nieuw Amerongen AV. A monoclonal antibody directed against high M_r salivary mucins recognizes the SO_3-3Galβ1-3GalNAc moiety of sulfo-Lewis[a]: a histochemical survey of human and rat tissue. Glycobiology 1997;7:37–43.

11. van der Reijden WA, van der Kwaak JS, Vissink A, Veerman ECI, Nieuw Amerongen AV. Treatment of xerostomia with polymer-based saliva substitutes in patients with Sjögren's syndrome. Arthritis Rheum 1996;39:57–63.
12. Ruissen ALA, van der Reijden WA, van 't Hof W, Veerman ECI, Nieuw Amerongen AV. Evaluation of the use of xanthan as vehicle for cationic antifungal peptides. J. Control Release 1999;60:49–56.
13. Veerman ECI, Ligtenberg AJM, Schenkels LCPM, Walgreen-Weterings E, Nieuw Amerongen AV. Binding of human high-molecular-weight salivary mucins (MG1) to *Hemophilus parainfluenzae*. J Dent Res 1995;74:351–7.
14. Veerman ECI, Bank CMC, Namavar F, Appelmelk BJ, Bolscher JGM, Nieuw Amerongen AV. Sulfated glycans on oral mucin as receptors for *Helicobacter pylori*. Glycobiology 1997;7:737–43.
15. Bolscher JGM, Nazmi K, Ran LJ, van Engelenburg FAC, Schuitemaker H, Veerman ECI, Nieuw Amerongen AV. Inhibition of HIV-1 IIIB and clinical isolates by human parotid, submandibular, sublingual and palatine saliva. Eur J Oral Sci 2002;110:149–56.
16. Tabak LA. In defense of the oral cavity: structure, biosynthesis, and function of salivary mucins. Annu Rev Physiol 1995;57:547–64.
17. Sreebny LM. Saliva in health and disease: an appraisal and update. Int Dental J 2000;50:140–61.
18. Kalk WWI, Vissink A, Stegenga B, Bootsma H, Nieuw Amerongen AV, Kallenberg CGM. Sialometry and sialochemistry. A non-invasive approach for diagnosing Sjögren's syndrome. Ann Rheum Dis 2002;61:137–44.
19. Nieuw Amerongen AV, Veerman ECI. Current therapies for xerostomia and salivary gland hypofunction associated with cancer therapies. Support Care Cancer 2003;11:226–31.
20. Dodds MWJ, Johnson DA, Yeh CK. Health benefits of saliva: a review. J Dent 2005;33:223–33.
21. Osterberg T, Landahl S, Hedegard B. Salivary flow, saliva pH and buffering capacity in 70-year old men and women. Correlation to dental health, dryness in the mouth, disease and drug treatment. J Oral Rehabil 1984;11:157–70.
22. Närhi TO, Meurman JH, Ainamo A. Xerostomia and hyposalivation. Causes, consequences and treatment in the elderly. Drugs Aging 1999;15:103–16.
23. Tenovuo J, Grahn E, Lehtonen OP, Hyppe T, Karhuvaara L, Vilja P. Antimicrobial factors in saliva: ontogeny and relation to oral health. J Dent Res 1987;66:475–79.
24. Nieuw Amerongen AV, Veerman ECI. Saliva—the defender of the oral cavity. Oral Dis 2002;8:12–22.
25. Nieuw Amerongen AV, Bolscher JGM, Veerman ECI. Salivary proteins: protective and diagnostic value in cariology? Caries Res 2004;38:247–53.
26. Bolscher JGM, Groenink J, van der Kwaak JS, et al. Detection and quantification of MUC7 in submandibular, sublingual, palatine, and labial saliva by antipeptide antiserum. J Dent Res 1999;78:1362–9.
27. Ligtenberg AJM, Veerman ECI, Nieuw Amerongen AV. A role for Lewis a antigens on salivary agglutinin in binding to *Streptococcus mutans*. Antonie van Leeuwenh 2000;77:21–30.

28. Bikker FJ, Ligtenberg AJM, Nazmi K, et al. Identification of the bacteria-binding peptide domain on salivary agglutinin (gp-340/DMBT1), a member of the scavenger receptor cysteine-rich superfamily. J Biol Chem 2002;277:32109–15.
29. Van 't Hof W, Veerman ECI, Helmerhorst EJ, Nieuw Amerongen AV. Antimicrobial peptides: properties and applicability. Biol Chem 2001;382:597–619.

Saliva collectors

Arjan Vissink, Andy Wolff, and Enno C.I. Veerman

4

INTRODUCTION

Accurate measurement of salivary flow rate and composition is essential for many clinical, experimental, and diagnostic protocols. Saliva collection is a noninvasive means of assessing a variety of disease activities and the level of certain drugs and hormones. As in every clinical investigation, the value of salivary collection is bounded by several limitations including the following:

- Saliva wets and lubricates the oral surfaces. Collection of whole saliva means gathering the fluid that will flow outside the mouth, which is not the entire amount of saliva, since part of it will remain coating the oral surfaces.
- Collection of a null amount of saliva does not necessarily reflect a status of absolute absence of saliva secretion.
- Salivary fractions are lost in the collection process owing to evaporation and fluid retention in the collection devices.
- Saliva secretion varies during the day and is influenced by temperature, season, hydration status, actual health condition (including medication intake), and mood. Thus, same individuals will probably yield diverse secretory rates of saliva at different occasions.
- The collection conditions for saliva are not absolute. An unstimulated status may not be completely devoid of stimuli, since minor oral movements or the current state of mind of the subject may provide significant enhancing effects on salivary secretion. On the other hand, it is impossible to completely standardize the intensity of stimulation.

Nevertheless, the value of saliva as a diagnostic specimen is being increasingly recognized. Therefore, despite its limitations, saliva collection will become an growingly common diagnostic procedure, which will require standardization and accuracy.

GENERAL CONSIDERATIONS WHEN COLLECTING SALIVA

The high natural and condition-related variation in saliva secretion over the course of the day makes it important to use standardized conditions for its collection. The use of these uniformly standardized methods and conditions for collection of saliva greatly facilitates comparison of studies carried out by different research groups.

Factors that influence the secretion and composition of saliva are, among others, the time of day and duration of collection. Very short (<1 min) or very long (>15 min) collection periods tend to yield unreliable values for calculation of the mean salivary flow rate. Moreover, it has been frequently observed that during the first minutes of collection, for example, the left parotid (PAR) gland produces more saliva than the right PAR gland, but that in the remaining part of the collection period (typically 10 min) this difference disappears.[1] Other authors have shown that long and intensive stimulation might result in exhausting the submandibular (SM) salivary glands in particular and thus in lower flow rates.[2,3]

Thus, for reliable monitoring of the functional potency of a salivary gland, it is recommended to collect both unstimulated and stimulated saliva during an appropriate period. We feel that a 5-min collection period is on the short side, and therefore we would advise a collection period of 10 min for diagnostic and research purposes. For further standardization, patients must be instructed to refrain from eating and drinking at least 90 min prior to the test session, and to avoid swallowing and oral movements during collection.[1,4–6] To minimise the effects of diurnal variation, it is advised to collect all saliva samples at the same, fixed time of the day. In a clinical setting this is not always possible, and therefore, one has to collect subsequent saliva samples in the same patient at the same time of the day.

An important effect, particularly at very low flow rates, is the substantial evaporation of the saliva sample during the collection period. Thus, collection circumstances should be designed in such a way that evaporation of the sample is minimized, at least in patients with very low flow rates.[7]

Few studies have attempted to examine the association between climate and salivary flow rate.[8–12] Salivary secretion rate is higher in winter than in summer.[9,11] Flow rate also decreases as a result of increasing environmental temperature.[10] A recent study has found PAR and submandibular (SM)/sublingual (SL) secretion rates significantly higher in winter than in summer, while air-conditioning canceled the seasonal effect on salivary secretion rates. Thus, room temperature seems to be an important factor affecting salivary secretion rates. Ideally, temperature should be recorded and reported when assessing salivary flow rates in a non-air-conditioned environment.[13] Standardized sample conditions are given in Table 4.1.

Table 4.1 Proposal for standardized collection of whole and glandular saliva.

- Collect saliva samples always at the same time of day, preferably between 9:00 and 11:00 a.m.
- Refrain from eating and drinking at least 90 min before collection
- If applicable, stop the use of drugs that might affect salivary secretion for at least 1 day (or longer when the drug has a long half-life)
- Rinse mouth with deionised water prior to the collection to void the mouth of saliva
- Collect saliva for 10 min

WHOLE SALIVA

Whole saliva is a mixture of not only salivary secretions, but also fluids, debris, and cells not originating from the salivary glands. The main advantage of whole saliva as specimen material is the easy and noninvasive collection. The method is free of stress (as experienced in blood collection) and privacy issues (as in urine collection). There are different methods available for collecting whole saliva. Regardless of the method used, subjects should be instructed to void the mouth of saliva prior to collection, by rinsing the mouth thoroughly with deionised water. The subject should be seated comfortably with the eyes open, head tilted slightly forward (Fig. 4.1).[6]

Common methods for collecting whole saliva include the draining, spitting, suction, and swab (absorbent) method. Common stimuli are chewing on paraffin wax or chewing gum. Preferably, the number of chewing cycles per minute is set at a fixed rate, for example, using a metronome. Occasionally, gustatory stimuli such as citric acid are applied. However, such a stimulus might have a greater impact on salivary composition than chewing on paraffin wax or on unflavored chewing gum base.

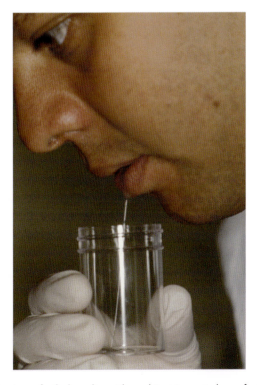

Figure 4.1 Collection of whole saliva. The subject is seated comfortably with the eyes open, head tilted slightly forward, and (for unstimulated saliva) instructed to rest for 5 min and to minimize oral movement.

A simple method for diagnosis of hyposalivation has been developed, which consists of measuring the weight loss of a candy after it has been passively incubated between the tongue and the palate for 3 min. This method is suggested for rapid screening of patients to discriminate which of them suffer from hyposalivation, before subjecting them to more intensive salivary testing. Candy weight loss correlated with glandular (PAR and SM/SL) secretion rates, particularly with the stimulated ones, and with subjective oral wetness/dryness reports.[14]

Draining method

Saliva is allowed to drip off the lower lip into a preweighed or graduated test tube or sampling container. The subject is instructed to expectorate into the test tube at the end of the collection period. The tube can be fitted with a funnel to ease collecting of saliva that drips from the lips or is expectorated. The amount of saliva is determined by weighing (assuming a specific gravity of 1 g/cm^3) or read from the scale on the graduated test tube.[6]

Spitting method

Saliva is allowed to accumulate in the floor of the mouth and the subject spits it out into the preweighed or graduated test tube or a sampling container every 60 s or when the patient experiences an urge to swallow the fluid accumulated in the floor of the mouth. The tube can be fitted with a funnel to ease collection of saliva. Again, the amount of saliva is determined by weighing or read from the scale on the graduated test tube.[6]

When aiming for collection of unstimulated saliva, one has to consider that the spitting action might have some stimulating effect on salivary flow. However, at very low flow rates the spitting method is preferred to the draining method, as less evaporation of saliva is thought to occur when applying the spitting as compared to the draining method, thus providing more reliable secretion data.[7]

A similar method is applied for collection of stimulated whole saliva. The patient is instructed to chew on paraffin wax or flavorless chewing gum or a piece of Parafilm at a fixed rate (Parafilm® M is a self-sealing, moldable, and flexible film for numerous uses in the laboratory such as sealing the openings of vessels). The patient has to spit the secreted saliva into a test tube or a cup. When applying a gustatory stimulus, one has to consider that the collected saliva will be contaminated with constituents originating from the gustatory agent.

Suction method

Saliva is continuously aspirated from the floor of the mouth into a graduated test tube or preweighed sampling container by a saliva ejector or aspirator. The amount of saliva is determined by weighing or read from the tube.[6]

Absorbent method

Saliva is collected (absorbed) by preweighed swab, cotton roll, or gauze sponge placed in the mouth at the orifices of the major salivary glands and is removed for reweighing at the end of the collection period.[6] In patients with severe xerostomia, an estimation of the degree of hyposalivation, thus not actual flow rate data, can also be obtained by a swab method.[15] The swab method is used to soak up all saliva in the mouth and on the teeth or dentures with a gauze sponge, which is weighed before and after the collection. The patients are asked not to take fluids or food for 2 h before the test. The weight difference provides an estimation of the degree of hyposalivation.

A commercially available absorbent method for collection of whole saliva is the Salivette method (Sarstedt, Nümbrecht, Germany) (Fig. 4.2). Using this method, saliva collection is carried out by chewing a cotton wool swab (this swab can be citric acid treated). Recovery of the saliva sample is achieved by returning the swab to the Salivette and centrifuging the container. The fluid sample obtained is used for analysis. This method is mainly used to investigate saliva constituents and, for example, drug, hormones, or steroids monitoring.

Reliability

For flow rate data of whole saliva, see Table 4.2, but mention that the flow rate data are dependent on the collection method applied. The suction and swab methods introduce some degree of stimulation and variability and thus are not recommended for unstimulated whole saliva collection. The swab method was found to be the least reliable.[16] Draining and spitting provided similar reproducible and reliable unstimulated whole saliva flow rates. The spitting method was also recommended for stimulated whole saliva collection.

Saliva flow can be stimulated by applying 0.1–0.2 mol/L citric acid (2–4% weight/volume) bilaterally to the tongue at fixed intervals (e.g., 15–60 s). Saliva is collected for at least 5 min, but preferably 10 min (at least in healthy controls, 5 min might be sufficient for a reliable estimation of salivary secretion and composition). Disadvantage of the use of gustatory stimulants is that they can interfere with some salivary analyses. Furthermore, stimulants may not elicit a constant flow rate because of a saliva diluting effect. On the contrary, mechanical (masticatory) stimulation, for example, standard size gum base, or paraffin wax (1.5 g, mp = 42°C) will not lead to contamination of saliva with exogenous substances. To standardize mechanical stimulation (mastication) throughout the collection period, the frequency of mastication can be controlled by using a metronome at about 70 chews/min.[6]

An important phenomenon that has to be taken into account when collecting whole saliva is the practice effect. Once people are familiar with collection of saliva, their unstimulated salivary flow rate will increase by about 15%, compared to the first time they were asked to salivate.[22,27] This practice effect does not occur when, for example, PAR saliva is collected under stimulated conditions. In addition to the practice effect, the sampling conditions might

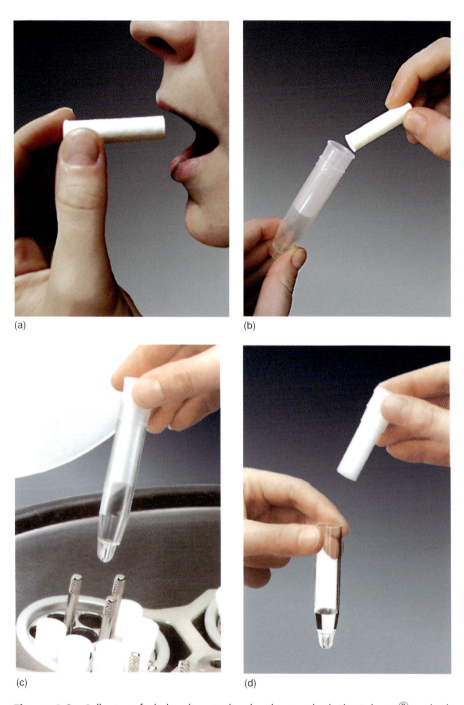

(a)

(b)

(c)

(d)

Figure 4.2 Collection of whole saliva via the absorbent method: The Salivette® method. (a) Saliva collection is carried out by chewing a cotton wool swab. (b) Recovery of the saliva sample is achieved by returning the swab to the Salivette. (c) Centrifuging the container. (d) Thereafter, cover is removed and saliva sample is ready for analysis.

Table 4.2 Flow rates of whole saliva.

| Author(s) | Flow rate | | Subjects | | | Stimulus |
	Unstim	Stim	Age	Sex	Health	
Navazesh and	0.50	2.38	18–32	M + F	H	Chewing (20/min)
Christensen (1982)[16]		2.64	18–32	M + F	H	2% citric acid
Shern et al. (1990)[17]	0.50	1.50	21–58	M + F	H	2% citric acid
Denny et al. (1991)[18]	0.38	0.90	18–35	M + F	H	Chewing (45/min)
	0.19	1.52	65–83	M + F	H	Chewing (45/min)
Navazesh et al. (1996)[19]	0.38	1.35	23–75	M + F	H	Chewing (45/min)
Bardow et al. (2000)[20]	0.49	1.57	25–30	M + F	H	Chewing (50/min)
		2.11				Chewing (100/min)
Won et al. (2001)[21]	0.44	–	23–28	M	H	
	0.33	–	23–28	F	H	
Lee et al. (2002)[4]	0.43	–	24–63	M + F	H	
Márton et al. (2004)[5]	0.36	–	Elderly	M + F	H	
Gotoh et al. (2005)[22]	0.23	2.06	Young	F	H	Chewing
Eliasson et al. (2006)[23]	0.4	2.1	20–64	M	H	Chewing
	0.3	2.0	18–64	F	H	
	0.2	2.5	65–82	M	H	Chewing
	0.2	1.6	65–81	F	H	
Inoue et al. (2006)[24]	0.50	–	20–31	M	H	
	0.35	–	20–32	F	H	
Márton et al. (2006)[25]	0.37	–	32–76	M + F	H	
Pijpe et al. (2007)[26]	0.33	–	23–58	M + F	H	

Unstim, unstimulated; Stim, stimulated; M, male; F, female; H, healthy.

also affect salivary flow and composition. For example, in children repetition of sampling results in a higher flow rate, but not buffer capacity.[28]

Application of an absorbent method might provide results that are dissimilar from those obtained with, for example, suction, drooling, spitting, or paraffin wax-stimulated collection methods. The cotton rolls applied might reduce, among other things, the content of Na^+, K^+, Cl^-, glycoprotein markers, IgA, lysozyme and lactoferrin, while increasing the concentrations of Ca^{2+}, inorganic phosphate, and thiocyanate.[29,30] Also, steroid levels obtained with, for example, the Salivette method do not correlate with levels in saliva obtained with the passive drooling method.[31] Use of polypropylene-coated cotton rolls solves this problem only in part. Furthermore, at very low flow rates, the absorbent method just might be of benefit to get an indication of general dryness of the oral surfaces.[15] Although not considered to be very reliable, the absorbent method might help the clinician to semiquantitatively assess the level of oral dryness when treating such patients.

PAROTID SALIVA

PAR saliva is the easiest glandular saliva to collect. The orifice of the PAR gland is very accessible for cannulation, but usually a (modified) Lashley or Carlsson–Crittenden cup is applied. Other methods include the use of a personalized plastic intraoral device[32] and a snail collector.[33]

Cannulation

The orifice of the main PAR excretory duct (Stensen's duct) is located in the buccal mucosa at the level of the first/second upper molar. The access to the duct can be tested using a blunt lacrimal probe. Next, a thin tube can be inserted in the duct via the orifice. If needed, the tube can be fixed with a suture so that no leakage will occur.

Lashley cup/Carlson–Crittenden cup

These cups are easily applied, even by untrained personnel. The inner chamber is attached to a rubber bulb or a suction device via plastic tubing and the cup is placed over Stensen's duct (Fig. 4.3).[1,6] As unstimulated flow rates of PAR saliva are very low or even absent, PAR saliva is usually collected under stimulated conditions. The most commonly applied stimulus is application of a 2–4% (weight/volume) citric acid solution to the lateral borders of the tongue at 30 or 60 s intervals using a cotton swab.

Reliability

For flow rate data of PAR saliva see Table 4.3.

Burlage et al.[1] showed a high correlation between flow rates from the left and right PAR glands ($r^2 = 0.79$; Fig. 4.4a). The variation in flow rates between the various measuring points was least pronounced for the lowest flow rates (Fig. 4.4a). In Sjögren's patients an even higher correlation between left and right flow rates was observed ($r^2 = 0.90$; Fig. 4.4b). The intravolunteer variation in PAR flow rate was $23.3 \pm 5.9\%$ (range 7.0–32.3%). Moreover, increasing the number of collections did not result in significant reduction of the intravolunteer variation or a more reliable (baseline) value. This was shown both in healthy persons and head and neck radiation patients.[1]

The results from a large number of studies.[6,34,37–43] demonstrate that salivary flow rates are not constant and exhibit considerable variation. Burlage et al.,[1] however, showed a large degree of similarity between flow rates of the left and right PAR glands in healthy subjects as well as in patients with Sjögren's syndrome. This is not surprising since in systemic diseases such as Sjögren's syndrome similar gland types are affected simultaneously. Similarly, high correlation between left and right PAR flow rates has been reported in healthy and drooling children.[44,45] This confirms our view that significant left and right differences occur only in cases of localized pathology or asymmetric exposure to radiotherapy.

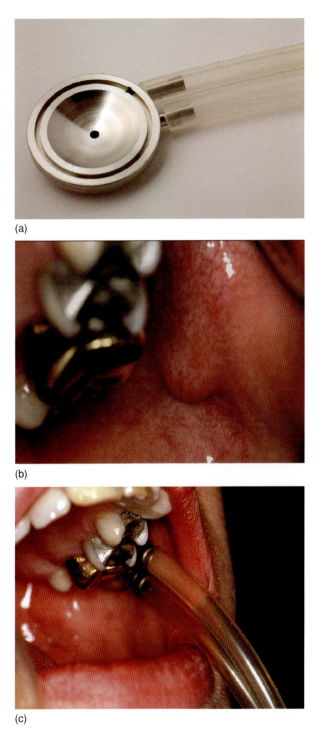

(a)

(b)

(c)

Figure 4.3   The Lashley cup for collection of parotid saliva. (a) The cup consists of an inner and outer chamber. The inner chamber serves as the collection chamber. (b) The orifice of the parotid duct in the cheek. The cup is placed over this orifice. (c) The cup in place over the orifice of the parotid duct. The flow of parotid saliva is clearly visible in the duct.

Table 4.3 Mean flow rates of parotid saliva (mL/min/gland).

Author(s)	Flow rate		Subjects			Stimulus[a]
	Unstim	Stim	Age	Sex	Health	
Ferguson et al. (1973)[34]	—	1.22	ND	M + F	H	Sucking on "sprangles acid drops"
Baum (1981)[35]	—	0.86	20–39	M + F	H	2% citric acid
	—	0.71	40–59	M + F	H	
	—	0.90	60–88	M + F	H	
Navazesh et al. (1996)[19]	—	0.65	23–75	M + F	H	3% citric acid
Veerman et al. (1996)[36]	—	0.23	25–49	M + F	H	3% citric acid
Fisher and Ship (1999)[37]	0.03	0.40	20–40	M + F	H	2% citric acid
	0.03	0.26	60–80	M + F	H	
Bardow et al. (2000)[20]	0.13	0.63	25–30	M + F	H	0.2% citric acid
		1.44				2% citric acid
Ghezzi et al. (2000)[38]	—	0.37	20–38	M + F	H	2% citric acid
	—	0.29	60–77	M + F	H	
Ghezzi and Ship (2003)[39]	—	0.34	20–38	M + F	H	2% citric acid
	—	0.29	60–77	M + F	H	
Burlage et al. (2005)[1]	—	0.33	30–60	M + F	H	2% citric acid

[a] Application of citric acid varied between every 15–60 s. Unstim, unstimulated; Stim, stimulated; ND, not described; M, male; F, female; H, healthy.

Ghezzi et al.[38] demonstrated that in establishing a standard endpoint, both intraindividual and interindividual variations over time must be taken into account. They suggested that a 45% decrease in stimulated PAR flow from "normal" levels can be considered as an objective measure of salivary hypofunction. In the study of Burlage et al.,[1] the greatest amount of intrasubject variation was 32.3% (mean 24%), indicating a somewhat lower variation in normal stimulated PAR flow levels. Bardow et al.[20] also reported a lower variation in the flow rate in healthy subjects (mean 22%). Therefore, we suggest that a 25–35% increase in the PAR flow rate from the baseline level highlights a "real" effect of a given therapy in dry mouth patients, this in addition to symptomatic improvement. Moreover, increasing the number of initial collections has only a negligible effect on the reliability of the baseline value. This is in line with the observations of Jongerius et al.[44] and Rotteveel et al.[45] Based on these data we would like to suggest that one reliable baseline sample, that is, a sample collected without any interference due to the technique applied, is sufficient for clinical studies evaluating the progression of a disease or the effect of a therapy. In healthy subjects and patients suffering from a systemic disease affecting all salivary glands, for example, Sjögren's syndrome, comparison of left and right flow rates might serve as an intraindividual control.

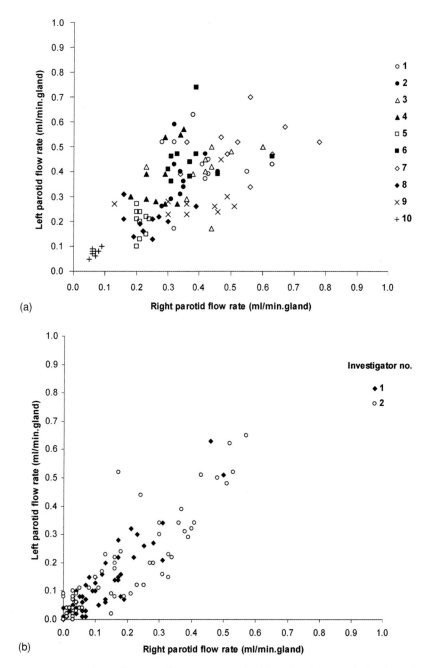

Figure 4.4 Correlation between flow rates from the left and right parotid glands (Burlage et al., 2005).[1] Note the clustering of the flow rates for the lower secretion rates while there is a wider spread in flow rates measured in subjects with higher flow rates, and the good agreement between the investigators. (a) Healthy volunteers. (b) Patients with Sjögren's syndrome.

SUBMANDIBULAR/SUBLINGUAL SALIVA

SM/SL glands contribute between 30 and 60% of volume of stimulated whole saliva, depending on the degree of stimulation.[46] While PAR saliva is relatively easy to collect by established methods, there are no universally accepted techniques for collection of SM/SL secretions. Most studies on saliva, therefore, have been limited to PAR or whole saliva. However, several studies have revealed more significant involvement of SM/SL glands as a result of various diseases. In this section, the major collection approaches for SM/SL saliva are described.

Cannulation

Secretions from the SM and SL glands often enter the oral cavity via a common duct, making it difficult to collect secretions from each gland separately. Tapered polyethylene tubing (~0.5–1.5 mm) may be used for cannulation of Wharton's duct. However, extreme caution must be used when placing the cannula because the wall of the duct is thin and may rupture.[6]

Segregator (individual prosthesis)

Schneyer[47] introduced a method for collection of separate SM and SL saliva in human. This custom-made segregator for collecting SM and SL saliva has a central chamber for collection of SM saliva and two lateral chambers for collection of SL saliva (Fig. 4.5). The collector is placed on the lower jaw. Polyethylene tubing connects the chambers to the collecting tube. Fabrication of such a collecting device is time-consuming because a mould of the floor of the subjects' mouth has to be made and the device has to be fabricated and adjusted

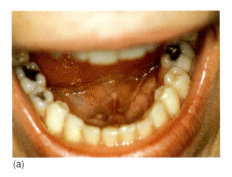
(a)

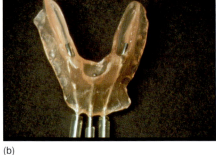
(b)

Figure 4.5 The segregator for collection of submandibular and sublingual saliva. (a) The segregator will be placed on the lower jaw with chambers covering the orifices of the submandibular and sublingual ducts. (b) Inner surface of the segregator. The central chamber will cover the orifices of the submandibular duct (Wharton's duct). Often the main duct of the sublingual gland (Bartholin's duct) also drains in this area or has already joined the main submandibular excretory duct. The lateral chambers will cover the ducts of the sublingual gland that directly drain into the floor of the mouth (ducts of Rivini).

on an individual basis. A modification of this method allowing for application of masticatory and gustatory stimuli by adding a masticatory plane to the Schneyer apparatus was introduced by Henriques and Chauncey.[48] Afterward, there have been many minor adjustments of this approach including those of Truelove et al.[49] and Coudert et al.[50]

Since the orifices of the main excretory ducts of the SM and SL glands are in close proximity, with the use of this collector mainly SM saliva, although slightly contaminated with SL saliva, is collected via the central chamber, while the fluid from the lateral chambers was shown to be predominantly SL saliva.[36] However, as this device has to be individually adapted, it is not feasible for routine use in general practice.

Suction method

A simple method for collection of mixed SM/SL saliva is blocking Stensen's duct, for example, with Lashley cups or cotton rolls, and thus isolating Wharton's, Bartholin's, and other SL ducts. Subsequently, the saliva on the floor of the mouth can be collected with a syringe (Fig. 4.6), micropipette, or with gentle suction (see Wolff apparatus). Using this method saliva from both the SM and SL ducts is collected together, as separate aspiration is rather difficult due to the close anatomical relationship between the orifices of both glands and the frequent presence of communicating ducts between the SM and SL main ducts. The glands can be stimulated with citric acid solution (2–4% weight/volume) applied with a cotton swab to the lateral borders of the tongue at 30–60 s intervals. Mixing of the acid solution applied to the tongue and SM/SL saliva pooling anteriorly on the floor of the mouth has to be carefully avoided.

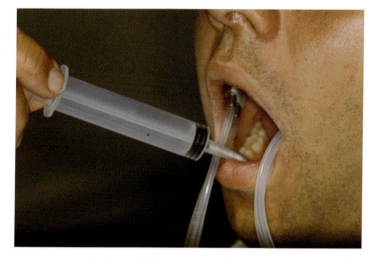

Figure 4.6 Suction method for collections of submandibular/sublingual saliva. The orifices of the parotid ducts can be blocked with, for example, Lashley cups or cotton rolls. The saliva collected in the floor of the mouth is now mainly submandibular/sublingual saliva and can be collected with a syringe.

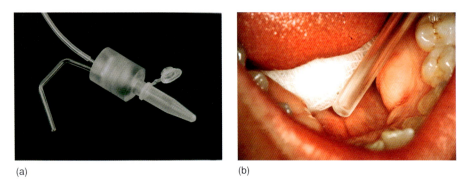

(a)   (b)

Figure 4.7 Submandibular/sublingual saliva collecting device. (a) Two lengths of tubing, one for saliva collection (left) and the other for suction (right), are connected to the top of the buffering chamber. An additional hole is provided for manual suction control. A 1.5 mL centrifuge tube (for saliva storage) is attached to the bottom of the chamber. (b) Use of the submandibular/sublingual saliva collection device on gauze-covered submandibular/sublingual duct openings.

Alternatively, the device introduced by Pedersen et al.[51] can be used, consisting of a Drummond micropipette holder fitted with a 2 mL amber latex dropper bulb, which can be placed over the orifices of the SM glands.

Wolff apparatus

The collecting system for SM/SL saliva developed by Wolff et al.[46] consists of collecting tubing, a buffering chamber, a storing tube, and a suction device (Fig. 4.7a). The collecting tube consists of cellulose acetate butyrate tubing (outer diameter 1/8 in.; inner diameter 1/16 in.), which is gas autoclavable and cold formable, facilitating adjustment of its shape for intraoral use. The storing tube is either a 1.5 mL centrifuge tube or a 5 mL polystyrene tube. The suction device is a vacuum pump. Attached to the pump is a piece of Tygon® tubing (outer diameter 1/16 in., inner diameter 1/32 in.) long enough to reach the collecting zone.

All components are connected to and securely fit into openings of a buffering chamber 4 cm long and 2.5 cm wide, constructed of polycarbonate (steam autoclavable). The interior is a hollow sphere with four openings: one at the bottom (where the storing tube is attached) and three at the top. The collecting tubing enters the buffering chamber through one of the top holes and exits at the bottom to deliver the collected saliva into the storing tube. Another orifice, to which the end of a 250 µL pipette tip is cemented, serves to connect the Tygon tubing. The third hole facilitates manual control of suction since only a finger is required to occlude and open it (Fig. 4.7b).

The main function of the buffering chamber is to avoid saliva being sucked into the suction device; thus, over 93% of the collected samples are recovered in the storing tube. Bubbles are frequent when SM/SL saliva is collected by suction. The buffering chamber provides space where bubbles can expand and

Table 4.4 Mean submandibular/sublingual flow rates (mL/min/gland) as measured by the various sampling devices in healthy subjects.

Author(s)	Flow rate		Subjects			
	Unstim	**Stim**	**Age**	**Sex**	**Health**	**Stimulus**[a]
Schneyer (1955)[47]	0.15	—	Young	M	ND	
Henriques and Chauncey (1961)[48]	—	0.61	ND	ND	ND	Chewing
Dawes (1975)[41]	0.16	—	Young	M + F	ND	
Pedersen et al. (1985)[51]	0.07	0.12	18–35	M	H	Lemon drops
	0.05	0.09	18–35	F	H	
Tylenda et al. (1988)[52]	0.15	0.47	26–39	M	H	2% citric acid
	0.21	0.41	26–39	F	H	
	0.23	0.45	40–59	M	H	
	0.12	0.33	40–59	F	H	
Oliveby et al. (1989)[53]	0.11	0.31	26–38	M + F	H	Xylitol + lycasin
Atkinson et al. (1990)[54]	0.11	0.41	22–72	F	NM	
Ship et al. (1991)[55]	0.11	0.33	22–72	M	H	
	0.10	0.33	20–90	F	H	
Nederfors and Dahlof (1993)[56]	—	2.25	20–46	M + F	H	3% citric acid
Veerman et al. (1996)[36]	0.15	—	25–49	M + F	H	
Wolff et al. (1997)[46]	0.17	0.49	25–41	M + F	H	2% citric acid
Ghezzi et al. (2000)[38]	—	0.32	20–38	M + F	H	2% citric acid
	—	0.30	60–77	M + F	H	
Kalk et al. (2001)[57]	0.12	0.46	23–58	M + F	H	2% citric acid
Ghezzi and Ship (2003)[39]	—	0.34	20–38	M + F	H	2% citric acid
		0.30	60–77	M + F	H	

[a] Application of citric acid varied between every 15–60 s. Unstim, unstimulated; Stim, stimulated; M, male; F, female; H, healthy; NM, nonmedicated; ND, not described.

break. Fluid eventually flows to the storing tube without leaking into the tubing connected to the suction device.

Reliability

For flow rate data of SM/SL saliva see Table 4.4. Moreover, no test/retest data are available in the literature. The Wolff apparatus shows high reproducibility both for intraexaminer (reliability of 0.92 for "normal" and 0.89 for xerostomic individuals) and interexaminer (0.93 for "normal" and 0.80 for xerostomic individuals) correlation measurements.[46] See further the section "Is the Saliva Collected by a Saliva Collection Method Indeed the Saliva Which Has Been Sought?"

MINOR SALIVARY GLANDS

Minor salivary gland secretions can be collected by pipette, absorbent filter paper, or special devised (individual) collectors. Secretions may also be determined by Periotron® (Oraflow, New York, USA), which measures small volumes of fluids. For collection of saliva from the minor salivary glands, the mucosa is dried first and, after a 2 min interval, saliva samples may be obtained by touching the developing drops of saliva with the absorbent paper. The quantity of saliva may then be determined by weight or utilizing a Periotron.[6,17] With a Periotron small volumes of fluids can be measured.

Labial and buccal saliva

Saliva from the minor labial and buccal glands can be collected by a paper strip absorption method. Either 2.2 × 4.4 mm filter-paper strips (Periopaper strips) or 6 × 16 mm high-purity chromatography paper (Whatman 3MM, Whatman International, Madistone, England) can be held with cotton pliers to a selected oral site for 5–30 s (dipstick method). Otherwise, frying pan-shaped filter paper strips (measuring area 31.7 mm^2, Sialopaper, Proflow) can be held flat to an oral tissue site in a blotting fashion for 30 s. The volume of saliva can be measured electronically with a Periotron device.[4,17,58] Flow rates can be calculated in units of μL/min/cm^2 of mucosal area.

Palatine saliva

Pipette

After rinsing the mouth with deionised water, the palatine (PAL) surface is dried with cotton wool. Saliva droplets that appear on the orifices of the PAL glands can subsequently be aspirated using a pipette.

Filtration paper

PAL flow can be measured with preweighed 8 mm diameter filter paper discs (Rundfilter MN 640d; Macherey-Nagel GmbH & Co KG, Duren, Germany) placed bilaterally in the region of the maxillary second molar, 15 mm palatally from the (e)dentulous ridge. Saliva collection occurs over 30 s. Data were recorded in μL/min/cm^2 after weight determination from the filter papers (electronic scale, Sartonius BA-110S), which had been stored in previously measured tubes (Eppendorf Microtube 0.5 mL with attached cup, No 72699; Sarsted Ltd, Leichester, UK) for complete isolation.[5] Similarly Periopaper, Sialopaper, or high-purity chromatography paper can be applied and the volume assessed with a Periotron.[4,17,58] Studies revealed that PAL secretions are very variable in the same subject and depend on the stimulation status of the PAL glands as PAL glands depleted of saliva may need considerable time to recover before saliva flow can be again observed from that gland.[36,59]

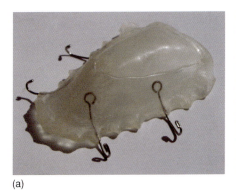
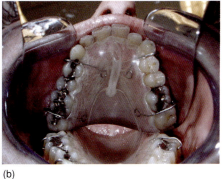

(a)   (b)

Figure 4.8 Collection of palatine saliva using an individual collection prosthesis. (a) Inner face of the palatine collector. The chamber covers most of the palatine glands on the hard palate and anterior third of the soft palate. (b) Palatine collector is worn.

Impression of palate

Instead of using filter paper or a pipette, PAL saliva can also be collected by making an individual impression of the upper jaw. When removing the mold filled with impression paste after setting of that paste, the impression surface facing the palate is often covered with a saliva film predominantly consisting of PAL saliva. This film can then be collected for, mainly, chemical analyses. This method is not reliable for assessing PAL flow rates.

Individual collection prosthesis

The custom-made segregator for collecting PAL saliva covers the hard and anterior third of the soft palate. PAL secretions accumulate in the chamber and flow out of the tube as a result of secretion pressure and of gentle suction with a syringe (Fig. 4.8). When using this device, the flow rate of "unstimulated" PAL saliva was comparable to that of stimulated PAR saliva.[36]

Reliability of collecting saliva from the minor salivary glands

For flow rate data of saliva from the minor salivary glands see Table 4.5, but it has to be considered that the flow rate data are dependent on the stimulus applied.

A striking finding by Veerman et al.[36] was the rather high flow rate of PAL saliva, which was comparable to that of SM saliva in this study. Sodium dodecyl sulfate polyacrylamide gel electrophoresis (SDS-PAGE) and immunoblotting indicated that protein patterns of PAR and PAL saliva were essentially different, indicating that no significant contamination had occurred with PAR saliva. Probably the high PAL secretion rate observed when using this collector was caused by mechanical stimulation due to the presence of the collection device on the palatal surface (in fact the segregator for collection of SM/SL saliva will also show such an effect). This was suggested also by the relatively high pH of PAL secretions. Nevertheless, these data show that under certain conditions,

Table 4.5 Mean flow rates of saliva from the minor salivary glands.

| Author(s) | Flow rate | | Subjects | | | Stimulus[a] |
	Unstim	Stim	Age	Sex	Health	
Palatine saliva						
Ship et al. (1990)[60]	0.74[b]	0.75[b]	21–58	M + F	H	Hard palate, 2% citric acid
Sivarajasingam and Drummond (1995)[62]	0.59[b]	—	17–81	M	H	Hard palate
	0.53[b]	—	17–81	F	H	
Eliasson et al. (1996)[61]	1.02[b]	—	22–89	M	H	Hard palate
	0.78[b]	—	22–89	F	H	
Veerman et al. (1996)[36]	0.21[c]	—	25–49	M + F	H	Soft + hard palate
Won et al. (2001)[21]	2.5[b]	—	23–28	M	H	Soft palate
	1.9[b]	—	23–28	F	H	
Lee et al. (2002)[4]	7.6[b]	—	24–63	M + F	H	Hard palate
	26.4[b]	—				Soft palate
Márton et al. (2004)[5]	1.7[b]	—	Elderly	M + F	H	Hard palate
Eliasson et al. (2006)[23]	0.7[b]	—	20–64	M	H	Hard palate
	0.8[b]	—	18–64	F	H	
	0.9[b]	—	65–82	M	H	Hard palate
	0.8[b]	—	65–81	F	H	
Márton et al. (2006)[25]	1.35[b]	—	32–76	M + F	H	Hard palate
Labial saliva						
Shern et al. (1990)[17]	0.96[b]	1.00[b]	21–58	M + F	H	Lower lip, 2% citric acid
Sivarajasingam and Drummond (1995)[62]	1.61[b]	—	17–81	M	H	Upper lip
	1.19[b]	—	17–81	F	H	
	2.38[b]	—	17–81	M	H	Lower lip
	2.00[b]	—	17–81	F	H	
Eliasson et al. (1996)[61]	5.12[b]	—	22–89	M	H	Lower lip
	4.83[b]	—	22–89	F	H	
Won et al. (2001)[21]	2.6[b]	—	23–28	M	H	Lower lip
	2.9[b]	—	23–28	F	H	
Lee et al. (2002)[4]	17.6[b]	—	24–63	M + F	H	Upper lip
	28.9[b]	—				Lower lip
Eliasson et al. (2006)[23]	3.0[b]	—	20–64	M	H	Lower lip
	2.7[b]	—	18–64	F	H	
	3.4[b]	—	65–82	M	H	Lower lip
	2.5[b]	—	65–81	F	H	
Buccal saliva						
Shern et al. (1990)[17]	2.64[b]	2.52[b]	21–58	M + F	H	2% citric acid
Sivarajasingam and Drummond (1995)[62]	3.02[b]	—	17–81	M	H	
	2.94[b]	—	17–81	F	H	
Eliasson et al. (1996)[61]	16.7[b]	—	22–89	M	H	
	15.2[b]	—	22–89	F	H	
Lee et al. (2002)[4]	48.8[b]	—	24–63	M + F	H	
Eliasson et al. (2006)[23]	14.6[b]	—	20–64	M	H	
	13.8[b]	—	18–64	F	H	
	15.9[b]	—	65–82	M	H	
	14.1[b]	—	65–81	F	H	

[a] Application of citric acid varied between every 15–60 s. [b]mL/min; [c]μL/min/cm^2; Unstim, unstimulated; Stim, stimulated; M, male; F, female; H, healthy.

PAL glands contribute much more to whole saliva than usually is assumed. Another striking phenomenon was that the PAL flow can be as high as SM or PAR flow, but the glands cannot keep up this flow for a very long period of time. After exhaustion it may take more than 24 h before the PAL glands were able to reach such a high flow rate again.

IS THE SALIVA COLLECTED BY A SALIVA COLLECTION METHOD INDEED THE SALIVA THAT HAS BEEN SOUGHT?

In contrast to the collection of PAR saliva, collecting PAL, SM, and SL saliva using the earlier-described devices intrinsically has the risk of potential cross-contamination of secretions from different glands. For some glands it is indeed inevitable to obtain secretions from more than one type of gland. For example, in the palate both serous and mucous glands are present, and since the device for PAL secretions covers the whole palate, a mixture of both serous and mucous PAL secretions will be collected using this device. Indeed, saliva collected with these devices contains components such as MUC5B and MUC7, which are characteristic for mucous glands, in addition to proteins such as amylase, which is typically secreted by serous glands. Moreover, placement of the device onto the palate presents a very strong stimulus for saliva secretion, which makes it impossible to monitor resting flow rates using this device.

The SM secretion collected by Schneyer's device to some extent will be contaminated with SL saliva, as the orifices of both glands are in very close proximity or even identical. In practice this may not be a very big problem, for example, when one is interested in monitoring the secretion rates of SM glands, since the SL glands contribute little if any to these secretions when collection times are 10–15 min. On the other hand, the SL secretion collected from the laterally situated orifices is solely derived from the SL gland, and not contaminated with SM secretions.

The Wolff apparatus appears to collect relatively pure SM/SL fluids, since contamination of the collected sample by a stimulant solution swabbed repeatedly over the tongue during saliva collection was found in 50% of the tested subjects at a titer of 1:32 or 1:16, while no contamination was detected in the other individuals.[46]

REFERENCES

1. Burlage FR, Pijpe J, Coppes RP, et al. Variability of flow rate when collecting stimulated human parotid saliva. Eur J Oral Sci 2005;113(5):386–90.
2. Vissink A, Spijkervet FK, Van Nieuw Amerongen A. Aging and saliva: a review of the literature. Spec Care Dentist 1996;16(3):95–103.
3. Wu AJ, Baum BJ, Ship JA. Extended stimulated parotid and submandibular secretion in a healthy young and old population. J Gerontol 1995;50A(1):M45–8.

4. Lee SK, Lee SW, Chung SC, Kim YK, Kho HS. Analysis of residual saliva and minor salivary gland secretions in patients with dry mouth. Arch Oral Biol 2002;47(9):637–41.
5. Márton K, Boros I, Fejerdy P, Madlena M. Evaluation of unstimulated flow rates of whole and palatal saliva in healthy patients wearing complete dentures and in patients with Sjögren's syndrome. J Prosthet Dent 2004;91(6):577–81.
6. Navazesh M. Methods for collecting saliva. Ann N Y Acad Sci 1993;694:72–7.
7. Schmidt-Nielsen B. The solubility of tooth substance in relation to the composition of saliva (thesis). Acta Odontol Scand 1946;7(Suppl 2):1–88.
8. Kariyawasam AP, Dawes C. A circannual rhythm in unstimulated salivary flow rate when the ambient temperature varies by only about 2 degrees C. Arch Oral Biol 2005;50(10):919–22.
9. Kavanagh DA, O'Mullane DM, Smeeton N. Variation of salivary flow rate in adolescents. Arch Oral Biol 1998;43(5):347–52.
10. Louridis O, Demetriou N, Bazopoulou-Kyrkanides E. Environmental temperature effect on the secretion rate of "resting" and stimulated human mixed saliva. J Dent Res 1970;49(5):1136–40.
11. Shannon IL. Climatological effects on human parotid gland function. Arch Oral Biol 1966;11(4):451–3.
12. Shannon IL, Chauncey HH. A parotid fluid collection device with improved stability characteristics. J Oral Ther Pharmacol 1967;4(2):93–7.
13. Elishoov H, Wolff A, Schnur Kravel L, Shipperman A, Gorsky M. The influence of season, environment temperature, and temperature perception on unstimulated parotid and submandibular/SL secretion rates. Arch Oral Biol 2008;53(1):75–8.
14. Wolff A, Herscovici D, Rosenberg M. A simple technique for the determination of salivary gland hypofunction. Oral Sur Oral Med Oral Pathol Oral Radiol Endod 2002;94(2):175–8.
15. Vissink A, s-Gravenmade EJ, Panders AK, et al. A clinical comparison between commercially available mucin- and CMC-containing saliva substitutes. Int J Oral Surg 1983;12(4):232–8.
16. Navazesh M, Christensen CM. A comparison of whole mouth resting and stimulated salivary measurement procedures. J Dent Res 1982;61(10):1158–62.
17. Shern RJ, Fox PC, Cain JL, Li SH. A method for measuring the flow of saliva from the minor salivary glands. J Dent Res 1990;69(5):1146–9.
18. Denny PC, Denny PA, Klauser DK, Hong SH, Navazesh M, Tabak LA. Age-related changes in mucins from human whole saliva. J Dent Res 1991;70(10):1320–27.
19. Navazesh M, Brightman VJ, Pogoda JM. Relationship of medical status, medications, and salivary flow rates in adults of different ages. Oral Surg Oral Med Oral Pathol Oral Radiol Endod 1996;81(2):172–6.
20. Bardow A, Madsen J, Nauntofte B. The bicarbonate concentration in human saliva does not exceed the plasma level under normal physiological conditions. Clin Oral Investig 2000;4(4):245–53.

21. Won S, Kho H, Kim Y, Chung S, Lee S. Analysis of residual saliva and minor salivary gland secretions. Arch Oral Biol 2001;46(7):619–24.

22. Gotoh S, Watanabe Y, Fujibayashi T. Validity of stimulated whole saliva collection as a sialometric evaluation for diagnosing Sjögren's syndrome. Oral Surg Oral Med Oral Pathol Oral Radiol Endod 2005;99(3):299–302.

23. Eliasson L, Birkhed D, Osterberg T, Carlen A. Minor salivary gland secretion rates and immunoglobulin A in adults and the elderly. Eur J Oral Sci 2006;114(6):494–9.

24. Inoue H, Ono K, Masuda W, et al. Gender difference in unstimulated whole saliva flow rate and salivary gland sizes. Arch Oral Biol 2006;51(12):1055–60.

25. Márton K, Boros I, Varga G, et al. Evaluation of palatal saliva flow rate and oral manifestations in patients with Sjögren's syndrome. Oral Dis 2006;12(5):480–86.

26. Pijpe J, Kalk WW, Bootsma H, Spijkervet FK, Kallenberg CG, Vissink A. Progression of salivary gland dysfunction in patients with Sjögren's syndrome. Ann Rheum Dis 2007;66(1):107–12.

27. Miyawaki S, Torikai K, Natsume I, et al. Evaluation of two quantitative tests for salivary secretion–the chewing gum test and the Saxon test in normal subjects and in patients with Sjögren's syndrome. Ryumachi 1991;31(1):22–7.

28. Le Bell Y, Soderling E, Karjalainen S. Effect of repeated sampling and prestimulation on saliva buffer capacity and flow rate values in children. Scand J Dent Res 1991;99(6):505–509.

29. Aufricht C, Tenner W, Salzer H, Khoss A, Wurst E, Herkner K. Salivary IgA concentration is influenced by the saliva collection method. Eur J Clin Chem Clin Biochem 1992;30(2):81–3.

30. Lenander-Lumikari M, Johansson I, Vilja P, Samaranayake LP. Newer saliva collection methods and saliva composition: a study of two Salivette kits. Oral Dis 1995;1(2):86–91.

31. Gallagher P, Leitch MM, Massey AE, McAllister-Williams RH, Young AH. Assessing cortisol and dehydroepiandrosterone (DHEA) in saliva: effects of collection method. J Psychopharmacol (Oxford, England) 2006;20(5):643–9.

32. Wagner SA, Slavik M. An individualized plastic intraoral device for the collection of human parotid saliva. Int J Clin Pharmacol Ther Toxicol 1984;22(5):236–9.

33. Morales I, Dominguez P, Lopez R. Devices for saliva collection from the major salivary glands. Results in normal subjects. Rev Med Chil 1998;126(5):538–47.

34. Ferguson DB, Fort A, Elliott AL, Potts AJ. Circadian rhythms in human parotid saliva flow rate and composition. Arch Oral Biol 1973;18(9):1155–73.

35. Baum BJ. Evaluation of stimulated parotid saliva flow rate in different age groups. J Dent Res 1981;60(7):1292–6.

36. Veerman EC, van den Keybus PA, Vissink A, Nieuw Amerongen AV. Human glandular salivas: their separate collection and analysis. Eur J Oral Sci 1996;104(4 (Pt 1)):346–52.

37. Fisher D, Ship J. Effect of age on variability of parotid salivary gland flow rates over time. Age Aging 1999;28:447–561.
38. Ghezzi EM, Lange LA, Ship JA. Determination of variation of stimulated salivary flow rates. J Dent Res 2000;79(11):1874–8.
39. Ghezzi EM, Ship JA. Aging and secretory reserve capacity of major salivary glands. J Dent Res 2003;82(10):844–8.
40. Dawes C. Circadian rhythms in human salivary flow rate and composition. J Physiol 1972;220(3):529–45.
41. Dawes C. Circadian rhythms in the flow rate and composition of unstimulated and stimulated human submandibular saliva. J Physiol 1975;244(2):535–48.
42. Ferguson DB, Botchway CA. Circadian variations in flow rate and composition of human stimulated submandibular saliva. Arch Oral Biol 1979;24(6):433–7.
43. Ferguson DB, Fort A. Circadian variations in human resting submandibular saliva flow rate and composition. Arch Oral Biol 1974;19(1):47–55.
44. Jongerius PH, van Limbeek J, Rotteveel JJ. Assessment of salivary flow rate: biologic variation and measure error. Laryngoscope 2004;114(10):1801–804.
45. Rotteveel LJ, Jongerius PH, van Limbeek J, van den Hoogen FJ. Salivation in healthy schoolchildren. Int j pediatr otorhinolaryngol 2004;68(6):767–74.
46. Wolff A, Begleiter A, Moskona D. A novel system of human submandibular/SL saliva collection. J Dent Res 1997;76(11):1782–6.
47. Schneyer L. Method for the collection of separate submaxillary and SL salivas in man. J Dent Res 1955;34:257–61.
48. Henriques BL, Chauncey HH. A modified method for the collection of human submaxillary and SL saliva. Oral Surg Oral Med Oral Pathol 1961;14:1124–9.
49. Truelove EL, Bixler D, Merritt AD. Simplified method for collection of pure submandibular saliva in large volumes. J Dent Res 1967;46(6):1400–403.
50. Coudert JL, Lissac M, Parret J. A new appliance for the collection of human submandibular saliva. Arch Oral Biol 1986;31(6):411–13.
51. Pedersen W, Schubert M, Izutsu K, Mersai T, Truelove E. Age-dependent decreases in human submandibular gland flow rates as measured under resting and post-stimulation conditions. J Dent Res 1985;64(5):822–5.
52. Tylenda CA, Ship JA, Fox PC, Baum BJ. Evaluation of submandibular salivary flow rate in different age groups. J Dent Res 1988;67(9):1225–8.
53. Oliveby A, Lagerlof F, Ekstrand J, Dawes C. Studies on fluoride concentrations in human submandibular/SL saliva and their relation to flow rate and plasma fluoride levels. J Dent Res 1989;68(2):146–9.
54. Atkinson JC, Travis WD, Pillemer SR, Bermudez D, Wolff A, Fox PC. Major salivary gland function in primary Sjögren's syndrome and its relationship to clinical features. J Rheumatol 1990;17(3):318–22.
55. Ship JA, Patton LL, Tylenda CA. An assessment of salivary function in healthy premenopausal and postmenopausal females. J Gerontol 1991;46(1):M11–15.
56. Nederfors T, Dahlof C. A modified device for collection and flow-rate measurement of submandibular-SL saliva. Scand J Dent Res 1993;101(4):210–14.

57. Kalk WW, Vissink A, Spijkervet FK, Bootsma H, Kallenberg CG, Nieuw Amerongen AV. Sialometry and sialochemistry: diagnostic tools for Sjögren's syndrome. Ann Rheum Dis 2001;60(12):1110–16.
58. Disabato-Mordarski T, Kleinberg I. Use of a paper-strip absorption method to measure the depth and volume of saliva retained in embrasures and occlusal fussae of the human dentition. Arch Oral Biol 1996;41(8–9):809–20.
59. Makinen KK, Virtanen KK, Soderling E, Kotiranta J. Effect of xylitol-, sucrose-, and water-rinses on the composition of human palatine gland secretions. Scand J Dent Res 1985;93(3):253–61.
60. Ship JA, DeCarli C, Friedland RP, Baum BJ. Diminished submandibular salivary flow in dementia of the Alzheimer type. J Gerontol 1990;45(2):M61–6.
61. Eliasson L, Birkhed D, Heyden G, Stromberg N. Studies on human minor salivary gland secretions using the Periotron method. Arch Oral Biol 1996;41(12):1179–82.
62. Sivarajasingam V, Drummond JR. Measurements of human minor salivary gland secretions from different oral sites. Arch Oral Biol 1995;40(8):723–9.

Salivary secretion in health and disease

Michael D. Turner and Jonathan A. Ship

NORMAL SALIVARY SECRETION

The salivary glands are primarily divided into two classifications: the major glands, consisting of three pairs of major salivary glands (parotid, submandibular, and sublingual), and a multitude of minor glands, which are located in the buccal, labial, and palatal tissues. The salivary glands can also be classified secondary to function, with the parotid glands being primarily serous in secretion, the submandibular with a mixed serous and mucous secretion, and the sublingual and minor salivary glands being primarily mucous.[1,2]

These glandular secretions combine together to form whole saliva. Whole saliva also contains nonsalivary portions such as desquamated cells, bacteria, bacterial byproducts, extraneous debris, and various blood components from various oral diseases.[2] Normal whole saliva secretory rates vary between 800 and 1,500 mL/day with a pH in the range of 6.0–7.0. This pH range is effective for activating the digestive enzyme of amylase, which is found in serous saliva and catalyzes the breakdown of starches. Saliva contains the ions of potassium, sodium, bicarbonate, and chloride, which are important for the activation of the gustatory receptors located on the taste buds. Two major mucins, mucin 1 (MG1) and mucin 2 (MG2), play an important part in the lubrication of the mucosal surfaces. Saliva also has a rich secretion in antimicrobial and immunomodulatory proteins, which contribute to mucosal lubrication and tissue coating, tooth remineralization, and buffering. They include histatins, proline-rich proteins, statherins, carbonic anhydrases, secretory IgA, lactoferrin, lactoperoxidase, lysozyme, amylases, and a protein with purported anti-HIV capabilities (secretory leukocyte protease inhibitor or SLPI).

The parasympathetic nervous pathway stimulates salivary secretion. The neurotransmitter acetylcholine is released and binds to muscarinic receptors, predominantly the muscarinic 3 receptors. These receptors cause the activation of phospholipase C, which creates the secondary messenger inositol trisphosphate (IP3). IP3 migrates to receptors on the endoplasmic reticulum, which serves as the intracellular calcium storage site. Once the IP3 binds to this receptor, the ionized calcium is released.[3] This controlled elevation in cytosolic calcium activates the potassium and chloride channels, forming a salt gradient and eventually secretion of fluid (Fig. 5.1).

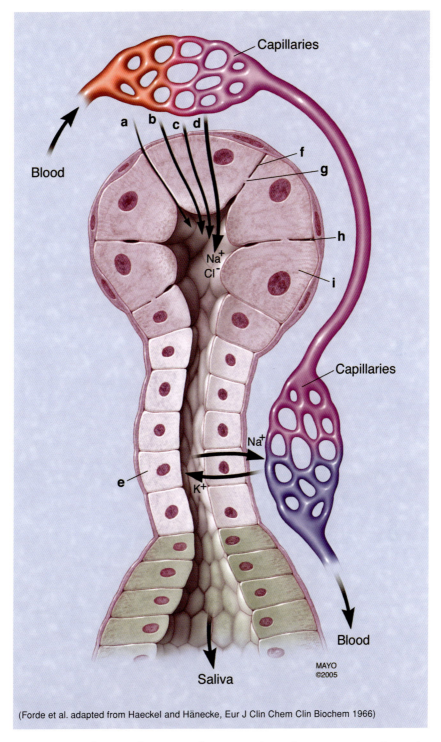

Capillaries

Blood

a b c d

f

g

h

Na$^+$
Cl$^-$

i

Capillaries

Na$^+$

e

K$^+$

Blood

Saliva

MAYO
©2005

(Forde et al. adapted from Haeckel and Hänecke, Eur J Clin Chem Clin Biochem 1966)

Figure 5.1 Mechanism of transport of protein and ions from serum into salivary ducts. a, active transport; b, passive diffusion; c, simple filtration; e, duct cells pump Na$^+$ to blood; f, cell membrane; g, pore; h, intracellular space; i, acinar cell. (Reference 4. By permission of Mayo Foundation for Medical Education and Research. All rights reserved.)

The secretion from the acinar cell, in addition to fluid, contains amylase and mucin in a solution of ions similar to the other extracellular fluids. A loop diuretic-sensitive sodium–potassium–chloride transport protein assists the migration of chloride into the acinar cells in opposition to its apparent electrochemical gradient.[5] Concurrently, one molecule of chloride leaves the cell by a calcium-activated chloride channel in the cellular membrane. To maintain electrical neutrality, sodium from the interstitium seeps out through the tight junctions of the acinar region. This elevated sodium chloride concentration directly produces an osmotic gradient across the acinar cell membranes, drawing water into the lumen.

As the secretion flows through the ductal pathways, two major active transport processes transform the ionic composition of the fluid in the saliva. First, sodium ions are absorbed from all the salivary ducts and potassium ions are secreted. However, there is a larger absorption of sodium in comparison to potassium secretion, which results in an osmotic gradient of -70 mV. Bicarbonate ions are then secreted by the ductal epithelium into the lumen of the duct (Fig. 5.1). The net result of these transport processes is that under resting conditions the concentrations of salivary sodium and chloride ions are only about 15 mEq/L, roughly one-seventh to one-tenth their concentrations in plasma. Conversely, the concentration of potassium ions is about 30 mEq/L, seven times as great as in plasma, and the concentration of bicarbonate ions is 50–70 mEq/L, which is about two to three times that of plasma.

The route that water moves through the acini has not been clearly established, but recent studies suggest that specific water channels, termed aquaporins (AQPs), are involved.[2] At least ten AQP types have been identified; AQP 5 has been localized to acinar cell luminal membranes in salivary glands, although the AQP isoform on the basolateral salivary membranes is not currently known.[6]

SALIVARY FUNCTION ACROSS THE HUMAN LIFESPAN

Most adolescents and adults are not aware of their own salivary function, similar to tear output. However, when salivary function is diminished by approximately 50%, the subjective symptoms of xerostomia begin to arise. Salivary hypofunction and xerostomia are common in the geriatric population. It was previously hypothesized that salivary function declined with age, although studies have now demonstrated that the secretory output from the major salivary glands does not undergo clinically significant decreases in healthy individuals.[7–11] Salivary components also appear to be stable in the absence of disease and xerostomia-inducing medications.[12] The majority of cases of xerostomia are likely due to polypharmacy, systemic diseases (e.g., Sjögren's syndrome), and head and neck radiation.[2]

What does occur with increasing age in the salivary glands is that acinar cell volume diminishes and ductal and connective tissue volume increases, decreasing the functional capacity of the gland.[13] Fortunately, there is a large secretory capacity of the gland that permits function to be maintained throughout the human lifespan. However, with age-associated physiologic insults (systemic medical disorders, dehydration, medications, head and neck radiotherapy), secretory reserve, and functional capacity is impaired significantly, reducing salivary output and leading to xerostomia and a host of oral-pharyngeal disorders.[14]

DISORDERS OF THE SALIVARY GLANDS

Salivary hyperfunction/sialorrhea

Salivary hyperfunction is either due to an increase in saliva production, a decrease in salivary clearance, or both. Hypersalivation can be caused by medications, hyperhydration, heavy metal poisoning, idiopathic paroxysmal hypersalivation, organophosphorous (acetylcholinesterase) poisoning, obstructive esophagitis, gastroesophageal reflux disease, nausea, cerebral vascular accident, neuromuscular diseases, neurologic diseases, and central neurologic infections (Table 5.1). Minor causes of hypersalivation can occur from local irritations, such as infant teething, aphthous ulcers, or a poorly adapted oral prosthesis.

Hypersalivation can impair the ability to clear oral secretions and, in severe cases, could produce a partial or total airway obstruction. This can result in aspiration of oral contents, aspiration pneumonia, and asphyxiation.

Table 5.1 Causes of salivary gland hyperfunction.

Drugs
  Bethanechol
  Cevimeline
  Clozapine
  Lithium
  Nitrazepam
  Physostigmine
  Pilocarpine
  Risperidone
Oral conditions
  Teething
  Ill-fitting prostheses
  Mucosal ulcerations (aphthous ulcers)
Other conditions
  Cerebral vascular accident
  Gastroesophageal reflux disease
  Heavy metal poisoning
  Hyperhydration
  Idiopathic disorders
  Nausea
  Obstructive esophagitis
  Parkinson's disease
  Secretory phase of menstruation

Hypersalivation also causes perioral traumatic irritations and ulcerations that can result in a secondary fungal or bacterial infection.

Because of the plethora of etiologic causes of hypersalivation, it is essential to obtain a thorough past history of the hypersalivation as well as a complete past medical history. A systematic oral evaluation must be performed, focusing on salivary gland enlargements, oral ulcerations, head/neck/oral masses, neuromuscular function, and condition of removable intraoral prostheses. Since most cases of hypersalivation are a secretion clearance issue, a swallowing study should be obtained early in the diagnostic work-up.

In the event of a normal swallowing study, a salivary flow rate can be obtained. The normal rate of unstimulated salivary output from all glands is approximately 2.0–3.5 mL/5 min. Collection of unstimulated whole saliva (~60 min after any eating, drinking, chewing, or oral hygiene) using a nonexpectorating technique that results in more than 5.0 mL in 5 min suggests greater than normal saliva production.

Heavy metals and organophosphate poisoning should be considered and appropriate blood samples, especially blood lead levels should be drawn. In levels between 5 and 14 µg/dL, erythrocyte protoporphyrin levels should be monitored to assist in determining the duration and timing of the exposure.

Premenopausal women should be assessed for possible pregnancy, and in postmenopausal or male patients, androgen levels should be evaluated for an androgen-excreting tumor. In an acute onset, a CT of the brain should be obtained to exclude a cerebral vascular accident or a central nervous system mass.

Salivary hypofunction/xerostomia

It is complicated to determine global estimates of xerostomia and salivary gland hypofunction due to limited epidemiological studies and confounding variables, yet it is probable that approximately 30% of the population aged 65+ years experiences these disorders.[15] Medication-induced xerostomia is the most probable cause, since 70% of all adults are taking at least one medication that can cause xerostomia. The prevalence of xerostomia is nearly 100% among patients with Sjögren's syndrome and head and neck radiation for the treatment of cancer.[2,16]

The cause of xerostomia and salivary hypofunction in older adults is most likely due to numerous systemic conditions (e.g., Sjögren's syndrome, diabetes, Alzheimer's disease, and dehydration) and their treatments (medications, head and neck radiation, chemotherapy)[2,17] (Table 5.2). Older salivary glands are more vulnerable to the deleterious effects of disease, medication, and radiotherapy, which probably explains why the prevalence of xerostomia and salivary hypofunction increases with age.[15,18]

The most common cause of salivary dysfunction is prescription and nonprescription medications. It has been determined that over 1,000 medications have been reported to cause xerostomia, as an adverse side effect.[18]

The most common classes of medications that cause salivary dysfunction are associated with anticholinergic consequences. However, any medication that hinders acetylcholine binding through direct or indirect inhibition, or that

Table 5.2 Causes of salivary gland hypofunction.

Drugs
  Anticholinergics
  Antihistamines
  Antihypertensives
  Anti-Parkinsonian
  Antiseizures
  Oncological chemotherapy
  Sedatives
  Tranquilizers
  Tricyclic antidepressants
Radiation and radioisotopes
  External beam radiation
  Internal radionuclide therapy
  Radioactive iodine (I-131)
Oral conditions
  Salivary gland benign tumors
  Salivary gland microbial infections
  Salivary gland malignant tumors
Other conditions
  Amyloidosis
  Bell's palsy
  Cystic fibrosis
  Diabetes
  Graft-versus-host disease
  Granulomatous diseases (sarcoidosis, tuberculosis)
  Human immunodeficiency virus infection
  Idiopathic disorders
  Late-stage liver disease
  Malnutrition (anorexia, bulimia, dehydration)
  Psychological factors (affective disorder)
  Sjögren's syndrome (primary and secondary)
  Thyroid disease (hyper- and hypofunction)

interferes with the ion transport pathways in the acinar cell, may change the amount and constituents of salivary output (Table 5.2).

Chemotherapy has also been implicated with salivary disorders that occur during and immediately after treatment. The majority of patients report a return of salivary function to pretreatment levels, although permanent changes have been reported.[10] Finally, radioactive iodine (I-131) used in the treatment for thyroid tumors may cause parotid, but not submandibular dysfunction in a dose-dependent fashion.

Radiation for the treatment of head and neck cancers can, if the salivary glands are within the field of treatment, cause severe and irreversible salivary hypofunction.[19] The serous acini that produce saliva are radiosensitive and undergo cell death by apoptosis when exposed to external beam radiotherapy. Within 1 week of the start of irradiation (after 10 Gy have been delivered), salivary output declines by 60–90%, with later return of function if the total dose to the salivary tissue is ≤25 Gy.[19] The majority of patients receive therapeutic dosages that exceed 60 Gy, resulting in complete atrophic fibrosis of their salivary glands.

Sjögren's syndrome (SS) is a systemic autoimmune disorder that is associated with inflammation of epithelial tissues, and is the most common medical disorder that is directly associated with xerostomia and salivary dysfunction.[20] SS occurs in primary and secondary forms. Primary SS involves the salivary and lacrimal glands and is related with a decrease in the production of saliva and tears. Secondary Sjögren's syndrome occurs in conjunction with other autoimmune diseases. The American European Consensus Group revised the classification criteria for SS, and it can be used for diagnosing SS.[21] Secondary Sjögren's syndrome manifests in the disease processes of rheumatoid arthritis, primary biliary cirrhosis, systemic lupus erythematosus, ankylosing spondylitis, and juvenile idiopathic arthritis.[22]

Sjögren's syndrome remains a frequently encountered autoimmune, connective tissue disorder, with prevalence in the population of approximately 0.6%.[23] One study reported the average annual incidence rate for physician-diagnosed primary SS in one Minnesota (USA) county at about 4 cases per 100,000 population, which could be an underestimate of actual cases.[20] The onset of disease symptoms is often subtle, and accordingly, diagnosis may be delayed until severe symptoms manifest. The female to male ratio has been estimated to be 9:1, although reported ratios vary.

The pathogenesis of SS remains unknown.[2,24] Multiple theories have been postulated, but even the classification of the disease as a B-cell versus a T-cell disorder is controversial. It has been postulated that an environmental agent (e.g., virus) may trigger events in a genetically susceptible host, resulting in the development of SS. Alternatively, decreased function of the hypothalamic–pituitary–adrenal axis may cause SS, as it also occurs in other autoimmune rheumatic diseases. Hormonal factors may influence the pathogenesis, since females with SS are far more common than males. Finally, SS has a genetic component—the prevalence of SS and autoantibodies (e.g., anti-Ro/SSA) may be higher in family members than the general population.[2]

There is also a reported 44-fold increase in the frequency of B-cell lymphomas among SS patients.[24] Laboratory tests will frequently be positive for rheumatoid factor (90%), anti-Ro/SSA or anti-La/SSB (50–90%), with the presence of hypergammaglobulinemia.[22] Antinuclear antibodies are present in approximately 80% of cases. Autoantibodies that precipitate anti-Ro/SSA are associated with systemic manifestations, including anemia, leukopenia, thrombocytopenia, purpura, cryoglobulinemia, hypocomplementemia, lymphadenopathy, and vasculitis.

REFERENCES

1. Guyton AC. *Text Book of Medical Physiology*, 11th edn. Philadelphia: Elsevier; 2006.
2. Ship JA, Pillemer SR, Baum BJ. Xerostomia and the geriatric patient. J Am Geriatr Soc 2002;50:535–43.

3. Ambudkar IS. Regulation of calcium in salivary gland secretion. Crit Rev Oral Biol Med 2000;11:4–25.

4. Wong DT. Salivary diagnostics powered by nanotechnologies, proteomics, and genomics. J Am Dent Assoc 2006;137(3):313–21.

5. Turner RJ. Mechanisms of fluid secretion by salivary glands. Ann N Y Acad Sci 1993;694:24–35.

6. Agre P, Bonhivers M, Borgnia MJ. The aquaporins, blueprints for cellular plumbing systems. J Biol Chem 1998;273:14659–62.

7. Baum BJ. Evaluation of stimulated parotid saliva flow rate in different age groups. J Dent Res 1981;60:1292–6.

8. Baum BJ, Kuyatt BL, Takuma T. Adrenergic regulation of protein synthesis in rat submandibular salivary gland cells. Arch Oral Biol 1984;29:499–502.

9. Challacombe SJ, Percival RS, Marsh PD. Age-related changes in immunoglobulin isotypes in whole and parotid saliva and serum in healthy individuals. Oral Microbiol Immunol 1995;10:202–207.

10. Ship JA, Nolan NE, Puckett SA. Longitudinal analysis of parotid and submandibular salivary flow rates in healthy, different-aged adults. J Gerontol A Biol Sci Med Sci 1995;50:M285–9.

11. Ship JA, Baum BJ. Is reduced salivary flow normal in old people? Lancet 1990;336:1507.

12. Wu AJ, Atkinson JC, Fox PC, Baum BJ, Ship JA. Cross-sectional and longitudinal analyses of stimulated parotid salivary constituents in healthy, different-aged subjects. J Gerontol 1993;48:M219–24.

13. Scott J, Flower EA, Burns J. A quantitative study of histological changes in the human parotid gland occurring with adult age. J Oral Pathol 1987;16:505–510.

14. Ghezzi EM, Ship JA. Aging and secretory reserve capacity of major salivary glands. J Dent Res 2003;82:844–8.

15. Centers for Disease Control and Prevention. Public health and aging: trends in aging—United States and worldwide. JAMA 2003;289:1371–3.

16. Baum BJ, Ship JA, Wu AJ. Salivary gland function and aging: a model for studying the interaction of aging and systemic disease. Crit Rev Oral Biol Med 1992;4:53–64.

17. Porter SR, Scully C, Hegarty AM. An update of the etiology and management of xerostomia. Oral Surg Oral Med Oral Pathol Oral Radiol Endod 2004;97:28–46.

18. Smith RG, Burtner AP. Oral side-effects of the most frequently prescribed drugs. Spec Care Dentist 1994;14:96–102.

19. Shiboski C H, Hodgson TA, Ship JA, Schiodt M. Management of salivary hypofunction during and after radiotherapy. Oral Surg Oral Med Oral Pathol Oral Radiol Endod 2007(103 Suppl);S66:e61–19.

20. Pillemer SR, Matteson EL, Jacobsson LT, et al. Incidence of physician-diagnosed primary Sjogren syndrome in residents of Olmsted County, Minnesota. Mayo Clin Proc 2001;76:593–9.

21. Vitali C, Bencivelli W, Mosca M, Carrai P, Sereni M, Bombardieri S. Development of a clinical chart to compute different disease activity indices for systemic lupus erythematosus. J Rheumatol 1999;26:498–501.

22. von Bultzingslowen I, Sollecito TP, Fox PC, et al. Salivary dysfunction associated with systemic diseases: systematic review and clinical management recommendations. Oral Surg Oral Med Oral Pathol Oral Radiol Endod 2007(103 Suppl);S57:e51–15.

23. Fox RI, Stern M, Michelson P. Update in Sjogren syndrome. Curr Opin Rheumatol 2000;12:391–8.

24. Fox PC. Autoimmune diseases and Sjogren's syndrome: an autoimmune exocrinopathy. Ann N Y Acad Sci 2007;1098:15–21.

6

Processing and storage of saliva samples

Enno C.I. Veerman, Arjan Vissink, David T. Wong, and Arie van Nieuw Amerongen

INTRODUCTION

Human saliva is a complex biological fluid, which contains a large number of inorganic (e.g., Ca^{2+}, K^+, Na^+, phosphate, and bicarbonate) and organic (e.g., (glyco)proteins and peptides) constituents with important functions for the maintenance of oral health. The relatively easy and noninvasive collection of saliva (see Chapter 4) and the good correlation of concentrations of certain constituents between saliva and plasma make saliva an attractive diagnostic fluid for monitoring of general health, early disease detection, biomonitoring of pesticides, monitoring of drugs and smoking,[1] and various forensic and clinical applications.[2] However, due to logistic, financial, practical, and methodological reasons, it is not always possible to analyze samples immediately after collection. Thus, storage and stabilization prior to analysis of the salivary samples is often needed. In this chapter, several issues related to the collection, processing storage, and stabilization of salivary samples are discussed.

SALIVARY COLLECTION PROCEDURES

As discussed extensively in Chapter 4, there are various methods available for collecting whole and glandular saliva. Regardless of the method used for whole or glandular saliva (unless the saliva sample is directly collected from the orifice of a particular salivary gland), subjects should be instructed to void the mouth of saliva by rinsing the mouth thoroughly with deionised water. Then, saliva can be collected into ice-cooled vials by the draining, the spitting, or the suction method for whole saliva by one of the described methods in Chapter 4 for collection of glandular saliva. Collection of saliva into ice-cooled vials is recommended to slow down the activity of hydrolytic enzymes present in saliva. Further, collection in vials containing a cocktail of protease inhibitors, including ethylene diamine tetraacetic acid (EDTA), phenylmethanesulfonylfluoride (PMSF), soy bean trypsin inhibitor, and E-64, is in particular useful when saliva is collected for protein purification purposes to prevent proteolysis. Addition of protease inhibitors may also be used as an alternative for collection into ice-cooled vessels, but it should be verified that these

compounds do not interfere with the analysis of the biomarker. To stimulate secretion, saliva can be collected while the patient is chewing on paraffin wax or
a nonflavored chewing gum base. Masticatory stimulation is particular useful
in cases when the biomarker originates from serum and where the biomarker
can only enter the mouth fluid via minute wounds in the mucosa. The touching
of mucosa by pieces of paraffin or chewing gum will enhance or promote leakage of serum-derived material through the mucosa, and thus increases their
concentration.

Bacteria and cellular debris have to be removed directly after collection.
This can be done by centrifugation (5 min, 10,000 g, or 20 min, 3,000 g) or by
filtration. Use of cotton-based filters is not recommended, since hormones and
proteins readily adsorb to these matrices, which will compromise the analysis.

For stabilization of salivary DNA and RNA, optimized protocols have recently been developed. Salivary DNA stabilization was best optimized by the
commercial vendor DNA Genotek (www.dnagenotek.com). On average, approximately 110 µg of genomic DNA can be isolated from 2 mL of whole saliva,
making saliva a very attractive, noninvasive source for obtaining human DNA
for a variety of research and clinical applications. For the emerging field of
salivary RNA, we have optimized research protocols tailored for transcriptomic biomarker discovery in saliva. This involves the initial separation of the
cell-free portion of saliva at 4°C, followed by the addition of "Superase Inhibitor (SI)" that is an RNase inhibitor (Ambion, Austin, TX) at 100 U/mL. We
have found this to be the most effective way of preserving RNA in salivary
supernatant.[3]

It is of interest to note that the discovery of salivary RNA has heralded the
commercialization of two salivary RNA stabilizers. QIAGEN in 2006 launched
RNAprotect Saliva, while DNA Genotek launched Oragene-RNA in the third
quarter of 2007. Both these RNA-stabilizing products further claim to be ambient temperature compatible, requiring no special refrigeration, making it ideal
for field application research in epidemiology and health services.

GENERAL CONSIDERATIONS ON PROCESSING

From a practical perspective one validated, generally accepted method for collection, processing, and storage of saliva samples, which is compatible with all
biomarker types, would be ideal. It should be realised, however, that the chemical stability of the biomarker, as well as the diagnostic purpose, to a large extent
determine the way the sample should be processed and stored. For instance,
collection, processing, and storage of samples for analysis of ions such as Na^+
and K^+ is less critical than for analysis of a highly labile enzyme. Even reliable
measurement of a simple ion such as H^+ in a salivary sample poses a problem,
and in fact can only be done in freshly collected salivary samples. Conditions
or treatments such as freezing/thawing, or prolonged storage, will result in
partial or complete removal of the bicarbonate via CO_2 evaporation, causing a
change in pH. Another type of analysis that is only feasible in freshly collected
saliva is determination of the rheological (viscoelastic) properties of saliva.
Manipulations such as stirring, vortexing, and centrifugation will lower the

viscosity irreversibly, because of the breaking up of mucin aggregates, which are responsible for the viscoelastic properties of saliva. Also, freezing and thawing or prolonged storage at low temperature will influence the viscoelasticity of saliva since it often gives rise to cryoprecipitation of insoluble calcium salts and/or mucin complexes.

Another factor that has to be taken into account is the bacterial load, particularly in whole saliva, which is typically in the order of 10^7 cells/mL. Bacteria are a rich source of hydrolytic enzymes, including proteinase and glycosidases, which can break down salivary biomarkers. Therefore, whole and glandular saliva samples should be collected on ice to reduce the enzymatic activity. As soon as possible, removal of the bacterial cells by centrifugation or by filtration is required for keeping a sample stable.

The noninvasive nature of saliva collection enables saliva specimens to be gathered under circumstances (e.g., large-scale surveys, remote locations, and absence of medically trained personnel) when it is not feasible to sample blood. At the same time those circumstances induce restrictions on how salivary samples can be handled and stored after collection, for instance, the availability of high-speed centrifuges to remove bacterial and cellular debris, and access to refrigeration. Typically, once a saliva sample has been collected, it should be kept on ice or frozen in an attempt to maintain the stability of the biomarker and slow down proteolytic breakdown of biomarkers by bacterial and/or host enzymes. When this is not possible, often sodium azide is added to retard bacterial growth. It has to be borne in mind, however, that sodium azide is an inhibitor of heme-containing enzymes, for example, peroxidases, and henceforth can interfere with horse-radish peroxidase-based enzyme-linked immunosorbent assays (ELISAs). Furthermore, sodium azide does not protect against degradation by proteases or glycosidases. When designing a protocol for handling salivary samples, the intrinsic properties of the biomarker and the diagnostic purpose have to be taken into account. For instance, when decisions will be drawn on basis of either a positive or a negative outcome of a test, for instance, in testing HIV seropositivity, the processing of the saliva sample is less critical (within certain limits) than when decisions will be based on the absolute quantity of a salivary biomarker. Once a choice has been made for a particular method of processing, in either case it is important that the researcher will adhere to that method to minimize fluctuations. In the following sections, some processing and storage methods, in relation to various biomarkers that currently are tested in saliva, are discussed.

FREEZING, THAWING, AND STORAGE

After collection in ice-cooled vessels, salivary samples must be snap frozen, preferentially in liquid nitrogen. Especially when samples have to be stored for a prolonged period of time, storage at $-80°C$ is preferred over storage at $-20°C$, since at the latter temperature a gradual breakdown of some salivary proteins will occur.[4] To maintain the integrity of the proteins, the deep-frozen sample must be thawed as quickly as possible, for example, by transferring the sample vial to hot water for a short period of time. Contrary to what is sometimes believed, slowly thawing a deep-frozen sample, for example at 4°C, not only can affect the activity and structure of labile proteins, but also can lead to cryoprecipitation of mucin-protein complexes, and thus induce a general, irreversible loss of protein biomarkers. To avoid repetitive freezing and thawing of saliva samples, they can be stored in 100 μL aliquots. Alternatively, the potential detrimental effects of freezing and thawing can also be obviated by storing the sample at −80°C, 1:1 diluted in glycerol.

Storage of salivary DNA and RNA follows similar guidelines. What is of interest is our recent finding that, similar to serum and plasma RNA, salivary RNA exhibits unusual stability when compared to in vitro transcribed RNA due to complexing by macromolecular entities that confer stability.[5]

MONITORING OF STEROID HORMONES

Collection of saliva for assessment of hormone levels provides a convenient method of measuring the unbound fraction of a hormone, since it can be collected multiple times at the subject's own home. Examples of hormones that are tested in saliva are steroid hormones, including cortisol,[6] testosterone, progesterone,[7] and dehydroepiandrosterone (DHEA).[8] As the number of studies assessing salivary hormones has increased, knowledge has accumulated indicating that the process by which salivary flow rate is stimulated and saliva samples have been collected potentially influences the validity of salivary immunoassays.

Cortisol is an example of a stable hormone for which saliva is optimally suited as a diagnostic fluid. Salivary cortisol levels were found to be useful in identifying patients with Cushing's syndrome and Addison's disease and also for monitoring the hormone response to physical exercise and the effect of acceleration stress. Levels of salivary cortisol, which is in equilibrium with the unbound fraction of plasma cortisol, are unaffected by salivary flow rate and display the same diurnal variation as plasma cortisol. Salivary measures of cortisol correlate well with plasma cortisol levels for normal people of all ages and in states of abnormal adrenal function.[6,9] Cortisol is fairly stable in saliva for up to 6 weeks at room temperature, and for extended periods of time when frozen.

Whembolua et al.[10] have investigated the effect of bacterial load in saliva on the measurement of salivary testosterone, DHEA, and cortisol and found that testosterone, but not cortisol or DHEA-levels, decreased on storage at room temperature. Furthermore, these authors found that filtering of the samples to lower the bacterial load decreased the levels of DHEA, particularly when the sample had been stored at −80°C. Also, a study by Shirtcliff et al.[11] warns against the popular practice of cotton-based sampling methods to collect saliva and remove particulate material. An alternative is centrifugation of salivary samples. To facilitate precipitation of bacteria and other debris, it is recommended to lower the viscosity of the sample by homogenization using a vortex mixture.[12] Another advantage of lowering the viscosity is that this will improve the handling of the sample and prevent clogging of automated analysers.

For measurement of steroid hormones, which enter saliva by passive diffusion through the acinar cells, such as cortisol, parotid saliva could be a feasible alternative for whole saliva. Since parotid saliva is low viscous and semisterile, removal of bacteria by filtration or centrifugation is not needed. Another advantage in the context of steroid hormone measurement is that parotid saliva, compared to whole saliva, contains hardly any serum contaminants if collected by Lashley cups. Depending on the oral health of the donor, whole saliva may be substantially contaminated with serum components that enter the oral fluid by outflow of the gingival crevicular fluid or from oral wounds. This will compromise the quantitative estimates of free hormones, since in plasma the larger fraction of, for example, cortisol is protein bound.

SALIVARY IMMUNOGLOBULINS AS BIOMARKERS FOR MONITORING OF VIRAL INFECTIONS

The antibody response to infection is the basis for many diagnostic tests in virology. Salivary immunoglobulins originate mainly from the salivary glands (predominantly S-IgA) and from serum (mainly IgG). Analysis of antibodies in saliva as a diagnostic test for HIV or other infections offers several advantages when compared with serum. Saliva can be collected noninvasively, which eliminates the risk of infection for the healthcare worker who collects the blood sample. Furthermore, transmission of HIV via saliva is unlikely, since infectious virus particles are rarely isolated from saliva.[13,14] Saliva collection also simplifies the diagnostic process in special populations in whom blood drawing is difficult, that is, individuals with compromised venous access (e.g., injecting drug users), patients with hemophilia, children, and elderly people. Diagnostic tests for detection of viral infections (HIV, hepatitis B) are essentially qualitative, that is, they should reliably detect either the absence or the presence of specific antibodies. In order to optimize sensitivity, handling of salivary samples, therefore, must primarily be aimed at prevention of breakdown of the biomarker. Although immunoglobulins are intrinsically stable, the low level of, particularly, serum-derived IgG in saliva requires that when the test cannot be conducted on the spot salivary samples be optimally prepared and stabilized to prevent proteolytic breakdown. For this purpose, it is recommended that samples be stored at $-20°C$ or below. Storage at higher temperatures will result in proteolytic breakdown and false negative results.

SALIVARY PROTEINS: GENERAL CONSIDERATIONS

The effect of processing conditions, including storage time and temperature, centrifugation speed, and freeze thawing, has been comprehensively studied by Schipper et al.[4] using a proteomic approach based on analysis of saliva by surface-enhanced laser desorption ionization–matrix-assisted laser desorption ionization–time of flight (SELDI-MALDI-TOF). Delayed processing time experiments show certain new peptides evolving 3 h postsaliva donation, and quantitative analyses indicate relative intensity of other proteins and peptides changing with time. The addition of proteinase inhibitors partly counteracted the destabilization of certain protein/peptide mass spectra over time suggesting that some proteins in saliva are subject to digestion by intrinsic salivary proteinases. Surface-enhanced laser desorption ionization–time-of-flight–mass spectrometry(SELDI-TOF-MS) profiles were also changed by varying storage time and storage temperature, whereas centrifugation speed and freeze–thaw cycles had minimal impact. Based on these results, storage at −80°C seems better than at −20°C, since after storage of saliva at −20°C the intensity of many peaks substantially was decreased. Stable and reproducible storage of samples is of uttermost importance when saliva is used in tests in which elevation of a protein marker is a diagnostic criterion, such as in the diagnosis and monitoring of breast tumor, which is based on levels of c-erb B and CA-125 in saliva.[15]

DNA/RNA ANALYSIS

The use of salivary DNA and RNA has many applications. An important consideration is whether the source of the DNA/RNA is from whole saliva or from cell-free portion of saliva. DNA and RNA from whole saliva are likely to be a complex mixture from cellular and microbial origins. This is a logical source of human DNA/RNA from a noninvasive source. However, the whole saliva source of DNA and RNA is unlikely to be of diagnostic value as the disease-associative DNA or RNA will be masked by the overwhelming background of normal healthy cellular DNA/RNA. The cell-free or supernatant portion of saliva, on the other hand, has been found to be highly disease associative. Four salivary RNA biomarkers[16] and five proteomic biomarkers[17] from the saliva supernatant fractions have exceedingly high discriminatory values for oral cancer detection (~90% clinical accuracy). At this time it is not clear if there is significant salivary DNA that is of disease discriminatory value. It is with this in mind that we advocate special precaution to maximally preserve the integrity of salivary RNA in the supernatant of saliva, particularly when used for biomarker discovery studies. It should be noted that the two commercially available systems for salivary RNA stabilization are designed for whole saliva stabilization and cannot be used for saliva supernatant applications, unless there is a prior removal of cells, for example, by centrifugation.

PROCESSING AND STORAGE OF SALIVA: GENERAL GUIDELINES

Based on the literature, for multipurpose usage the following protocol for processing saliva samples is recommended:

1. Standardized collection of whole or glandular saliva in ice-cooled vials:
   (a) by drooling that is really without any stimulus;
   (b) by spitting, method of Navazesh[18] with low muscular stimulation;
   (c) by one of the methods described in Chapter 4 for collection of glandular saliva.

2. Vortexing (2 min, maximal speed). Note: Not advised for rheological measurements and not needed for glandular saliva directly collected from the orifice of a particular gland using cannulation or a Lashley cup.
3. Centrifugation (5 min, $10,000 \times$ g, or 20 min, $3,000 \times$ g). Note: Not needed for glandular saliva directly collected from the orifice of a particular gland using cannulation or a Lashley cup. Snap freezing of supernatant of the whole or glandular saliva sample in liquid nitrogen.
4. Storage at -20°C or below, but preferentially at -80°C.

Remarks:

- Centrifugation can also be performed afterward, before analysis, provided that immediately after collection the samples are frozen in liquid nitrogen.
- Caution dictates that salivary samples can best be stored in the frozen state until analysis. Only one freezing and thawing cycle is advised. Therefore, it is advised that the samples be frozen and stored in small aliquots.
- For salivary RNA, while ambient temperature stabilizers are available, they are primarily optimized for whole saliva applications. For biomarker discovery applications, it is still advisable to use special precautions as the disease-associative biomarkers reside in the cell-free portion of saliva. Superase inhibitor is the ideal sample storage and stabilization protocol for saliva supernatant stored at -20°C.
- Freezing in dry ice is a practical choice if liquid nitrogen or a -80°C freezer is not available when samples are collected.
- For immunochemical analysis (ELISA), the sample can be stored frozen after appropriate dilution (e.g., 1:100) in the assay buffer, usually PBS -0.5% Tween-20.
- Most important: The collection, processing, and storage of salivary samples should be identical and consistent within one type of study.

REFERENCES

1. Schneider NG, Jacob III P, Nilsson E, Leischow SJ, Benowitz L, Olmstead RE. Saliva cotinine levels as a function of collection method. Addiction 1997;92:347–51.
2. Zimmermann BG, Park NJ, Wong DT. Genomic targets in saliva. Ann N Y Acad Sci 2007;1098:184–91.
3. Park NJ, Yu T, Nabili V, et al. RNAProtect Saliva: an optimal room-temperature stabilization reagent for the salivary transcriptome. Clin Chem 2007;52(12):2303–304.
4. Schipper R, Loof A, de Groot J, Harthoorn L, Dransfield E, van Heerde W. SELDI-TOF-MS of saliva: methodology and pre-treatment effects. J Chrom B 2007;847:45–53.
5. Park NJ, Li Y, Yu T, Brinkman BM, Wong DT. Characterization of RNA in saliva. Clin Chem 2006;52(6):988–94.

6. Kirschbaum C, Hellhammer DH. Salivary cortisol in psychoneuroendocrine research: recent developments and applications. Psychoneuroendocrinology 1994;19:313–33.
7. Banerjee S, Levitz, M. On the processing of saliva samples for progesterone assay. Steroids 1983;42:539–47.
8. Gallagher P, Leitch MM, Massey AE, McAllister-Williams RH, Young AH. Assessing cortisol and dehydroepiandrosterone (DHEA) in saliva: effects of collection method. J Psychopharmacology 2006;20:643–9.
9. Laudat MH, Cerdas S, Fournier, Guiban D, Guilhaume B, Luton JP. Salivary cortisol measurement: a practical approach to assess pituitary-adrenal function. J Clin Endocrinol Metab 1988;66:343–8.
10. Whembolua G-LS, Granger DA, Singer S, Kivlighan KT, Marguin JA. Bacteria in the oral mucosa and its effects on the measurement of cortisol, dehydroepiandrosterone, and testosterone in saliva. Hormon Behav 2006;49:478–83.
11. Shirtcliff EA, Granger DA, Schwartz E, Curran MJ. Use of salivary biomarkers in biobehavioral research: cotton-based sample collection methods can interfere with salivary immunoassay results. Psychoneuroendocrinology 2001;26:165–73.
12. Veerman ECI, Valentijn-Benz M, Nieuw Amerongen AV. Viscosity of human salivary mucins: effect of pH and ionic strength and role of sialic acid. J Biol Buccale 1989;17:297–306.
13. Shugars DC, Sweet SP, Malamud D, Kazmi SH, Page-Shafer K, Challacombe SJ. Saliva and inhibition of HIV-1 infection: molecular mechanism. Oral Dis 2002;8:169–75.
14. Bolscher JG, Nazmi K, Ran LJ, et al. Inhibition of HIV-1 IIIB and clinical isolates by human parotid, submandibular, sublingual and palatine saliva. Eur J Oral Sci 2002;110:149–56.
15. Streckfus C, Bigler L. The use of soluble, salivary c-erbB-2 for the detection and post-operative follow-up of breast cancer in women: the results of a five-year translational research study. Adv Dent Res 2005;18:17–24.
16. Li Y, St John MA, Zhou X, et al. Salivary transcriptome diagnostics for oral cancer detection. Clin Cancer Res 2004;10(24):8442–50.
17. Hu S, Arellano M, Boontheung P, et al. Salivary proteomics for oral cancer biomarker discovery. Clin Cancer Res, in press.
18. Navazesh M. Methods for collecting saliva. Ann N Y Acad Sci 1993;694:72–7.

Part II

Saliva Diagnostics

Historical perspectives and present

Frank G. Oppenheim

INTRODUCTION

Oral fluid or whole saliva (WS) is a complex biological fluid since several contributors are responsible for its production. This renders diagnosis of disease by the analysis of saliva challenging on one hand and attractive on the other. The bulk of the fluid portion of WS (600–1,200 mL/day) derives from the major salivary glands comprising two parotid, two submandibular (SM), and two sublingual (SL) glands. In addition, there are a variety of minor salivary glands located on the inner aspect of the lip, the palate, the tongue and the buccal mucosa. In toto these glands represent the exocrine portion of WS, which has a protein concentration ranging between 150 and 400 mg%. Nonexocrine contributors can be divided into host-derived entities such as desquamated epithelial cells, intact and remnants of blood cells, gingival fluid, and possibly fluid entering the oral cavity through mucosal seepage. Nonhost-derived components are for the most part microorganisms and food residues. There are significant differences between the exocrine and the nonexocrine sources. All exocrine contributions from salivary glands are synthesized locally by specialized cells and secreted upon stimulation. Salivary flow is controlled predominantly by the sympathetic and parasympathetic nervous branches, resulting in a range of salivary flow rates and concomitant differences in the concentrations of individual salivary constituents. Nonexocrine WS constituents may also derive from local sites, but many are synthesized elsewhere in the body. For example, gingival fluid is a serum transudate rich in protein, which reflects the protein pattern of serum and enters the oral cavity through the gingival crevice. Anatomically, the oral cavity is also connected to other parts of the body. It is the portal of entry to the gastrointestinal tract and also communicates with the posterior nasal passage and upper respiratory tract. Indeed, gastric and pulmonary pathogens have been shown to be present in the oral cavity in a variety of clinical conditions.[1–4] Therefore, the quality of WS can reflect the addition of components from sites other than the oral cavity, and such components could point toward a variety of systemic diseases. It is therefore understandable that the oral environment is a mirror of oral and systemic health, which could be exploited to monitor and diagnose specific clinical parameters.[4]

MAJOR SALIVARY CONSTITUENTS

Classic biochemical separation techniques have been applied over the last three decades to isolate and characterize proteins secreted by the major human salivary glands. Early efforts in this area led to the development of a uniquely suited first separation step of salivary proteins present in major glandular secretions.[5] The proteins contained in parotid secretion (PS) can be separated by anion exchange chromatography into several fractions. Each of these fractions has been used for final purification of individual components. Such work has led to the discovery and characterization of the major salivary proteins comprising amylases,[6,7] acidic, basic, and glycosylated proline-rich proteins,[8–11] statherins,[12] histatins,[13–15] peroxidases,[16] cystatins,[17,18] and mucins.[19–21] A unique feature of many of these major proteins is that they display genetic polymorphisms and therefore constitute several families of structurally and functionally closely related molecules.[22,23] The basis for these polymorphisms can be related to gene duplication, differential mRNA splicing events, posttranslational modifications, and proteolysis.[24,25] In some cases, polymorphic forms differ significantly in size, while in other instances polymorphic forms show only minimal changes that do not affect the mass of the polymorphic molecules. For instance, among the family of acidic proline-rich proteins PRP1 and PIFs share their full 150-residue sequence, including their two phosphorylation sites, but differ only in the reversed locations of one Asp and one Asn residue at positions 4 and 50.[24,26] Overall, the preponderance of polymorphisms in glandular salivary secretions poses daunting challenges, not only for separating structurally related molecules, but also for their subsequent characterization. Importantly, as we enter into the era of high-throughput technologies such as mass spectrometry, the limitations introduced by polymorphism remain, albeit in a different fashion and form than those encountered using classical methods.

SALIVA AS A DIAGNOSTIC FLUID

Discovery of serum components in saliva

As noted earlier, whole saliva contains numerous nonexocrine macromolecules that, on a percent basis (v/v), do not add more than 4–5% to the composition of whole saliva (Fig. 7.1). Nevertheless, in some cases, their protein contributions are clearly noticeable. Early salivary protein studies led to the identification of an unknown component in whole saliva, called component C at the time. While this component C was clearly a dominant constituent of WS, it could only be detected at low or negligible levels in the main glandular secretions of PS and SM/SL (Fig. 7.2a). Considering that the PS and SM/SL secretions are the main fluid constituents of whole saliva, this observation strongly pointed toward a nonexocrine origin of component C. Comparison of the WS protein profiles with those in gingival crevicular fluid (GCF) subsequently revealed high doses of component C in GCF (Fig. 7.2b), which was later identified by immunological methods to be serum albumin.[27,28]

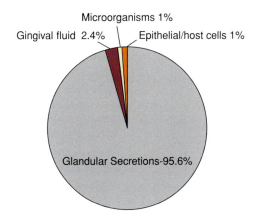

Figure 7.1 Percent (v/v) contributions of exocrine and nonexocrine contributors to whole saliva fluid.

Significant levels of albumin in WS can be explained by the fact that albumin levels are very high in serum and GCF (3,500–4,000 mg%). A small volume of GCF entering the oral cavity even in gingivally healthy subjects at approximately 5–20 μL/h thus would result in measurable levels of this serum component in saliva.[29] It was hypothesized that the gingival fluid flow rate would ultimately determine the levels of albumin found in WS, and that the state of gingival health may therefore affect this parameter. An experiment was designed to test this hypothesis using a classical experimental gingivitis approach. Healthy volunteers were subjected to oral examination, and their gingival health was maximized by scaling and root planning to reach a low gingival index ranging between 0.1 and 0.2. Over a period of 20 days, the subjects abstained from any home care procedures and resumed brushing and flossing at day 21. Patients were monitored with respect to both their mean gingival index (GI) and their whole saliva albumin levels at various time points during the gingivitis phase and 9 days after resumption of oral hygiene. The two parameters showed an excellent correlation (Fig. 7.2c). Whole saliva albumin levels increased concomitant with an increase in gingival index over the first 20 days. Both experimental variables decreased over the next 9 days to pre-experimental values as oral health was regained after resumption of oral hygiene. This study was a first demonstration of how the quantity of blood-derived components in WS could be of diagnostic value with respect to gingival health. Furthermore, the leakage of serum components into whole saliva via the gingival crevice links the oral cavity to the blood circulation, which has many useful implications for the detection of diseases that release biomarkers into the blood compartment.

Contemporary diagnostic parameters in saliva

The use of saliva is attractive to monitor parameters of health and disease not only because of its multiple contributors, but also since it is noninvasive, easy to obtain, painless, and there is no need to employ specially trained personnel for sample collection. The possibility to identify and measure biomarkers in

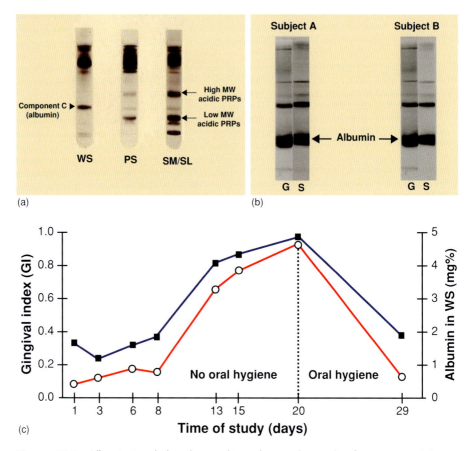

Figure 7.2 Albumin in whole saliva and its role as a biomarker for gingivitis. (a) Anionic PAGE of whole saliva supernatant (WS), parotid secretion (PS), and submandibular/sublingual secretion (SM/SL). Note: Protein C (albumin) in WS that is present at only low levels in PS and SM/SL. (b) comparison of protein patterns in gingival crevicular fluid (G) and in serum (S) of the same subject. (c) Gingival index and albumin levels in WS during experimentally induced gingivitis (days 1–20) and after resumption of oral hygiene (days 21–29).

saliva opens the avenue for diagnosis, early detection, monitoring progression of disease, and compliance to treatment modalities.[30] There are many studies reported with the goal to use oral fluids for clinical diagnostic purposes, and there are several reviews on the subject.[4,31–35] Salivary levels of the bacteria *Streptococcus mutans* and *Lactobacilli*[36] correlated with cariogenic activity, whereas the presence of *Porphyromonas gingivalis* correlated with periodontal infections.[37] An immunological assay for *Helicobacter pylori* in saliva has been developed to monitor patients suffering from gastric ulcers.[38] Salivary markers for viral infections including HIV,[39,40] hepatitis B[41] and hepatitis C,[42] Epstein-Barr,[43] herpes virus,[44] and cytomegalovirus[45] have been identified. For oral cancer, specifically oral squamous cell carcinoma, promising results have been obtained through analysis of the salivary transcriptome[46,47] and the oral microbial flora.[48] The concentrations of steroids, cortisol, estradiol, and progesterone in saliva have been evaluated to monitor ovarian function, stress levels, and progression of Cushing's syndrome.[33,35] Periodontal disease and possibly cardiovascular disease show correlations with levels of C-reactive protein in saliva.[49] In kidney patients salivary creatinine has been used for diagnostic purposes.[50] Furthermore, the efficacy of renal dialysis can be efficiently monitored through the assessment of a variety of salivary analytes.[51] Many of these studies are of interest since they show correlations between disease and salivary parameter(s) that could form the basis for new diagnostic tests.

MODERN PROTEOMICS APPROACHES IN SEARCH FOR BIOMARKERS

The emergence of mass spectrometry (MS) technologies combined with the human genome databases has rejuvenated the search for biomarker proteins. In recent years, some powerful new proteomics technologies have been employed that include multidimensional chromatographic and electrophoretic separation of proteins in conjunction with an arsenal of MS techniques. Similar to advances in "DNA-chip" technology for analysis of gene expression, modern proteomics has ushered in revolutionary new approaches for characterization and primary sequence determination of small amount of proteins and peptides in complex mixtures.

Advancements in mass spectrometric instrumentation

Advances made in this field of protein/peptide characterization have been due to improved microseparation techniques as well as to advances in the technology of MS. Both matrix-assisted laser desorption ionization-time-of-flight (MALDI-TOF) and nanoflow liquid chromatography-electrospray ionization tandem (LC-ESI-MS/MS) mass spectrometers have been the center of extensive use in variety of biological fields.[52,53] In the field of microseparation technologies, progress has been made in the area of two-dimensional polyacrylamide gel electrophoresis (2-D PAGE),[54] capillary electrophoresis,[55] and capillary high performance liquid chromatography (HPLC) technology.[56] The latter has been particularly valuable when used in concert with MS. With this technology, individual components in protein/peptide mixtures can be resolved and introduced by electrospray ionization (ESI) into the mass spectrometer allowing determination of the size of components and the degree of complexity of mixtures. When coupled with collision-induced dissociation, analysis of fragments can provide complete amino acid sequences of components.[53] The automation and combined microcapillary reverse-phase LC and tandem MS/MS capacity of these instruments have permitted large-scale identification of global proteomes to be carried out without prior purification of complex samples. In addition, peptides can be separated by sequential liquid chromatography steps followed by MS analysis. This is commonly referred to as

PS   SM/SL   WS

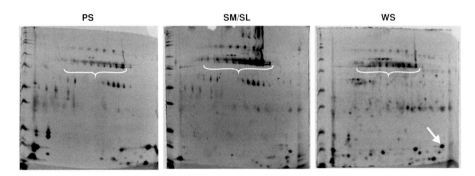

Figure 7.3   2-D gel electrophoretograms (1st dimension, IEF, pH 5–8; 2nd dimension, SDS-PAGE) of proteins contained in PS, SM/SL, and WS. Horizontal half parentheses indicate amylase isoforms. Arrow points to a spot identified by subsequent MS analysis to be cystatin SN.

multidimensional protein identification technology (MudPIT) and has become increasingly popular to establish comprehensive proteomes.[57]

Application of MS to the saliva field

The application of MS technology to human whole saliva and glandular secretions led to new insights of their characteristics and to the identification of proteins that were not known at the time to be part of this body fluid.[58–60] Protein identifications were achieved following the combined use of 2-D PAGE with in-gel tryptic fragmentation and MS (MALDI and ESI) to identify proteins/peptides in acquired enamel pellicle, WS, PS, and SM/SL secretions. Complications arising from the presence of multiple components in an apparent single electrophoretic band were resolved by applying the protein mixture to 2-D PAGE. An example of the 2-D PAGE patterns of the proteins and peptides in WS, PS, and SM/SL is shown in Figure 7.3. 2-D PAGE separation of salivary proteins has since been used by other groups[61–64] and has allowed for the separation of not only different molecules with apparently similar molecular weights, but also of different modification patterns or isoforms of the same protein. Significant interest in developing saliva-based biomarkers for diagnostics has fueled the establishment of various saliva proteome projects.[61–68]

The characterization of the full salivary proteome promises to lead to the identification of as yet unknown biomarkers for oral and systemic disease. Findings related to the absence or presence of a given protein may reveal involvement of that protein in health or a specific disease state. However, the mere identification of a specific protein, glycoprotein, phosphoprotein, or group of such proteins at a qualitative level is rarely sufficient for diagnostic exploitation. This is because frequently such proteins are present at elevated or decreased levels relative to normal levels, and such quantitative differences can be critical for diagnostics. Therefore, if MS analysis were to be used directly in oral diagnostics, then such approaches must incorporate quantitative measurements. The application of MS technology to establish quantitative proteomes has become feasible, and developments in this area have been ongoing for the past decade with continuing improvements and success,[69–71] including in the field of oral biology.[72]

Posttranslational protein modifications in oral diagnostics

In some cases simply identifying up-/downregulated protein(s) may not necessarily translate into understanding biological function, disease state, or progression. This is because biological function may rather be due to changes in the state of posttranslational modifications such as phosphorylation and glycosylation. These protein modifications can and do occur without changes in the protein level.[73,74] Many functional alterations in proteins are known to result from changes of posttranslational modifications such as phosphorylation, glycosylation, acetylation, and methylation.[75–77] The potential value of defining posttranslationally modified proteins, for example, phosphoproteins, in identifying biomarkers for diagnostics, can be illustrated by recent developments through the use of specific MS-based strategies targeted to the identification of the salivary phosphoproteome (Salih et al., unpublished observations). This work has led to the identification of a very intriguing set of phosphoproteins. Interestingly, about 95% of the phosphoproteins identified by MS analysis had not been identified by any of the saliva proteomics work carried out to date. This can be explained by specific enrichment procedures that were used to capture specifically the tryptic phosphopeptides. One of the phosphoproteins identified was tuftelin, also known as enamelin.[78] Figure 7.4 shows the MS/MS

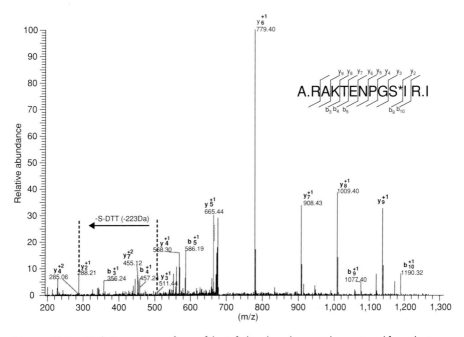

Figure 7.4 MS/MS spectrum of one of the tuftelin phosphopeptides captured from the tryptic digest of WS after 1,4-dithiothreitol (DTT) derivatization and covalent chromatography. The series of b and y fragmentation ions are labeled and the precise site of phosphorylation indicated by an asterisk within the identified sequence, A.RAKTENPGS*IR.I. *Note*: Loss of 223 Da is indicative of the presence of an S-DTT adduct pointing towards a phosphorylation site.

data of one of the phosphopeptide regions of tuftelin identified in whole saliva with the sequence A.RAKTENPGS*IR.I, where asterisks following the residue denotes phosphoserine. Tuftelin is an acidic protein synthesized by ameloblasts at the very early stages of enamel development and persists in extracellular matrix of enamel throughout development and mineralization.[78] Since its first discovery in ameloblasts, tuftelin has been localized in a wide range of soft tissues, but in almost all cases it has been related to abnormal developmental states such as tumors and carcinomas. These include kidney renal cell adenocarcinoma, germ cell tumors, ovary tumors, stomach adenocarcinoma, lung squamous cell carcinoma, lung carcinoid, and promyelocytes.[79] The appearance of tuftelin in many different "epithelial carcinomas" triggers a special interest within the context of saliva-based diagnostics because the fluid sample, which contained tuftelin, originated from the oral cavity. This shows that selective enrichment strategies may prove to be crucial for the identification of low-abundance diagnostic biomarkers in saliva.

MONO- VERSUS MULTIANALYTE MODELS

Potential pitfalls of diagnostic tests such as described earlier are related to the fact that they are based on the measurement of a single parameter. The best results with single biomarkers are obtained if the disease is clearly reflected in the mere presence of a biomarker, while absence of the biomarker indicates absence of a particular disease. It is therefore not surprising that the few FDA-approved salivary diagnostic tests are based on the detection of a single variable such as viral antibodies found in HIV infection[80] or the monitoring of a specific drug or its metabolite.[81] Since many diseases are multifactorial, detection and even quantitation of a single biomarker have resulted in relatively few useful diagnostic tests. For example, serum prostate-specific antigen (PSA) used for the diagnosis and monitoring of prostate cancer and CA125 for ovarian cancer are tests with poor sensitivity and specificity and have to be complemented with other analyses. One problem associated with salivary diagnostics is that the normal variation for levels of individual salivary proteins is not known.[33] This and the fact that many oral and nonoral diseases have a multifactorial etiology indicate that the univariate model is highly unlikely to provide adequate results. Indeed, most of the candidate biomarkers identified using the single marker approach fail in population studies. It has therefore been recognized that the multivariate model is more promising. The ability to screen and discover multiple biomarkers simultaneously may provide a more valid clinical diagnosis and may be more useful to recognize molecular patterns predictive for disease development. This multibiomarker approach has progressed by recent advances in clinical proteomics.

Cluster analysis of MS/MS data

High-throughput technologies such as LC-MS/MS have the ability to identify large numbers of proteins in samples of body fluids. The simultaneous analysis of the population of proteins present in complex biological body fluids can yield a profile unique to that specific sample. When the analysis is expanded to many hundreds of samples, population-specific protein expression profiles can be deduced that are characteristic of a particular group of subjects.

Cluster analyses can provide a characteristic fingerprint pattern indicative of health or disease. There is no need for the identification of individual biomarkers since the pattern of multiple biomarkers is more discriminatory and useful for clinical exploitation. Biomarker patterns are frequently not obvious to the human eye, and therefore the discovery of such patterns requires sophisticated data mining and learning algorithm software programs.[82,83] The employment of such bioinformatics and class prediction algorithms can be used to define known clinical pedigrees in terms of biomarker patterns.

Role of microfiber array technology in salivary diagnostics

MS technology not only has the capacity to identify and highlight specific protein biomarkers, it can also provide a list of critical protein(s) that can subsequently be targeted for diagnostics using other high-throughput technologies such as microsensors/microfluidics. Quite distinct from the MS analysis, the latter technologies utilize chromophoric fluorescent and immunoreactivity detection systems.[84] Optical fiber array methodology is uniquely suited for application in a multivariate model. Much of what has been said about proteomics is also applicable for the fiber array methodology. High-density arrays for multianalyte sensing provide a tool not only to identify but also to quantify simultaneously multiple specific biomarkers at the femto- to nanomole level. In addition, this technology has proved to be amenable to arrays with sensors reacting with more than one analyte, each triggering different signal outputs. This "cross-reactive" mode of the optical fiber array methodology may also be applied to pattern recognition in clinical samples obtained from different clinical phenotypes. It has been feasible to successfully identify markers in saliva that correlate with end-stage renal disease and to apply the multianalyte sensing methodology to monitor the efficiency of the dialysis procedure in these patients.[51]

CONCLUDING REMARKS

Technological developments both in MS and multiplex platforms have provided novel opportunities for the identification of biomarkers for diagnostics and drug discovery. These technologies continue to develop, and improvements are to be expected in protein quantitation and in the identification of posttranslational protein modifications. Advances in the distinguishing power between seemingly identical proteins may prove to be of ultimate importance in the discovery of biomarkers for disease. Saliva is a uniquely suited body fluid for diagnostic purposes, since it contains serum components and does not require invasive means for its collection. However, the dynamics of whole saliva composition, due to the presence of multiple enzymes, is frequently underestimated[85] and calls for stricter standardization in collection procedures. Advancements made recently in salivary protein research have shown that saliva contains in addition to the major salivary protein families hundreds of constituents present at low abundance. It also has become clear that these low-abundance proteins/peptides will likely be critical for the development of saliva-based diagnostic tools. The modern arsenal of high-throughput proteomics and multianalyte platforms represent an excellent basis to make salivary diagnostics a reality.

Acknowledgments

The author acknowledges thankfully the contributions made by Drs Erdjan Salih and Eva J. Helmerhorst. The author also acknowledges his support from NIH/NIDCR Grants DE05672, DE7652, DE17788.

REFERENCES

1. Mills CC. Occurrence of *Mycobacterium* other than *Mycobacterium tuberculosis* in the oral cavity and in sputum. Appl Microbiol 1972;24:307–310.
2. Scannapieco FA, Haraszthy GG, Cho MI, Levine MJ. Characterization of an amylase-binding component of *Streptococcus gordonii* G9B. Infect Immun 1992;60:4726–33.
3. Fourrier F, Duvivier B, Boutigny H, Roussel-Delvallez M, Chopin C. Colonization of dental plaque: a source of nosocomial infections in intensive care unit patients. Crit Care Med 1998;26:301–308.
4. Slavkin HC. Toward molecularly based diagnostics for the oral cavity. J Am Dent Assoc 1998;129:1138–43.
5. Oppenheim FG, Offner GD, Troxler RF. Phosphoproteins in the parotid saliva from the subhuman primate *Macaca fascicularis*. Isolation and characterization of a proline-rich phosphoglycoprotein and the complete covalent structure of a proline-rich phosphopeptide. J Biol Chem 1982;257:9271–82.
6. Keller PJ, Kauffman DL, Allan BJ, Williams BL. Further studies on the structural differences between the isoenzymes of human parotid-amylase. Biochemistry 1971;10:4867–74.
7. Beeley JA, Sweeney D, Lindsay JC, Buchanan ML, Sarna L, Khoo KS. Sodium dodecyl sulphate-polyacrylamide gel electrophoresis of human parotid salivary proteins. Electrophoresis, 1991;12:1032–41.
8. Oppenheim FG, Hay DI, Franzblau C. Proline-rich proteins from human parotid saliva. I. Isolation and partial characterization. Biochemistry 1971;10:4233–38.
9. Bennick A, Connell GE. Purification and partial characterization of four proteins from human parotid saliva. Biochem J 1971;123:455–64.
10. Levine M, Keller PJ. The isolation of some basic proline-rich proteins from human parotid saliva. Arch Oral Biol 1977;22:37–41.
11. Hay DI, Oppenheim FG. The isolation from human parotid saliva of a further group of proline-rich proteins. Arch Oral Biol 1974;19:627–32.
12. Schlesinger DH, Hay DI. Complete covalent structure of statherin, a tyrosine-rich acidic peptide which inhibits calcium phosphate precipitation from human parotid saliva. J Biol Chem 1976;252:1689–95.

13. Baum BJ, Bird JL, Millar DB, Longton, RW. Studies on histidine-rich polypeptides from human parotid saliva. Arch Biochem Biophys 1976;177:427–36.
14. Oppenheim FG, Xu T, McMillian FM, et al. Histatins, a novel family of histidine-rich proteins in human parotid secretion. Isolation, characterization, primary structure, and fungistatic effects on *Candida albicans*. J Biol Chem 1988;263:7472–7.
15. Oppenheim FG, Yang YC, Diamond RD, Hyslop D, Offner GD, Troxler RF. The primary structure and functional characterization of the neutral histidine-rich polypeptide from human parotid secretion. J Biol Chem, 1986;261:1177–82.
16. Mansson-Rahemtulla B, Rahemtulla F, Humphreys-Beher MG. Human salivary peroxidase and bovine lactoperoxidase are cross-reactive. J Dent Res 1990;69:1839–46.
17. Isemura S, Saitoh E, Sanada K. Characterization of a new cysteine proteinase inhibitor of human saliva, cystatin SN, which is immunologically related to cystatin S. FEBS Lett 1986;198:145–9.
18. Thiesse M, Millar SJ, Dickinson DP. The human type 2 cystatin gene family consists of eight to nine members, with at least seven genes clustered at a single locus on human chromosome 20. DNA Cell Biol 1994;13:97–116.
19. Loomis RE, Bergey EJ, Levine MJ, Tabak LA. Circular dichroism and fluorescence spectroscopic analyses of a proline-rich glycoprotein from human parotid saliva. Int J Pept Protein Res 1985;26:621–9.
20. Bobek LA, Tsai H, Biesbrock AR, Levine MJ. Molecular cloning, sequence, and specificity of expression of the gene encoding the low molecular weight human salivary mucin (MUC7). J Biol Chem 1993;268:20563–9.
21. Troxler RF, Offner GD, Zhang F, Iontcheva I, Oppenheim FG. Molecular cloning of a novel high molecular weight mucin (MG1) from human sublingual gland. Biochem Biophys Res Commun 1995;217:1112–19.
22. Azen EA, Oppenheim FG. Genetic polymorphism of proline-rich human salivary proteins. Science 1973;180:1067–69.
23. Oppenheim FG, Salih E, Siqueira WL, Zhang W, Helmerhorst EJ. Salivary proteome and its genetic polymorphisms. Ann N Y Acad Sci 2007;1098:22–50.
24. Maeda N. Inheritance of the human salivary proline-rich proteins: a reinterpretation in terms of six loci forming two subfamilies. Biochem Genet 1985;23:455–64.
25. Maeda N, Kim HS, Azen EA, Smithies O. Differential RNA splicing and post-translational cleavages in the human salivary proline-rich protein gene system. J Biol Chem 1985;260:11123–30.
26. Wong RS, Hofmann T, Bennick, A. The complete primary structure of a proline-rich phosphoprotein from human saliva. J Biol Chem 1979;254:4800–808.
27. Oppenheim, F. G. Preliminary observations on the presence and origin of serum albumin in human saliva. Helv Odontol Acta, 1970;14:10–17.
28. Oppenheim FG, Hay DI. Further studies of human serum albumin in oral fluid. Helv Odontol Acta 1972;16:22–26.
29. Goodson JM. Gingival crevice fluid flow. Periodontol 2000 2003;31:43–54.

30. Slaughter YA, Malamud D. Oral diagnostics for the geriatric populations: current status and future prospects. Dent Clin North Am 2005;49:445–61.

31. Kefalides PT. Saliva research leads to new diagnostic tools and therapeutic options. Ann Intern Med 1999;131:991–2.

32. Mandel ID. Salivary diagnosis: promises, promises. Ann N Y Acad Sci 1993;694:1–10.

33. Tabak LA. A revolution in biomedical assessment: the development of salivary diagnostics. J Dent Educ 2001;65:1335–9.

34. Kaufman E, Lamster IB. The diagnostic applications of saliva—a review. Crit Rev Oral Biol Med 2002;13:197–212.

35. Streckfus CF, Bigler LR. Saliva as a diagnostic fluid. Oral Dis 2002;8:69–76.

36. Larmas M. Saliva and dental caries: diagnostic tests for normal dental practice. Int Dent J 1992;42:199–208.

37. Kaufman E, Lamster IB. Analysis of saliva for periodontal diagnosis—a review. J Clin Periodontol 2000;27:453–65.

38. Tiwari SK, Khan AA, Ahmed KS, et al. Rapid diagnosis of *Helicobacter pylori* infection in dyspeptic patients using salivary secretion: a non-invasive approach. Singapore Med J 2005;46:224–8.

39. Frerichs RR, Htoon MT, Eskes N, Lwin S. Comparison of saliva and serum for HIV surveillance in developing countries. Lancet 1992;340:1496–9.

40. Hodinka RL, Nagashunmugam T, Malamud D. Detection of human immunodeficiency virus antibodies in oral fluids. Clin Diagn Lab Immunol 1998;5:419–26.

41. van der Eijk AA, Niesters HG, Gotz HM., et al. Paired measurements of quantitative hepatitis B virus DNA in saliva and serum of chronic hepatitis B patients: implications for saliva as infectious agent. J Clin Virol 2004;29:92–4.

42. van Doornum GJ, Lodder A, Buimer M, van Ameijden, EJ, Bruisten, S. Evaluation of hepatitis C antibody testing in saliva specimens collected by two different systems in comparison with HCV antibody and HCV RNA in serum. J Med Virol 2001;64:13–20.

43. Ikuta K, Satoh Y, Hoshikawa Y, Sairenji, T. Detection of Epstein-Barr virus in salivas and throat washings in healthy adults and children. Microbes Infect 2000;2:115–20.

44. Spicher VM, Bouvier P, Schlegel-Haueter SE, Morabia A, Siegrist CA. Epidemiology of herpes simplex virus in children by detection of specific antibodies in saliva. Pediatr Infect Dis J 2001;20:265–72.

45. Lucht E, Brytting M, Bjerregaard L, Julander I, Linde A. Shedding of cytomegalovirus and herpesviruses 6, 7, and 8 in saliva of human immunodeficiency virus type 1-infected patients and healthy controls. Clin Infect Dis 1998;27:137–41.

46. Li Y, St John MA, Zhou X, et al. Salivary transcriptome diagnostics for oral cancer detection. Clin Cancer Res 2004;10:8442–50.

47. Li Y, Zhou X, St John MA, Wong DT. RNA profiling of cell-free saliva using microarray technology. J Dent Res 2004;83:199–203.

48. Mager DL, Haffajee AD, Devlin PM, Norris CM, Posner MR, Goodson JM. The salivary microbiota as a diagnostic indicator of oral cancer: a

descriptive, non-randomized study of cancer-free and oral squamous cell carcinoma subjects. J Transl Med 2005;3:27.

49. Christodoulides N, Floriano PN, Acosta SA, et al. Toward the development of a lab-on-a-chip dual-function leukocyte and C-reactive protein analysis method for the assessment of inflammation and cardiac risk. Clin Chem 2005;51:2391–5.

50. Lloyd JE, Broughton A, Selby C. Salivary creatinine assays as a potential screen for renal disease. Ann Clin Biochem 1996;33(Pt 5):428–31.

51. Walt DR, Blicharz TM, Hayman RB, et al. Microsensor arrays for saliva diagnostics. Ann N Y Acad Sci 2007;1098:389–400.

52. Hillenkamp F, Karas M. Mass spectrometry of peptides and proteins by matrix-assisted ultraviolet laser desorption/ionization. Methods Enzymol 1990;193:280–95.

53. Aebersold R, Mann M. Mass spectrometry-based proteomics. Nature 2003;422:198–207.

54. Dunn MJ, Corbett JM. Two-dimensional polyacrylamide gel electrophoresis. Methods Enzymol 1996;271:177–203.

55. Heegaard NH, Kennedy RT. Identification, quantitation, and characterization of biomolecules by capillary electrophoretic analysis of binding interactions. Electrophoresis 1999;20:3122–33.

56. Nice EC, Aguilar MI. Micropreparative HPLC of peptides and proteins. Methods Mol Biol 2004;251:165–76.

57. Washburn MP, Wolters D, Yates JR, III. Large-scale analysis of the yeast proteome by multidimensional protein identification technology. Nat Biotechnol 2001;19:242–7.

58. Leymarie N, Berg EA, McComb ME, et al. Tandem mass spectrometry for structural characterization of proline-rich proteins: application to salivary PRP-3. Anal Chem 2002;74:4124–32.

59. Yao Y, Berg EA, Costello CE, Troxler RF, Oppenheim FG. Identification of protein components in human acquired enamel pellicle and whole saliva using novel proteomics approaches. J Biol Chem 2003;278:5300–308.

60. Yao Y, Grogan J, Zehnder M, et al. Compositional analysis of human acquired enamel pellicle by mass spectrometry. Arch Oral Biol, 2001;46:293–303.

61. Ghafouri B, Tagesson C, Lindahl M. Mapping of proteins in human saliva using two-dimensional gel electrophoresis and peptide mass fingerprinting. Proteomics 2003;3:1003–1015.

62. Hardt M, Thomas LR, Dixon SE, et al. Toward defining the human parotid gland salivary proteome and peptidome: identification and characterization using 2D SDS-PAGE, ultrafiltration, HPLC, and mass spectrometry. Biochemistry 2005;44:2885–99.

63. Walz A, Stuhler K, Wattenberg A, et al. Proteome analysis of glandular parotid and submandibular-sublingual saliva in comparison to whole human saliva by two-dimensional gel electrophoresis. Proteomics 2006;6:1631–9.

64. Vitorino R, de Morais Guedes S, Ferreira R, et al. Two-dimensional electrophoresis study of in vitro pellicle formation and dental caries susceptibility. Eur J Oral Sci 2006;114:147–53.

65. Hu S, Loo JA, Wong DT. Human body fluid proteome analysis. Proteomics, 2006;6:6326–53.
66. Vitorino R, Lobo MJ, Ferrer-Correira AJ, et al. Identification of human whole saliva protein components using proteomics. Proteomics 2004;4:1109–115.
67. Wilmarth PA, Riviere MA, Rustvold DL, Lauten JD, Madden TE, David LL. Two-dimensional liquid chromatography study of the human whole saliva proteome. J Proteome Res 2004;3:1017–23.
68. Xie H, Rhodus NL, Griffin RJ, Carlis JV, Griffin TJ. A catalogue of human saliva proteins identified by free flow electrophoresis-based peptide separation and tandem mass spectrometry. Mol Cell Proteomics 2005;4:1826–30.
69. Gygi SP, Rist B, Aebersold R. Measuring gene expression by quantitative proteome analysis. Curr Opin Biotechnol 2000;11:396–401.
70. Oda Y, Huang K, Cross FR, Cowburn D, Chait BT. Accurate quantitation of protein expression and site-specific phosphorylation. Proc Natl Acad Sci U S A 1999;96:6591–6.
71. Zhou H, Boyle R, Aebersold, R. Quantitative protein analysis by solid phase isotope tagging and mass spectrometry. Methods Mol Biol 2004;261:511–18.
72. Hardt M, Witkowska HE, Webb S, et al. Assessing the effects of diurnal variation on the composition of human parotid saliva: quantitative analysis of native peptides using iTRAQ reagents. Anal Chem 2005;77:4947–54.
73. Charette SJ, Lavoie JN, Lambert H, Landry J. Inhibition of Daxx-mediated apoptosis by heat shock protein 27. Mol Cell Biol 2000;20:7602–612.
74. Mori S, Popoli M, Brunello N, Racagni G, Perez J. Effect of reboxetine treatment on brain cAMP- and calcium/calmodulin-dependent protein kinases. Neuropharmacology 2001;40:448–56.
75. Hubbard MJ, Cohen P. On target with a new mechanism for the regulation of protein phosphorylation. Trends Biochem Sci 1993;18:172–7.
76. Hunter T. Signaling—2000 and beyond. Cell 2000;100:113–27.
77. Uy R, Wold F. Posttranslational covalent modification of proteins. Science 1977;198:890–96.
78. Deutsch D, Palmon A, Fisher LW, Kolodny N, Termine JD, Young MF. Sequencing of bovine enamelin ("tuftelin") a novel acidic enamel protein. J Biol Chem 1991;266:16021–28.
79. Deutsch D, Leiser Y, Shay B, et al. The human tuftelin gene and the expression of tuftelin in mineralizing and nonmineralizing tissues. Connect Tissue Res 2002;43:425–34.
80. Branson BM. FDA approves OraQuick for use in saliva. On March 25, the FDA approved the first rapid test for HIV in oral fluids. AIDS Clin Care 2004;16:39.
81. Kacinko SL, Barnes AJ, Kim I, et al. A. Performance characteristics of the Cozart RapiScan Oral Fluid Drug Testing System for opiates in comparison to ELISA and GC/MS following controlled codeine administration. Forensic Sci Int 2004;141:41–8.
82. Drake RR, Cazare LH, Semmes OJ, Wadsworth JT. Serum, salivary and tissue proteomics for discovery of biomarkers for head and neck cancers. Expert Rev Mol Diagn 2005;5:93–100.

83. Pusch W, Flocco MT, Leung SM, Thiele H, Kostrzewa M. Mass spectrometry-based clinical proteomics. Pharmacogenomics 2003;4:463–76.

84. Walt DR. Fiber optic array biosensors. Biotechniques 2006;41:529,531,533 passim.

85. Helmerhorst EJ, Oppenheim FG. Saliva: a dynamic proteome. J Dent Res 2007;86:680–93.

Diagnostics other than blood

Sudhir Srivastava and Karl E. Krueger

INTRODUCTION

Recent advances in genetics and molecular biology have led to a better understanding of the biological basis of disease causation and progression. Diagnostic testing, for example, often involves measurement of specific molecular markers along with other physical devices such as X-ray, magnetic resonance imaging, and ultrasound that have found their way into clinical application. Molecular testing, however, is likely to be more acceptable to clinicians and patients as these tests can be performed using biological fluids, such as serum, and at much lower cost. The choices for what type of fluid should be collected and the test to be implemented are based on several considerations. Priority is generally placed on body fluids that can be collected by the least invasive means, accurate tests that are relatively inexpensive to perform, and measurement of biomarkers that show specificity for a defined site of clinical interest. This chapter discusses the different physiological fluids that are of diagnostic significance, how they can be used for clinical investigation of the functioning of various organ systems, and the special attributes that saliva is endowed with to make relatively simple tests amenable for a wide array of clinical indications.

THE ADVANTAGES AND DISADVANTAGES OF BLOOD

Current clinical practice for a plethora of tests from routine physical examinations to diagnostic assessment of physiological function or indication of a disease involves phlebotomy. The choice of blood as a biofluid for clinical testing is clear-cut considering its close relationship to the homeostasis of the body. Blood collection is minimally invasive and rapid causing at worst slight, momentary discomfort to the subject. Because blood circulates throughout all organs, its chemical makeup is a composite of nearly all metabolic processes occurring in the individual. Blood is paramount in delivery of nutrients and oxygen to tissues, transport of metabolites, hormones, and protein complexes between organ systems, and mediates removal of metabolic waste products. In many respects blood can be considered to exhibit a molecular panorama contributed by all organs. Thus in a diagnostic sense, one would expect to find molecular biomarkers for virtually any disease in blood.

The variety of molecules that can be measured in blood is extensive. Proteins normally found in circulation and secreted by tissues are self-evident components one would expect to find. Small molecule metabolites, nutrients, and hormones are other molecules intrinsic to the primary function of blood to transport these chemicals throughout the body. It is somewhat surprising that separate from the circulatory and immune cellular components, remnants from other tissues can also be detected such as exfoliated cells, as in the case of malignant cancer.[1] Furthermore, free circulating DNA and RNA is also found possibly representing debris from necrotic tissue.[2,3] The detection of somatic mutations and hypermethylated DNA in circulation is evidence that this DNA is partly derived from dying neoplastic cells rather than ruptured white blood cells.[4,5]

Quantitation of most small molecule metabolites is readily feasible in blood because the repertoire of molecular diversity is relatively low (estimated to be less than 2,000 molecules). Highly specific tests can normally be designed for each molecule of interest. The story with proteins in the blood is very different. Work initiated as part of the HUPO Plasma Proteome Project identified over 9,500 distinct proteins in blood with over 3,000 species proposed as definitive serum proteins with a high level of confidence.[6] This latter number probably represents an underestimate since most low-abundance protein species are not detected by this analysis. The dynamic concentration range of proteins in blood covers 12 orders of magnitude.[7–9] Most proteins found within the upper 4–5 orders are constitutive plasma proteins that would not be useful for many diagnostic tests. Those proteins that would reflect a certain disease or physiological state would lie in the lower abundance categories of the plasma proteome (Fig. 8.1).

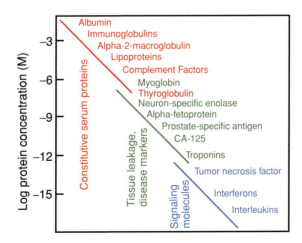

Figure 8.1 Dynamic concentration range of proteins found in serum. Relative levels of several proteins of diagnostic importance in blood are shown in relation to the levels of other integral blood proteins. The concept of this figure was adapted from Anderson and Anderson.[7]

The advent of new mass spectral techniques such as matrix-assisted laser desorption ionization-time of flight-mass spectrometry (MALDI-TOF-MS) and surface-enhanced laser desorption ionization-time of flight-mass spectrometry (SELDI-TOF-MS) permitted the serum or plasma proteome to be readily interrogated with minimal sample-handling requirements. These technology platforms which initially showed promise prompted the search for protein-based biomarkers of disease in blood. Although TOF-MS can only be effectively used for lower-molecular-weight proteins, it has relatively high resolution where thousands of polypeptide peaks can be analyzed in each profile. In most studies where protein identification of specific "diagnostic" peaks was made, the discovery of acute-phase reactants resulted in a rather disappointing outcome.[10–13] The diagnostic markers observed represent the host response to the disease rather than a direct byproduct of the disease.

This experience highlights how the inherent protein complexity of blood can confound biomarker discovery. Despite the fact that TOF-MS techniques are able to penetrate several orders of magnitude into the serum proteome, this is apparently still not sufficient to detect the most informative protein disease markers. The identification of acute-phase reactants such as markers of inflammation or immunological response is not likely to be specific to a disease, yet these would be among the more abundant proteins in blood. Discovery efforts for disease markers in blood will have to transcend this concentration barrier to interrogate proteins at the lower-abundance ranges.

Another issue that is often confronted with proteins in blood is that many proteins are not free, but are primarily bound to other proteins. Serum albumin, the most abundant extracellular protein found in blood, is complexed with many other polypeptides in a rather nonspecific manner[14] (also see Chapter 7 for serum albumin in saliva). This scenario holds for many of the other more prominent serum proteins. These macromolecular associations may obscure protein biomarker investigational efforts where the free form of the molecule is required.

Beyond the phase of biomarker discovery, test developments for validated biomarkers are engineered to be highly selective for the molecules of interest. For protein markers these tests typically involve the use of antibodies. The issue of detecting proteins at very low abundance in blood is thus overcome with specific, high-affinity antibodies accounting for many of the diagnostic enzyme-linked immunosorbent assays (ELISAs) in clinical use today. While blood poses significant hurdles for biomarker discovery, it is often found to be a convenient medium for well-established tests that have been developed for select molecules.

CONSIDERATION OF OTHER BODY FLUIDS

Whereas blood permeates all tissues and therefore can contain molecular constituents arising from all organs of the body, other body fluids are more restricted in their association with select organs. This privileged association of certain organs with certain biofluids offers the advantage of providing a

Table 8.1 Types of specimens are categorized according to the relative degree of invasiveness required to obtain samples.

Specimen type	Privileged organ system(s)	Special remarks
Noninvasive		
Exhaled breath	Lungs, respiratory airways	Volatile or aerosolized markers
Nipple aspirate fluid	Mammary glands	Requires special device
Saliva	Nasopharyngeal structures, upper aerodigestive tract	Stimulated and unstimulated collection methods
Sputum	Lungs, respiratory airways	Spontaneous or induced
Stool	Gastrointestinal tract	
Tears	Lacrimal glands	
Urine	Genitourinary tract	Exhibits diurnal variations
Minimally invasive		
Amniotic fluid	Fetal/placental tissues	
Cervical smears	Cervix	
Mildly invasive		
Bronchoalveolar lavage	Lungs, respiratory airways	Releases loosely adherent and inflammatory cells
Cerebrospinal fluid	Central nervous system	Turnover rate is >3 times per day
Endoscopy-derived specimens	Site specific	
Fine needle aspirates	Site specific	
Synovial fluid	Site specific for joints	Highly viscous

"Site specific" refers samples being collected from organs targeted by that procedure.

medium from which its molecular composition is more directly tied to its affiliated organ sites.

Table 8.1 provides a list of most body fluids that have been exploited for diagnostic tests. The organ systems that show a biological relationship or proximal location with each fluid type highlight how different specimen sources might provide a convenient window to probe the biological status of select organs. Most of these physiological fluids do not show the proteome complexity evident in blood. The origins of nucleic acids, secreted glycoproteins, exfoliated cells, and shedding of cellular remnants in these fluids are likewise integrated more directly with the organ systems with which the fluids are in immediate physical contact. Biomarker discovery efforts are therefore likely to be less complicated, given the relative simplicity in molecular profiles contributed by a limited group of organs. In fact, one of the paradigms currently being explored by numerous laboratories is to first identify biomarkers in fluid directly from the tissue of interest (usually collected by fine needle aspiration) or in cultured cells isolated from the involved site and then search for the equivalent molecular marker(s) in blood as a potential diagnostic.[15,16] A major advantage of using these other body fluids is that diagnostic tests will tend to be more specific for markers derived from a select number of tissues unlike blood where literally all organ systems can shed molecules into circulation. Wherever a marker may arise from multiple tissues, the use of these other body fluids should in principle show preference for markers derived primarily from the pertinent organ system as listed in Table 8.1.

A major consideration for diagnostic testing is to obtain specimens by the least invasive means feasible. The least invasive collection procedures pose lower risk and discomfort to the patient, and this generally reduces special preparation and care by clinical personnel during sample collection. Fluids or material that is excreted or discharged from the body can be collected by noninvasive means. Samples that can be readily accessed via an opening (oral, vaginal, or rectal) will likely require a minimal level of intrusion into the body, while other methods (typically requiring endoscopy) allow deeper penetration to achieve more direct access to more internally situated organs. Excisional surgery represents the most invasive means for sample or biopsy collection; however, to avoid this measure and to minimize tissue trauma, samples from the site under investigation can be drawn using a needle as is done with fine needle aspiration or removal of cerebrospinal fluid.

Examples of diagnostic tests used today or currently under development using specimens collected by these different routes are provided in Table 8.2. It is of particular interest to note those tests corresponding to the detection of molecules that are not selectively derived from the corresponding organ system(s) from which the biofluid is obtained. These likely represent markers that are transported systemically through the circulation and manage to enter other biofluid compartments by mechanisms involving passage through the epithelial linings of the appropriate organ system.

THE DIAGNOSTIC POTENTIAL OF SALIVA

Saliva fulfills several of the chief diagnostic concerns for a diagnostic biofluid inasmuch as it is obtained noninvasively requiring no special skill. Several saliva collection kits are already marketed and some have gained FDA approval for various diagnostic tests. Because of the ease, safety, and low cost of saliva collection, its promise for current and future diagnostics warrants special consideration. Table 8.3 lists different classes of biomarkers that are present in saliva which are being currently analyzed or investigated as potential tests for a multitude of clinical tests. Other chapters of this book discuss in greater detail these innovative applications on the use of saliva.

The principal components of saliva are produced by the salivary glands and thus any molecular markers derived from these glands, whether derived through secretion or passive diffusion, would be expected to be present in this biofluid. One recent study that was initiated through work on *Drosophila* reported the intriguing finding that amylase or its mRNA levels in human saliva may be a marker for sleep deprivation.[17] This unusual finding may hint

Table 8.2 Examples of diagnostic tests and their associated markers found in biofluids other than blood.

Specimen type	Marker(s)	Diagnostic indication
Amniotic fluid	Acetylcholinesterase	Neural tube defects
	Exfoliated cells	Chromosomal defects
	Bilirubin/Rh factor	Rh sensitivity
Cerebrospinal fluid	Infectious agents	Meningitis
	HSE DNA	Encephalitis
Cervical smears	PAP test (cytology)	Cervical intraepithelial neoplasia
	HPV	Cervical cancer risk
	Chlamydia DNA	Chlamydia infection
Fine needle aspirate	Cytological exam	Cellular pathology
Saliva	Viral DNA/antibodies	Various viral pathogens
	Bacterial DNA and antibodies	*Helicobacter. pylori* infection
		Caries susceptibility
	Steroid hormones	Endocrine function
	Drugs	Monitoring drug abuse
	c-erbB-2 protein	Breast cancer
Sputum	Eosinophils	Asthma
	Bacterial markers	Pathogen infection
	Exfoliated epithelial cells	Lung cancer risk
Stool	Stool cultures	Gastrointestinal infection
	Pancreatic enzymes	Cystic fibrosis
	DNA mutations	Inflammatory bowel disease/colorectal cancer
	FOBT	Colorectal cancer
Tears	Lysozyme	Keratoconjunctivitis sicca
Urine	Glucose	Diabetes
	Drugs	Monitoring drug abuse
	Metabolites	Metabolic parameters
	Albumin	Renal failure
	Bacteria	Urinary tract infections
	Exfoliated cells	Bladder cancer

FOBT, fecal occult blood test; HPV, human papillomavirus; HSE, herpes simplex encephalitis; PAP, Papanicolaou.

at some level of autonomic nervous system control over the serous lobules of salivary glands to elicit this unusual response detected in saliva.

Aside from material secreted from salivary glands, additional components from the oral cavity can be suspended or dissolved in saliva, most notably gingival crevicular fluid. In this respect saliva could be considered to exhibit preferential representation of markers derived from any tissues in direct contact with the oral cavity to include the tongue, teeth and gums, dermal linings inside the mouth, and the nasal-pharyngeal compartments. Specifically, buccal

Table 8.3 The different classes of markers found in saliva are listed with their potential uses, many of which are currently being explored for development of an effective test.

Biomarker class	Potential applications
DNA	Standard genotyping Bacterial infection Head and neck cancer diagnosis Forensics
RNA	Viral/bacterial identification Oral cancer diagnosis
Proteins	Periodontitis diagnosis Cancer diagnosis Caries susceptibility
Mucins/glycoproteins	Head and neck cancer diagnosis Caries susceptibility
Immunoglobulins	Viral infection (HIV, hepatitis B and C)
Metabolites	Various endocrine conditions Stress, psychological status Periodontitis diagnosis Cystic fibrosis diagnosis
Drugs and their metabolites	Monitor drug abuse Monitor patient compliance to therapy
Viruses	Epstein-Barr virus reactivation (mononucleosis)
Bacteria	Oral cancer diagnosis Caries susceptibility
Cellular material	Head and neck cancer diagnosis

or squamous cells shed from the dermal linings inside the mouth, microflora residing on the teeth and gingival surfaces or other upper aerodigestive tract structures, and secretions from any tissues in this proximity all contribute to the primary constituents that are found in saliva.

The diagnostic potential of saliva goes well beyond serving as a status indicator for the nasal-pharyngeal and upper aerodigestive regions. Constituents from within the entire respiratory tract are expelled through this route, and these can also become incorporated in saliva. Cellular waste products or secretions and exfoliated cells or their remnants from the airways can be expelled toward the oral cavity and thus be found in saliva.[18,19]

The implications of using saliva for the diagnosis of disease are enticing. The likelihood that oral cancer can be detected by testing saliva is not far-fetched, given the direct contact these neoplastic cells have with saliva[20]; however, it is also feasible that saliva may provide a window into the deeper stretches of the respiratory tract through the principles described in the preceding paragraph. The leading risk factor for lung as well as head and neck cancer is smoking history. Epithelial cells of the entire respiratory tract from the mouth to the alveoli of the lungs are subjected to the carcinogenic insults of smoke.

Most cells exposed to these agents might then undergo similar chromosomal changes setting them on a path toward malignant transformation. This concept is termed the field effect where cells over a large area exhibit similar preneoplastic changes.[21] The field effect is currently being exploited as a tool to diagnose lung cancer in patients with smoking history by examining the transcriptomic profiles of bronchial epithelial cells removed by brushing during bronchoscopy of the airways. Although neoplastic transformation may not have yet occurred in the bronchi, it is suggested that cancer in the lung can be effectively diagnosed through the field effect since the bronchi exhibits parallel cellular transformations, similar to those observed in the lung where cancer has already started.[22] Due to the field effect, it is plausible that markers derived from epithelial cells of the oral cavity, or cells dislodged from the airways, may provide diagnostic information for lung disease that might be detected in saliva.

The principle of the field effect holds for other etiological risk factors for head and neck cancers such as human papillomavirus[23,24] and alcohol consumption.[25] The basic paradigm for diagnosis remains the same as for smoking where cellular responses or exposure to carcinogenic agents are monitored from material released by the exposed cells within the oral cavity, from which the level of risk for disease can be determined.

The use of saliva as a diagnostic fluid described to this point has been mostly from the standpoint of measuring markers produced from local tissues (upper aerodigestive tract) or slightly more distal sites, but still in close contact with the oral cavity (lower respiratory system). However, saliva has a long history of showing diagnostic utility for conditions that have no direct relevance to upper respiratory function. Saliva has been demonstrated to be an excellent test material for many types of systemic markers including those for endocrine function, stress or psychological state, exposure to infectious agents, use or metabolism of drugs or other xenobiotics, and other cancers.[26,27] While the markers in each of these cases are not produced in, nor do they necessarily play an integral role in the biology of the tissues that line the oral cavity, they are still conveniently found to make their way into saliva apparently through passive diffusion, paracellular transit, or other unknown mechanisms. Perhaps the most profound example is development of a diagnostic test for malignant breast cancer based on salivary c-erbB-2.[28] Whatever the mechanism, clinicians and scientists have taken advantage of these findings to develop simple and noninvasive tests in saliva.

CONCLUDING REMARKS

Blood will always be a primary biofluid for diverse diagnostic tests, but it has distinct limitations and disadvantages. Other body fluids collected noninvasively and without the need for skilled personnel can fulfill select niches for different diagnostic purposes. Saliva has shown its value for a number of tests already being widely implemented, but current research suggests the full potential of this biofluid remains to be explored further. The presence of a wide array of biological markers such as proteins, glycoproteins, DNA, RNA, small molecule metabolites and messengers, drug metabolic byproducts, bacteria, viruses, exfoliated cells, and antibodies highlight the promise that saliva diagnostics offers for the future of clinical testing.

REFERENCES

1. Riethdorf S, Fritsche H, Muller V, et al. Detection of circulating tumor cells in peripheral blood of patients with metastatic breast cancer: a validation study of the CellSearch system. Clin Cancer Res 2007;13(3):920–28.
2. Gal S, Fidler C, Lo YM, et al. Quantitation of circulating DNA in the serum of breast cancer patients by real-time PCR. Br J Cancer 2004;90(6):1211–15.
3. Swaminathan R, Butt AN. Circulating nucleic acids in plasma and serum: recent developments. Ann N Y Acad Sci 2006;1075:1–9.
4. Hoque MO, Feng Q, Toure P, et al. Detection of aberrant methylation of four genes in plasma DNA for the detection of breast cancer. J Clin Oncol 2006;24(26):4262–9.
5. Schmidt K, Diehl F. A blood-based DNA test for colorectal cancer screening. Discov Med 2007;7(37):7–12.
6. Omenn GS, States DJ, Adamski M, et al. Overview of the HUPO Plasma Proteome Project: results from the pilot phase with 35 collaborating laboratories and multiple analytical groups, generating a core dataset of 3020 proteins and a publicly-available database. Proteomics 2005;5(13):3226–45.
7. Anderson NL, Anderson NG. The human plasma proteome: history, character, and diagnostic prospects. Mol Cell Proteomics 2002;1(11):845–67.
8. Hortin GL, Jortani SA, Ritchie JC, Jr, Valdes R, Jr, Chan DW. Proteomics: a new diagnostic frontier. Clin Chem 2006;52(7):1218–22.
9. Thadikkaran L, Siegenthaler MA, Crettaz D, Queloz PA, Schneider P, Tissot JD. Recent advances in blood-related proteomics. Proteomics 2005;5(12):3019–34.
10. Check E. Proteomics and cancer: running before we can walk? Nature 2004;429(6991):496–7.
11. Diamandis EP. Analysis of serum proteomic patterns for early cancer diagnosis: drawing attention to potential problems. J Natl Cancer Inst 2004;96(5):353–6.
12. Petricoin EF, Ardekani AM, Hitt BA, et al. Use of proteomic patterns in serum to identify ovarian cancer. Lancet 2002;359(9306):572–7.
13. Ransohoff DF. Lessons from controversy: ovarian cancer screening and serum proteomics. J Natl Cancer Inst 2005;97(4):315–19.
14. Petricoin EF, Belluco C, Araujo RP, Liotta LA. The blood peptidome: a higher dimension of information content for cancer biomarker discovery. Nat Rev Cancer 2006;6(12):961–7.
15. Omenn GS. Strategies for plasma proteomic profiling of cancers. Proteomics 2006;6(20):5662–73.
16. Sardana G, Marshall J, Diamandis EP. Discovery of candidate tumor markers for prostate cancer via proteomic analysis of cell culture-conditioned medium. Clin Chem 2007;53(3):429–37.

17. Seugnet L, Boero J, Gottschalk L, Duntley SP, Shaw PJ. Identification of a biomarker for sleep drive in flies and humans. Proc Natl Acad Sci U S A 2006;103(52):19913–18.
18. Franzmann EJ, Reategui EP, Carraway KL, Hamilton KL, Weed DT, Goodwin WJ. Salivary soluble CD44: a potential molecular marker for head and neck cancer. Cancer Epidemiol Biomarkers Prev 2005;14(3):735–9.
19. Jiang WW, Masayesva B, Zahurak M, et al. Increased mitochondrial DNA content in saliva associated with head and neck cancer. Clin Cancer Res 2005;11(7):2486–91.
20. Wong DT. Salivary diagnostics. J Calif Dent Assoc 2006;34(4):283–5.
21. Kopelovich L, Henson DE, Gazdar AF, et al. Surrogate anatomic/functional sites for evaluating cancer risk: an extension of the field effect. Clin Cancer Res 1999;5(12):3899–905.
22. Spira A, Beane JE, Shah V, et al. Airway epithelial gene expression in the diagnostic evaluation of smokers with suspect lung cancer. Nat Med 2007;13(3):361–6.
23. McKaig RG, Baric RS, Olshan AF. Human papillomavirus and head and neck cancer: epidemiology and molecular biology. Head Neck 1998;20(3):250–65.
24. Smith EM, Ritchie JM, Summersgill KF, et al. Human papillomavirus in oral exfoliated cells and risk of head and neck cancer. J Natl Cancer Inst 2004;96(6):449–55.
25. Riedel F, Goessler UR, Hormann K. Alcohol-related diseases of the mouth and throat. Dig Dis 2005;23(3–4):195–203.
26. Streckfus CF, Bigler LR. Saliva as a diagnostic fluid. Oral Dis 2002;8(2):69–76.
27. Kaufman E, Lamster IB. The diagnostic applications of saliva—review. Crit Rev Oral Biol Med 2002;13(2):197–212.
28. Streckfus C, Bigler L. The use of soluble, salivary c-erbB-2 for the detection and post-operative follow-up of breast cancer in women: the results of a five-year translational research study. Adv Dent Res 2005;18(1):17–24.

Perceptions of saliva: Relevance to clinical diagnostics

Sreenivas Koka and David T. Wong

INTRODUCTION

The search for a resource that can be used to detect a broad range of diseases easily and reliably is akin to a search for the diagnostic Holy Grail. Indeed, inside our mouths may lie the key to a library of biomarkers representing disease and health. Saliva—the source of all this information—is the secretory product of glands located in or around the oral cavity. By cracking the saliva diagnostic codes, we recognize that the source of diagnostic information in saliva is blood and that the validity of both media is equal.

Ivan Pavlov's experiments demonstrate that salivation is closely associated with the thought of food, one of life's primary indulgences. Yet most people never appreciate the uniqueness of saliva. Throughout the world, saliva has positive and negative connotations and thoughts of saliva may be viewed as grotesque in one population while being the vehicle of blessing in another. These variations belie interesting cultural, social, behavioral, and psychological points about how saliva is perceived around world.

GLOBAL CULTURAL VIEWS

History

Some of the precedent for saliva's negative views stems from the discovery that saliva may carry airborne pathogens and respiratory diseases. Early in the mid-nineteenth century, spitting in public was commonplace, usually associated with chewing tobacco. The turn from its socially acceptable position toward being shunned started in the mid-nineteenth century when human saliva was placed under the light microscope and was found to contain microorganisms. The surge in placing saliva in a negative light continued during the late nineteenth century when the German physician Robert Koch discovered bacterium responsible for tuberculosis.[1] Influenza and other respiratory pathogens soon were discovered to be also transmissible through respiratory droplets originating from infected individuals. However, phlegm and mucous from the respiratory tract are the original source of bacteria and viruses, and

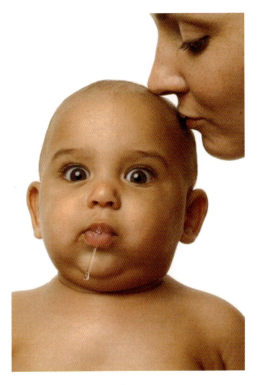

Figure 9.1 Infant salivating, a lovable sight to parent.

so saliva should not be automatically tied with germs and disease for being an innocent vehicle.

Social

Although approximately 1.5 L of saliva are produced daily, salivation, with the rare exception of infants and toddlers (Fig. 9.1), is often perceived as socially inappropriate. In America, accepted practices of spitting are usually reserved for sports athletes, for example, in baseball, spitting is a common practice within the dugout or on the field as a gesture of machismo. In addition, pitchers spit on the mound and batters spit onto their hands, attempting to gain good luck. The legendary Boston Celtic basketball player Larry Bird would spit on his hands for good luck at the beginning of every game.

Spitting in the general public, however, is seen as offensive behavior. In a motion of disrespect, spitting may also be used as the popular choice for an offensive gesture. Sayings such as "I spit on you" or "I spit on your grave" convey precisely those connotations. In the Mexican culture, "spitting on a parent" is a form of elder mistreatment, a form of family violence. However, in other cultures, saliva is much more intimately tied with their common beliefs and rituals.

In South America, a tradition that originated with the Incans persists even until today. Women in Peru, Bolivia, Venezuela, and countries along the Andes continue the process of fermenting manioc root, maize, or fruits into the intoxicating alcoholic "chicha," using the digestive and fermentative properties of their own saliva. In fact, the name "chichi" is derived from the Spanish word "chical," which is loosely translated as "to spit" or "saliva".[2] Hundreds of years ago, the drink was of great importance to the Incans; today, chicha is still used among Amazonians as a diet staple, as well as a work incentive and social drink.

Ritual

The Greeks have long-standing traditions with saliva and the act of spitting. Generally, the Greeks will spit to ward off bad luck in hopes of good luck and well-being. Spitting is commonly seen during ceremonious events including within the Greek Orthodox Church and during the ceremony of baptism where after the priest blesses a child with holy water he spits three times onto the ground to represent the holy trinity in renouncing the devil. During Greek weddings guests will gingerly spit on the bride to project their blessings and good fortune. It is also common in Greek culture to make three spitting gestures onto clothing and onto each other during greetings in order to ward off the infamous evil eye. Thus, the act of spitting is widely present in proper Greek etiquette.

Health and medicine

Nowhere is saliva more integrated within celebratory rituals and as a form of alternative medicine than in Africa. For example, the Somali use saliva as the primary remedy for an open blister.[3] To alleviate the pain and swelling of snakebites, the Somali usually treat the ailment with mixed butter and saliva.[4] Within other tribes such as the Azande of Sudan and the Masai of East Africa, saliva may be used alone as a first-aid astringent for minor wounds or mixed with herbal plants.[5] The Bena of Tanzania use saliva to treat boils and mothers of the Masia tribe use it to treat insect bites and swelling.[6] The primitive yet abundant source of saliva makes it an easy medicinal agent for common ailments.

In other parts of Africa, saliva carries a more spiritual meaning. Wolof tribesmen believe that saliva may confer blessings and curing properties from the source to the target[7] based on the belief that water is able to retain the memory and essence of its source. Therefore, following the birth of a child, it is common practice to invite the newborn's elders to bless him or her with their salivary secretion.[8] Similar rituals of direct salivary inoculations occur within the people of Ashanti in Ghana, where spiritual enlightenment of an infant is brought about through the grandfather spitting into the mouth of the newborn.[9]

In Asia, the act of spitting may date back to 4,000 years ago when the betel nut (an areca nut, betel leaf, and lime mixture) was habitually chewed in Thailand, India, Philippines, Taiwan, and Indonesia. The plant releases alkaloids, which are readily absorbed through the mucous membranes of the mouth, causing excessive secretions of saliva[10] and resulting in saliva reddish brown in color. The act of spitting is a traditionally accepted practice in Asia and regarded as a component of good personal hygiene. More recently, however, much is being done to decrease the act of spitting. After the SARS outbreak in 2003, China, Hong Kong, and Taiwan launched campaigns to discourage public spitting by issuing fines to public spitters. The desire to reduce this practice on public streets has resulted in strict government fines of up to $5,000 in Singapore.

PSYCHOLOGICAL ASPECTS

Darwin's theory

In nature, it is widely observed in various animals that a mother will inoculate her offspring within the first few hours of birth, to cover her offspring with her own saliva. This ensures the passing of vital bacteria and antibodies that will assist in the offspring's digestive and immune functions; without which, may lead to a loss of certain immune functions. Saliva may play an additional role during infancy by having a large influence on the development of an individual's future social behaviors.[11]

Perception

In any culture, a kiss is seen as a heavenly gentle gesture, shared during the most intimate of settings. People are generally willing to undergo the act with a loved one, yet are more reserved about the thought of kissing a stranger. Pet owners may allow their pets to lick them, yet the affection of other pets may be rejected. A certain amount of trust or an intimate bond between two entities is required to get over the idea of sharing saliva with another being.

A toothbrush, a spoon, and even a straw are all objects that are taboo to share, simply due to the fact that contact has been made with someone else's saliva. The psychological disconnection between saliva inside the mouth and saliva exposed to the outer environment may be due to the way our mind sees a difference between saliva that has passed beyond the mouth and saliva that remains within the confines of our bodies. Dr Gordon Allport, a social psychologist from Harvard, hypothesizes that saliva becomes nonself and alien to the mind the moment it exits the mouth. This modification in perception may be the leading factor in why people may have difficulties adjusting to the fact that saliva has true and viable diagnostic information about the internal body from which it came.[12]

In a study conducted on a broad range of patients at the Mayo Clinic in Rochester, Minnesota, perceptions of outpatients presenting for medical or dental care indicated that saliva was perceived as better than blood and urine in the categories of comfort and convenience of collection in a doctor's office and ease of home collection (Fig. 9.2). In addition, more subjects were interested in donating saliva for a research or medical test than blood or urine (Fig. 9.3). Men, a group who do not always seek diagnostic care to the same degree as women, and patients who had donated saliva before held particularly favorable views. These data are important as they confirm the often-expressed but hitherto

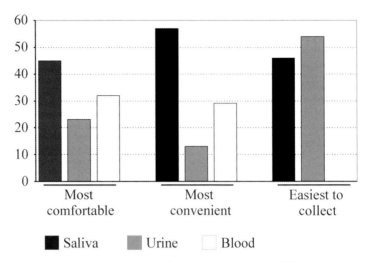

Figure 9.2 Percentage of outpatients selecting saliva, urine, and blood as most comfortable to give in doctor's office, most convenient to give in doctor's office, and easiest to collect at home. (Adapted from reference 13.)

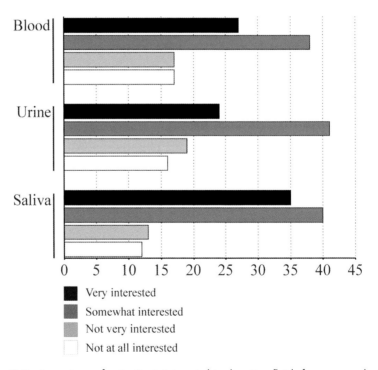

Figure 9.3 Percentage of outpatients interested in donating fluids for a research study if saliva, urine, or blood was to be collected. (Adapted from reference 13.)

unvalidated notion that saliva does indeed have advantages in terms of comfort (noninvasiveness) and convenience (no needle stick or urine cup filling).

SCIENCE AND THE FUTURE

The robust duties of saliva are commonly taken for granted and only truly appreciated when the precious medium is not found in abundance within the mouth, as in radiation or oral cancer patients. It is within these individuals where speech and severe eating difficulties routinely surface.[14] Along with sacrificing some of the comforts of life, functional pathologies within the oral cavity also quickly begin to emerge. The abundance of yeast growth topically on the tongue may also lead to halitosis and general bad oral health. Cavities are much more prevalent in patients with lowered salivary flow due to the loss of salivary bathing of the teeth, which normally confers a buffering role and antibacterial medium. Fittingly, Frank Oppenheim, chairman of the department of periodontology and oral biology at Boston University (author of Chapter 7), summarizes the importance of saliva's constituents with the statement, "If saliva were (merely) water, we would have little stumps of teeth or no teeth at all by age 20—we would have dissolved our teeth away."[15]

The functional value of saliva has long been thought to outweigh the diagnostic possibilities. However, research is fostering a transition from viewing saliva as a diagnostic outcast in comparison with blood or urine and promoting saliva as an abundant valuable resource. The advantages of using saliva testing as a diagnostic tool are due to its noninvasive nature, in addition to the quick and reliable results.[16] The current trend in the psychology of scientists is leaning toward saliva being seen in a positive light, with the potential for extracting data higher than ever. However, there may be cultural perceptions that form barriers against that which professionals already are beginning to discover, and those will slowly be overcome inevitably with time. The gap between saliva and other disease diagnostic biomedia (blood, urine, cerebral spinal fluid, tear, nipple aspirate, fecal matter) is rapidly closing. This is primarily due to the rapidity of the emerging sciences, sparked by the recent initiatives from the National Institute of Dental & Craniofacial Research (NIDCR). Scientific data to benchmark the diagnostic value of saliva against other biomedia will be necessary to assess the disease discriminatory value of saliva. It may well turn out that, similar to our recent finding that saliva is more accurate than blood for oral cancer detection,[17,18] saliva diagnostics may outperform other biomedia for other disease diagnostics as well.

In summary, it is clear that saliva has historically had a Dr Jekyll/Mr Hyde personality. However, when one closely and carefully examines the undesirable associations of saliva, one will conclude that the associations are largely mythical in origin and/or unscientific. The positive values of saliva, on the other hand, are scientifically based and are continuing to emerge. If the scientific values and diagnostic utilities of saliva is as good as or better than other bodily biomedia, it will be clear that its ease of obtainment, total noninvasiveness, ease, and pleasantness of use compared to other biomedia will eventually place saliva at the forefront of diagnostic biomedia choices. The day when saliva will be considered a diagnostically diverse and charismatic fluid should not be far away.

REFERENCES

1. Linsten J. *Robert Koch—Biography. Nobel Lectures.* Amsterdam: Elsevier; 1967.
2. Ridgely B. *Gold of the Aqllakuna: The Story of Chicha.* BarleyCorn; 1994.
3. Cerulli E. *New Notes on Islam in Somalia.* Rome: Ministero degli Affari Eseri, Instituto Poligrafico dello Stato P.V.; 1964.
4. Puccioni N. *Anthropology and Ethnography of the Peoples of Somalia.* Bologna: Nicola Zanichelli; 1936.
5. Anderson R. *Some Tribal Customs in Their Relation to Medicine and Morals of the Nyam-Nyam and Gour People Inhabiting the Eastern Bahr-El-Ghazal.* London: Bailiere, Tindall and Cox; 1911.
6. Merker M. *The Masai: Ethnographic Monograph of an East African Semite People.* Berlin: Dietrich Reimer; 1910.
7. Gamble DP. *A Wolof Naming Ceremony: Human Interaction and Its Aesthetic Significance.* London: International African Institute; 1957.
8. Wojcicki JM. Traditional behavioural practices, the exchange of saliva and HHV-8 transmission in sub-Saharan African populations. Br J Cancer 2003;89:2016–17.
9. Rattray R. *Ashanti.* Oxford: Clarendon Press; 1923.
10. Vinoy S, Mascai-Taylor C. The relationship between Areca nut usage and heart rate in lactating Bangladeshis. Ann Hum Biol 2002;29:488–94.
11. Block ML, Volpe LC. Saliva as a chemical cue in the development of social behavior. Science 1981;211:1062–4.
12. Allport G. The open system in personality theory. J Abnorm Soc Psychol 1960;61:301–10.
13. Koka S, Beebe TJ, Merry SP, et al. The preferences of adult outpatients in medical or dental care settings for giving saliva, urine or blood for clinical testing. J Am Dent Assoc 2008; 139(6):735–40.
14. Logemann JA, Pauloski BR. Xerostomia: 12-month changes in saliva production and its relationship to perception and performance of swallow function, oral intake, and diet after chemoradiation. Head Neck 2003;25:432–7.
15. Mestel R. *The Wonders of Saliva.* The Oral Cancer Foundation; 2005.
16. Dreifus C. *A Bloodless Revolution: Spit Will Tell What Ails You.* New York Times; 2005.
17. Li Y, Elashoff D, Oh M, et al. Serum circulating human mRNA profiling and its utility for oral cancer detection. J Clin Oncol 2006;24(11):1754–60.
18. Li Y, St John MA, Zhou X, et al. Salivary transcriptome diagnostics for oral cancer detection. Clin Cancer Res 2004;10(24):8442–50.

Saliva-based diagnostic technologies: Highlights of the NIDCR's program

Eleni Kousvelari, John T. McDevitt, Daniel Malamud, David T. Wong, and David R. Walt

INTRODUCTION

In medicine, many different types of body fluids have been used for analysis to help in monitoring or diagnosing a particular condition or treatment regimen. Only a few analytes are usually measured; however, a univariate measurement is highly unlikely to provide adequate results. With a multianalyte measurement system, analytes specific for a disease, as well as those that are not directly related to a disease mechanism but which yield useful data and provide disease signatures, can be measured. The ability to screen for multiple biomarkers simultaneously may provide a more valid clinical diagnosis and may be more useful for recognizing molecular patterns predictive for disease development. Both oral and nonoral diseases have a multifactorial etiology. For the latter class of diseases, saliva offers a sample matrix that could enable the rapid assessment and monitoring of health and disease states, exposure to environmental and occupational toxins, drugs of abuse, emerging and re-emerging diseases such as HIV/AIDS, and identification of the etiology of both oral and nonoral diseases that have multiple causative agents.[1–5] Saliva-based diagnostics may prove to be more accessible, accurate, less expensive, and present less risk than current methodologies. This chapter focuses on the NIDCR's project on the development of saliva-based diagnostic technologies.

EFFORT

The barriers to widespread implementation of saliva diagnostics derive from technological problems in achieving sensitivity, miniaturization, high throughput, automation, portability, low cost, high functionality, and speed to enable high-content chemical and biochemical analyses. Today, the potential of microsensor and microfluidic technologies[6–8] to facilitate the decentralization of medical testing is becoming accepted as one element in the next evolutionary stage of healthcare. Microfluidic systems can be designed to obtain and process measurements from small volumes of complex fluids, such as saliva, with efficiency and speed, and without the need for an expert operator. This unique set of capabilities is precisely what is needed to create portable point-of-care

111

medical diagnostic systems. These systems allow miniaturization, integration, and multiplexing of complex functions, which could move diagnostic tools out of the laboratory and closer to the patient. There is now renewed hope for achieving this goal.

The National Institute of Dental and Craniofacial Research (NIDCR) has initiated a concerted research effort in the area of saliva diagnostics, and progress is being made toward technologically viable systems moving toward commercial reality. The NIDCR, realizing the potential of new technologies and advanced instrumentation, held a workshop on "Development of New Technologies for Saliva and Other Oral Fluid-Based Diagnostics" in September 1999. The purpose of the workshop was to capitalize on recent developments in the diagnostics field and explore their potential to be employed for salivary diagnostics. More than 100 individuals from academia, government, and industry with expertise in salivary and oral biology, chemistry, instrumentation, engineering, and clinical sciences were brought together to exchange ideas. At the workshop, clinicians and oral biologists learned about new diagnostic technologies and engineers learned about the chemistry and biology of saliva. The charge to the participants was to develop a set of recommendations to help the NIDCR create a research program in the area of oral-based diagnostics.

In fiscal year 2002, NIDCR funded a series of grants to develop strategies to simultaneously measure and analyze multiple substances in saliva with great speed. Project teams, comprising multiple academic institutions as well as industry partners, are using a variety of technologies to develop diagnostic tests for a multitude of medical conditions. Seven projects were funded in 2002 employing different approaches for detecting analytes in saliva.

One system involves a parallel diffusion immunoassay in a polymeric laminated disposable format using an inexpensive and simple surface plasmon resonance optical system capable of imaging several surface-linked immunoassays in parallel.[9] The aim of this salivary diagnostic system is to measure small-molecule analytes such as hormones and drugs in whole saliva.

A second microfluidics project is aimed at developing an integrated platform that includes electrochemical sensors for oral cancer detection. Changes in electrical current depend on the concentration of target analytes and are measured amperometrically.

A third microfluidics platform, for detection of either a cytokine profile or oral bacteria, is based on a microchip electrophoretic immunoassay (μCEI) that relies on photolithographically fabricated molecular sieving gels to enrich the sample and a laser-induced fluorescence detector system.[10]

A fourth integrated microfluidic platform for the detection of multiple pathogens is based on an on-chip polymerase chain reaction/reverse transcriptase-polymerase chain reaction (PCR/RT-PCR) system. Detection of different nucleic acids will be accomplished using up-converting phosphors–inorganic luminescent materials that absorb infrared energy and subsequently emit it as visible light.

In addition to these microfluidics projects, two bead-based sensor arrays were supported under NIDCR funding. In these approaches, multiplexed arrays containing beads with different specificities will be used to perform salivary diagnostics. One array platform involves the fabrication of a prototype multibead channel interconnected chip. A macroporous sensing bead ensemble is inserted into a well etched Si-chip that contains flow through fluidic elements that serve to increase the rate of analyte binding. This bead-based microchip platform with fluorescence and optical detection capabilities has been adapted for a broad range of analyte classes including pH, electrolytes, metal cations, sugars, biological cofactors, toxins, proteins, antibodies, and oligonucleotides.[11–15] Initial focus for the saliva testing has been placed on cardiac risk assessment.

The second bead array is based on optical fibers.[16,17] The optical microfiber arrays contain different types of microsphere sensors placed into wells etched into the end of each fiber in an optical fiber bundle (containing up to ~50,000 wells). Both specific and cross-reactive sensing chemistries will be employed to obtain a global response pattern from the sensors. Detection of different analytes will be achieved by an optical imaging system. Initial work in this area has focused on renal and asthmatic patients.

Finally, the seventh project focuses on the validation of a first-generation oral chip for the identification and quantification of oral microbes. This platform comprises a high-throughput DNA microarray for rapid, reliable, and culture-independent detection of microbial biomarkers in oral fluids.

In phase II of the program (started in 2006), four projects were selected out of the seven originally funded projects. These four had demonstrated feasibility toward an integrated functional prototype of a handheld diagnostic system that could attract commercial interest. The currently supported projects include the two bead arrays: (Figs 10.1a and 10.1b)[11–17] the RT-PCR on-a-chip microfluidic system (Fig. 10.1c)[18] and the electrochemical sensing system (Fig. 10.1d).[19–21] These systems allow miniaturization, integration, and multiplexing of complex functions, enabling such systems to move closer to the patient.

At this stage of the research, the grantees are mainly focusing on refining the microfluidic platforms, examining different schemes for electrical or optical sensing, investigating innovative surface chemistries, and integrating the different components of the system into a miniaturized device. For example, the bead-based assay under development at Tufts University (in partnership with investigators at Boston University) has been focused on developing a portable system for diagnosing the underlying cause of an asthma exacerbation. During the discovery phase, saliva from asthmatics and controls was analyzed for a multitude of diagnostic markers including cytokines and chemokines, viral nucleic acids, and bacterial nucleic acids. The researchers screened a total of 17 cytokines and chemokines in saliva using commercially available enzyme-linked immunosorbent assays (ELISAs). These preliminary studies were performed to identify which analytes would be included for analysis on the portable system. The decision to select an analyte for future study was based on the analyte meeting one or more of the following criteria: (1) high salivary abundance, (2) biological relevance, (3) screening results distinguishing asthmatics from controls, and (4) screening results showing variability among asthmatics. Twelve analytes were determined to show promise as biomarkers and bead-based assays for these cytokines are being implemented in an optical fiber bead array format. Present efforts are focused on expanding the cytokine bead array to detect a larger number of proteins, which will significantly increase the

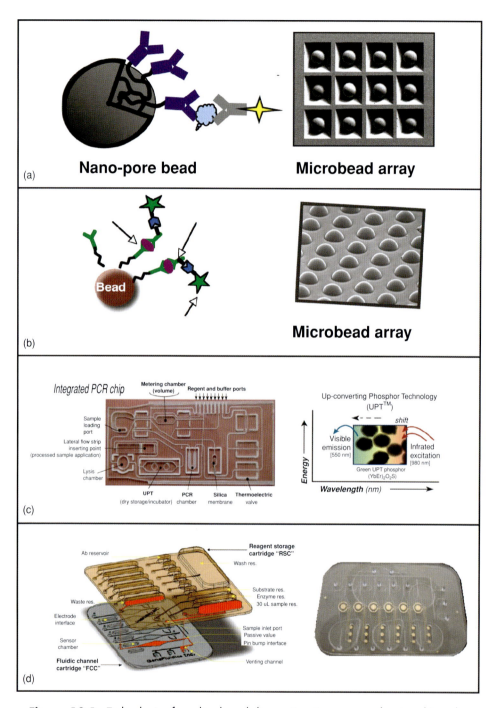

Figure 10.1 Technologies for saliva-based diagnostics: Four approaches to achieve the goal. (a) Microsphere-based nano-bio chip. (b) Microsphere-based optical fiber arrays. (c) On-chip PCR system. (d) Electrochemical sensing (left) reagent flow diagram between reagent storage cartridge (RSC) and fluidic channel cartridge (FCC), (right) disposable OFNASET-Cartridge for six multiplexed assays.

throughput of these initial screening studies. The multiplexed cytokine array will be used to create salivary cytokine/chemokine profiles for the asthmatic saliva samples that have been collected.

Viral infection has been implicated as one of the major causes of asthma exacerbation. The ability to identify a contracted pathogen at an early stage of infection would be highly beneficial to treatment. The first step in the development of salivary diagnostics for virus-induced asthma exacerbation is the screening of saliva samples for viruses and determining correlations between the presence of a particular virus and the disease state of asthma patients. Initial screening of asthmatic saliva from dozens of patients for viral RNA and DNA has identified a number of candidate viruses that correlate with an asthma exacerbation. In addition, bacterial nucleic acids have been screened with a number of organisms correlating with asthma exacerbation.

A microfluidic lab-on-a-chip device is being designed and developed that mates with these bead-based microarrays to detect cytokines/chemokines and nucleic acids in oral fluids. The ultimate objective is to demonstrate a fully self-contained, automated lab-on-a-chip device that attains the performance and functionality of a conventional microarray in a low-cost, easy-to-use microfluidic implementation. All sample preparation steps will be performed directly on the microfluidic device. A portable optical reader that will read the fluorescent signal from the bead arrays is being designed and developed. This portable reader will mate with the microfluidic device in the final prototype.

The second project (a consortium among four Universities—University of Texas at Austin, University of Kentucky, University of Louisville, University of Texas Health Science Center at San Antonio, and a company, LabNow) is based on a bead array pioneered at University of Texas at Austin. It is directed toward the development of a fully functional integrated platform that is capable of testing for both cellular and soluble analytes. In this system all aspects of the sample collection, sample processing, solid-state reagent dissolution, fluid delivery, waste storage, and detection components have been incorporated into a single disposable cartridge that interfaces with a portable analyzer unit.

During the initial phase of this program, the researchers examined three methods of oral fluid collection—stimulated whole saliva, unstimulated whole saliva, and OraSure collection device—with respect to their capacity to support the recovery of various analytes across multiple disease conditions. Over 30 biomarkers were explored in the areas of heart disease, sexually transmitted diseases, and cancer. These analyte recovery studies have provided information relative to the physiological range of these analytes in saliva, many of which had never been reported in saliva diagnostics previously. Further, these studies serve to provide firm expectations for the best modes of sample introduction into the final biochip elements, as well as help to define the best initial biomarker targets.

Using this information, the new microchip bead-array platform and the associated universal analyzer system, the investigators are now focusing on the development of saliva-based cardiac diagnostic tests. For the first time, CRP concentration levels have been measured in control and cardiac disease patient groups. A case-control comparison of CRP level is shown in Figure 10.2a. The receiver operating characteristic (ROC) curve analysis is used to explore the

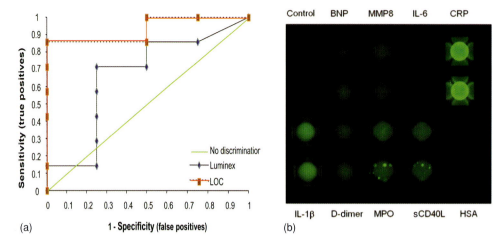

Figure 10.2 (a) Two receiver operating characteristic (ROC) curves are plotted showing the capacity of saliva-based CRP measurements to classify correctly control and cardiac heart disease patients. The red curve represents data obtained with the bead-based lab-on-a-chip system, while the blue curve represents data obtained with commercial Luminex instrument. Note that best possible prediction method would yield a point in the upper left corner or coordinate (0.1) of the ROC space, representing 100% sensitivity (all true positives are found) and 100% specificity (no false positives are found). A completely random guess would give a point along a diagonal line (the so-called line of no discrimination) from the left bottom to the top right corners. The data show that the bead array microchip provides superior clinical classification capabilities relative to that obtained with the commercially available Luminex system. (b) The image is showing the fluorescence signatures of an internal control and nine protein markers associated with cardiovascular disease present in saliva (sCD40L, soluble CD40 ligand; BNP, b-type natriuretic peptide; D-dimer, thrombosis marker; IL-1β, interleukin-1β; MPO, myeloperoxidase; CRP, C-reactive protein; MMP-8, matrix metalloproteases; and IL-6, interleukin-6).

sensitivity and selectivity of tests performed with the bead microchip platform as well as with the commercially available Luminex instrument. This bead microchip system yields a large ROC curve area along with a sensitivity value of 86% and specificity value of 100%, whereas the Luminex system elicits values of only 71 and 75%, respectively, for the case-control group classification. The increased ROC curve area indicates higher sensitivity, higher selectivity, and overall better classification accuracy for the bead microchip relative to the established methodology. These data strongly indicate the excellent analytical performance of the bead microchip system.

In addition to the single analyte studies, the bead-based microchip platform has been adapted for multiplexed protein detection for cardiac risk. Shown in Figure 10.2b are data acquired from nine cardiovascular disease-associated markers that have strong utility in the diagnosis of patients with such disease. Cardiac heart disease is the number one health problem in the United States with recurrent heart attacks being responsible for a large proportion of the deaths in this area. An accurate, sensitive, and reliable multianalyte diagnostic system once developed can help monitor recurrent heart attack victims.

The design of the third project (a consortium among four universities—New York University, University of Pennsylvania, Lehigh University, and Leiden University Medical Center) involves collecting and delivering an oral sample to a microfluidic cassette to be used for identifying multiple bacterial and viral pathogens. The cassette consists of a series of conduits that process the oral sample and then detect multiple antigens, nucleic acids, and antibodies. For proof of principle, the group has focused on HIV, *Bacillus cereus*, and *Streptococcus pyogenes*.[22] Oral fluid (~300 µL) is collected and directly inserted into the cassette where on-chip reagents are used to process the sample, which is then flowed onto a nitrocellulose strip. Immobilized antigens on the strip bind sample antibodies; immobilized antibodies capture specific pathogen-derived antigens; and a miniature PCR device amplifies RNA and/or DNA released from the viruses and bacteria. The PCR-produced amplicons are then flowed onto the nitrocellulose and are captured at specific sites on the nitrocellulose strip. These analytes are detected using a novel up-converting phosphor reporter (UPT). Analytes bind to the functionalized UPT and are detected by visible light emitted when the strips are interrogated with a red laser. The goal is to have a portable handheld point-of-care device capable of providing diagnostic results in less than 1 h. Progress to date has led to an oral collection device that is directly inserted into the microfluidic chip. Pouches on the chip store buffers and reagents and ultimately will be actuated by miniaturized solenoids for fully automated operation. All the individual steps in the analysis pathway have been developed and optimized using bench-top methods that are then modified, as necessary, for on-chip assays. It has been demonstrated that oral samples containing intact HIV and bacteria can be loaded into the system, lysed, the nucleic acids isolated and then amplified and both viral and bacterial amplicons detected simultaneously. This modular platform can be easily adapted for a variety of uses, for example, antibody or antigen detection only, nucleic acid only, or all analytes detected simultaneously. Additionally, the chips can be designed with specific capture zones for different applications, for example, the detection of sexually transmitted diseases, respiratory diseases, or agents of bioterrorism.

The fourth project is a consortium team at UCLA in partnership with Gene-Fluidics Inc. and Beckton Dickinson Diagnostics to develop the Oral Fluid NanoSensor Test (OFNASET). The two main pieces of the OFNASET are a reagent storage cartridge (RSC), which would house all the reagent and sample reservoirs, and a fluidic channel cartridge (FCC), which houses all the fluidic channels, reaction chambers, and valve structures. The two pieces are shown in (Fig. 10.1d). The design of the OFNASET is based on GeneFluidics' electrochemical technology platform and is intended for the quantitative, multiplex detection of saliva biomarkers by immunoassay and direct nucleic acid assay.

Once all individual components are fully integrated, the OFNASET instrument will have four primary modules including signal detection, fluidic handling, interfacing, and wireless connectivity. The signal detection module will include a potentiostat board to control and retrieve signal from the redox reaction of interest, a data acquisition board to convert the signal into digital data for exporting, and a smart phone (HP iPAQ) to control instrument operation

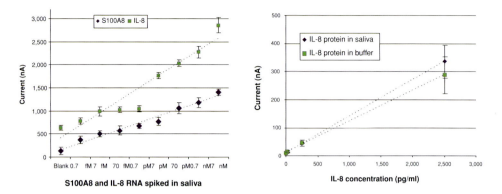

Figure 10.3 Electrochemical detection of (a) spiked saliva with in vitro transcribed (IVT) RNA for S100A8 (blue diamonds) and IL-8 (green squares); (b) immunoassay of IL-8 in buffer system (green squares) and in spiked saliva system (blue diamonds). Limit of detection (LOD) of IL-8 immunoassay in buffer system is 13 pg/mL. LOD of IL-8 spiked into saliva detection is 27 pg/mL.

(instead of a computer). The cartridge control module will include a fluidic control circuit board to provide sequential control signals to the pneumatic components, a manifold to interface the cartridge and the pneumatic components, a pneumatic source to supply positive and negative pressure for all valve mechanisms in the manifold. The interface module will include a portable smart phone, an imbedded bar code for reader to identify the cartridge type, and a USB (universal serial bus) 2.0 interface to enable data transfer. The intended clinical application of the OFNASET will be for the saliva-based molecular screening for oral cancer detection. This research group has identified five salivary proteins and seven salivary RNAs that are highly discriminatory for oral cancer.[23] The ROC values of the salivary oral cancer protein and RNA biomarkers are 0.93 and 0.95, respectively.[23] Studies are ongoing to determine if the combination of salivary proteomic and transcriptomic biomarkers will further elevate the discriminatory values for oral cancer detection. They have validated a proprietary electrochemical molecular analysis platform with spiked saliva samples for both IL8 RNA and protein detection as illustrated in Figure 10.3. For RNA detection in saliva, a specific hairpin probe was developed. Applying the hairpin probe, signals from RNA biomarkers are specifically amplified, while the nonspecific interferents generate a low signal. This probe greatly improves the signal-to-noise ratio. The current sensitivity is around 1–10 fM of RNA spiked into saliva with only 4 μL of sample (Fig. 10.3a). For protein detection, the saliva samples are directly delivered to the electrochemical sensor's surface precoated with capture antibody. After adding the reporter antibody, changes in current caused by the reaction are recorded. An effective protocol has been developed to address the signal-to-noise level of the immunosensor, which results from the strong interaction between the metal surface and the protein. With this optimized protocol, the device was able to detect specific IL8 levels in spiked saliva (Fig. 10.3b, blue diamonds). The signal level of IL8 in spiked saliva were similar to the signal detected in buffer system containing known levels of IL8. Limit of detection (LOD) of IL-8 in buffer (Fig. 10.3b, green squares) is 13 pg/mL, and the LOD of IL8 in spiked saliva is 27 pg/mL (Fig. 10.3b, blue squares). These data provide the support for salivary analyte detection without any preamplification process.

CHALLENGES

The NIDCR's program is groundbreaking in its attempt to bring integrated miniature systems to the clinic for salivary diagnostics. Salivary diagnostic tests have the potential to change medicine's reliance on blood sampling. Saliva offers the potential for painless and convenient sample collection. Advances in diagnostic technology promise inexpensive platforms for performing real-time analysis of a large number of proteins, nucleic acids, small molecules, and drugs in oral fluids. For example, the development of this technology would permit the Centers for Disease Control and Prevention and state health departments to perform health surveillance more effectively and monitor individuals' risk of exposure to harmful infectious or environmental agents. Ultimately, such surveillance could be carried out in the privacy of one's home.

In order for these new technologies to become a practical reality, strong partnerships with industry early in the development stage are of paramount importance. Quality control in such areas as manufacturing, packaging and storage, ease of use, reproducibility, and interpretation of results must be considered in the early design phases. Additionally, new techniques must be validated against existing standard procedures and approved for safety and efficacy by regulators. Financial considerations such as manufacturing and distribution costs, general availability, and price will determine their ultimate utility, especially in areas where screenings need to be performed both on a large scale and frequently (i.e., population monitoring). Clearly, implementation issues will have an impact on the effective deployment of these potentially revolutionary devices.

As diagnostic technology moves toward the home, how much access to medical data should individuals have without systems in place for interpreting the data into meaningful health information? In this regard, a daunting research task is the development of efficient computational methods as well as data and communications software and systems that are user-friendly, long-lasting, reliable, survivable, and programmable.

The translation and adoption of technological advances into saliva-based diagnostic platforms present challenges for the dental and medical communities, as well as the public at large. As new diagnostic technologies make it to the patient's bedside and home, they may challenge our current healthcare paradigms. Rapid, high-throughput, high-capacity, and inexpensive tools will accelerate the pace of discovery, and, ultimately, of the development of therapeutics. Early detection of oral and other diseases and conditions may force us to reconsider the professional boundaries that exist today among healthcare providers. For example, what will be the level of acceptance within the medical and dental communities for using saliva-based tests for monitoring disease and disease progression? These technologies have the potential to be used not only in the physician's office, but virtually in any setting—hospital, home, workplace, and battlefield. Shared decision-making among patients, health-care professionals, and society will be the standard of care in the twenty-first century.

The twenty-first century finds science and engineering facing increasingly complex ethical and social issues. Modern point-of-care diagnostic technologies are not an exception. In order to maximize the societal benefits of such technologies, ethical, legal, privacy, and cultural implications, as well as quality of life and national security issues, must be addressed. It is critical to address all these issues in order to maximize the societal benefits of these point-of-care diagnostic technologies.

REFERENCES

1. Sreebny LM. Saliva in health and disease: an appraisal and update. Int Dent J 2000;50(3):140–61.
2. Cope G, Nayyar P, Holder R, Brock G, Chapple I. Near-patient test for nicotine and its metabolites in saliva to assess smoking habit. Anal Clin Biochem 2000;37(5):666–73.
3. Liu H, Delgado MR. Therapeutic drug concentration monitoring using saliva samples—focus on anticonvulsants. Clin Pharmicokinet 1999;36(6):453–70.
4. Hodinka RL, Nagashunmugam T, Malamud D. Detection of human immunodeficiency virus antibodies in oral fluids. Clin Diagn Lab Immun 1998;5(4):419–26.
5. Miller SM. Saliva testing—a nontraditional diagnostic tool. Clin Lab Sci 1994;7(1):39–44.
6. Whitesides GM. The origins and the future of microfluidics. Nature 2006;442:368–73.
7. Vilkner T, Janasek D, Manz A. Micro total analysis systems. Recent developments. Anal Chem 2004;76:3373–86.
8. Liu RH, Yang J, Lenigk R, Bonanno J, Grodzinski P. Self-contained, fully integrated biochip for sample preparation, polymerase chain reaction amplification, and DNA microarray detection. Anal Chem 2004;76:1824–31.
9. Yager P, Edwards T, Fu E, et al. Microfluidic diagnostic technologies for global public health. Nature 2006;442:412–18.
10. Herr AE, Hatch AV, Throckmorton DJ, et al. Microfluidic immunoassays as rapid saliva-based clinical diagnostics. Proc Natl Acad Sci 2007;104:5268–73.
11. Christodoulides N, Tran M, Floriano PN, et al. A microchip-based multianalyte assay system for the assessment of cardiac risk. Anal Chem 2002;74(13):3030–36.
12. Christodoulides N, Mohanty S, Miller CS, et al. Application of microchip assay system for the measurement of C-reactive protein in human saliva. Lab Chip 2005;5(3):261–9.
13. Goodey A, Lavigne JJ, Savoy SM, et al. Development of multianalyte sensor arrays composed of chemically derivatized polymeric microspheres

localized in micromachined cavities. J Am Chem Soc 2001;123(11):2559–70.

14. Ali MF, Kirby R, Goodey AP, et al. DNA hybridization and discrimination of single-nucleotide mismatches using chip-based microbead arrays. Anal Chem 2003;75(18):4732–9.

15. Christodoulides N, Floriano PN, Acosta SA, et al. Towards the development of a lab on a chip dual function white blood cell and C-reactive protein analysis method for the assessment of inflammation and cardiac risk. Clin Chem 2005;51(12):2391–5.

16. Walt DR, Epstein J. Fluorescence-based fibre optic arrays: a universal platform for sensing. Chem Soc Rev 2003;32:203–14.

17. Song L, Walt DR. Fiber-optic microsphere-based arrays for multiplexed biological warfare agent detection. Anal Chem 2006;78(4):1023–33.

18. Wang J, Chen Z, Corstjens PLAM, Mauk GM, Bau HH. A disposable microfluidic cassette for DNA amplification and detection. Lab Chip 2006;6:46–53.

19. Huang TJ, Liu M, Knight LD, Grody WW, Miller JF, Ho CM. An electrochemical detection scheme for identification of single nucleotide polymorphisms using hairpin-forming probes. Nucleic Acids Res 2002;30:e55.

20. Gau JJ, Lan EH, Dunn B, Ho CM, Woo JC. A MEMS based amperometric detector for *E. coli* bacteria using self-assembled monolayers. Biosens Bioelectron 2001;16:745–55.

21. Wang TH, Peng YH, Zhang CY, Wong PK, Ho CM. Single-molecule tracing on a fluidic microchip for quantitative detection of low-abundance nucleic acids. J Am Chem Soc 2005;127(15):5354–9.

22. Abrams WR, Barber CA, McCann K, et al. Development of a microfluidic device for detection of pathogens in oral samples using up-converting phosphor technology (UPT). Ann NY Acad Sci 2007;1098:375–88.

23. Li Y, John MA, Zhou X, et al. Salivary transcriptome diagnostics for oral cancer detection. Clin Cancer Res 2004;10(24):8442–50.

Human salivary proteomics

Shen Hu, Markus Hardt, Susan J. Fisher, David T. Wong,
John R. Yates, James E. Melvin, and Joseph A. Loo

INTRODUCTION

The proteome is the protein complement to the genome, and proteomics offers the means for analyzing the portion of the genome that is expressed. The proteomes of biofluids are especially valuable due to their potential clinical importance as sources of disease biomarkers. In this context, saliva contains an array of peptides and proteins that play a wide variety of roles, including maintenance of the integrity of the oral cavity and teeth, lubrication of tissues, inhibition of microbial growth, aiding taste, and facilitating food digestion.[1]

A global analysis of the human salivary proteome can, in principle, provide a deeper understanding of oral biology and disease pathology. Because of its ready accessibility, saliva is also an attractive medium for noninvasive diagnosis and/or prognosis of human diseases.[2] Proteomic analysis of saliva over the course of disease progression could reveal valuable biomarkers for early detection and monitoring of disease status.

PROTEIN CHARACTERIZATION TECHNOLOGIES FOR DECIPHERING THE PROTEOME

A proteomics-based approach has been practiced for many years to monitor changes in protein expression. The primary readout of protein expression was based on analysis of proteins separated by one- and two-dimensional polyacrylamide gel electrophoresis (PAGE). However, the development of novel mass spectrometry (MS) methods made the identification of PAGE-separated proteins much more amenable and contributed greatly to expanding the range of proteomic-type applications.

Characterization of protein primary structure by MS was advanced by ionization methods such as electrospray ionization (ESI) and matrix-assisted laser desorption ionization (MALDI). Coupling ESI and MALDI with mass analyzers, such as quadrupole/linear ion trap, time-of-flight (TOF), quadrupole TOF (QTOF), Fourier transform ion cyclotron resonance (FT-ICR), and the OrbiTrap improved sensitivity, resolution, accuracy, and speed for protein sequence

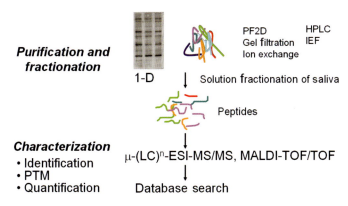

Figure 1.1 General strategy for bottom-up proteome characterization.

elucidation. The sensitivity of MS and MS/MS allows for the identification of proteins below the one picomole (10^{-12} mol) level and in many cases in the low femtomole (fmol, 10^{-15} mol) regime.

Bottom-up proteomics

"Bottom-up" and "top-down" proteomics are two fundamental strategies for MS-based proteome analysis. In the more commonly employed bottom-up approach, a complex protein sample is subjected to proteolytic cleavage (most often with trypsin and/or endoproteinase Lys-C), and the resulting peptides are sequenced/identified by tandem MS coupled with interrogation of a proteomic or genomic sequence database (Fig. 11.1). This strategy could be coupled with 1D- and 2D-PAGE through in-gel digestion of excised protein bands/spots. The 2D-PAGE approach is commonly used because it can provide direct information on protein abundance (through stain intensity), posttranslational modifications (PTMs), and isoforms.[3]

A gel-free embodiment of a "shotgun" proteomics philosophy includes multidimensional protein identification technology (MudPIT).[4] Peptide mixtures can be separated by reversed phase (RP) LC, or a first dimension of strong cation exchange chromatography (SCX) followed by a second dimension of RP-LC. The major advantage of this approach is that it circumvents the challenges inherent in protein separation and recovery by transforming the problem into one of more tractable peptide analysis.

Prefractionation of intact proteins and/or proteolytically derived peptides prior to LC-MS/MS measurements can help to achieve a more comprehensive analysis of complex samples such as body fluids (Fig. 11.2). This "divide and conquer" approach can be performed using a variety of separation techniques, including ion exchange chromatography, gel filtration chromatography, free flow electrophoresis (FFE),[5] gel IEF and liquid-phase IEF, capillary isoelectric focusing (CIEF),[6] and chromatofocusing coupled with RP-LC. Multiplexing of these techniques, especially of those based on orthogonal separation mechanisms can further enhance the resolving power of the fractionation. A common observation is that each of the different proteomics platforms identifies a

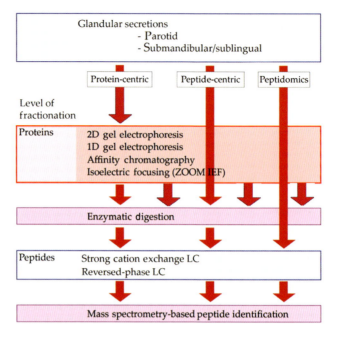

Figure 1.2 Proteomic workflows utilized in the salivary proteome cataloguing project. Fractionation methods used depend on whether a protein-centric (separation of intact proteins), peptide-centric (separation of proteolyzed proteins), or peptidomic (analysis of endogenous peptides) strategy is targeted.

different set of unique proteins. Therefore, different proteomics platforms may be used in parallel to further enhance the coverage of, for example, the saliva proteome.[7]

Top-down proteomics

Top-down proteomics refers to MS measurement of intact protein molecular weight and direct fragmentation of gas-phase proteins for their characterization.[8] This is most often accomplished with high-resolution FT-ICR, but other analyzers such as OrbiTrap and lower-resolution QTOF and linear ion trap instruments also have capabilities for top-down measurements. The ability of top-down MS to dissect different molecular forms of proteins will have a significant impact on characterization of PTMs. Recent developments of electron capture dissociation (ECD) and electron transfer dissociation (ETD) methods show promise in top-down MS and PTM characterization.[9]

Protein modifications

Posttranslational modifications of salivary proteins are an integral part of their structure and, in many cases, critical functional determinants. In this context, disease-associated alterations in protein structure and PTMs are potential targets for saliva-based diagnostics and new drug development. As in plasma/serum, many proteins in saliva are glycosylated. Analysis of glycoproteins may have clinical significance as changes in the extent of glycosylation could be linked to cancer and other disease states. Lectin affinity chromatography is commonly used for enrichment of glycoproteins prior to MS analysis.[10] Another approach is to capture glycoproteins using hydrazide chemistries and resins. Following the enzymatic cleavage of N-linked glycopeptides with N-glycosidase F and trypsin digestion, glycoproteins can be identified by LC-MS/MS analysis of the formerly N-linked glycopeptides.[11] Several classes of salivary proteins are phosphorylated, such as proline-rich proteins and statherin. Analysis and identification of phosphorylation sites is challenging because phosphorylation can be heterogeneous and be present in low abundance. Some approaches for enriching phosphopeptides/proteins prior to LC-MS/MS include immobilized metal ion affinity chromatography,[12] titanium dioxide-based capture resins,[13] and phosphospecific antibody-coupled resins.

CURRENT STATUS OF SALIVARY PROTEOME ANALYSIS

Whole saliva (WS) has been the focus for many of the early proteomic studies.[6,14–19] For example, the UCLA group used a combination of 2D-PAGE analysis and size-based fractionation schemes coupled with LC-QTOF-MS/MS to identify over 300 distinct proteins from WS.[14] Other varieties of prefractionation methods of intact proteins prior to trypsin digestion and subsequent LC-QTOF-MS/MS identified approximately 1,000 proteins from WS. Other research groups have used similar strategies to fractionate proteolytic peptides from whole saliva proteins based on the coupling of capillary isoelectric focusing or free flow electrophoresis with RP-LC-MS/MS to decipher the WS proteome[5,6]; again, approximately 1,000 proteins have been cataloged. In addition, 84 N-glycopeptides representing 45 unique N-glycoproteins have been identified in WS.[20]

As the next step, proteomic-type analyses of individual glandular secretions are important for understanding the biology of the parotid and submandibular/sublingual (SM/SL) glands and to provide clarity about the source of individual proteins. To this end, a consortium (Scripps Research Institute and University of Rochester; University of California, San Francisco; University of California, Los Angeles; and University of Southern California) funded by the NIH, National Institute of Dental and Craniofacial Research Human Salivary Proteome Initiative cataloged the proteins in human parotid and SM/SL secretions. Using a wide variety of fractionation tools and mass spectrometry platforms, in total, nearly 12,000 distinct peptides were identified, which were matched to 1,100 nonredundant proteins. Of these, approximately 900 separate protein identifications were made in both parotid and SM/SL saliva of which 60% were common to both glandular secretions. With regard to cellular location, gene ontology analysis suggested that a high proportion of the proteins in ductal saliva normally resides in the extracellular region, whereas others localized to various cellular compartments including the plasma membrane, cytoplasm, organelles, or cytoskeleton. The majority of the identified proteins served in binding, structural, and enzymatic activities; many formed complexes; and they participated in metabolic and regulatory pathways (unpublished results).

PROSPECTS FOR UNCOVERING DISEASE PROTEIN BIOMARKERS IN SALIVA

Saliva contains many proteins that are originated from either the parotid or the SM/SL glands. As such, the components of saliva are in large part distinct from the constituents of plasma/serum and are possible indicators of diseases that localize to the oral cavity. For example, Sjögren's syndrome (SS), a chronic autoimmune disorder that is clinically characterized by a dry mouth and eyes, is also accompanied by salivary changes, such as increased levels of inflammatory proteins and decreased levels of acinar proteins as compared with non-SS individuals.[21]

Published data also suggest that saliva is an important source of analytes that can be measured for diagnostic and prognostic purposes. In oral squamous cell carcinoma (OSCC) patients, combined testing of salivary levels of Cyfra 21-1, TPA, and CA125 had a similar diagnostic value as measuring the same markers in patient sera.[22] Using subtractive proteomics and immunoassays, additional candidate salivary protein biomarkers for OSCC, including Mac-2 binding protein, calgranulin B, profilin, and CD59, have been identified (unpublished results).

Moreover, salivary constituents may show promise for monitoring systemic conditions. Testing of saliva for antibodies to human immunodeficiency virus (HIV) has been practiced, and the assay is equivalent to serum in its accuracy with the advantage of being safer and easier to use.[23] Early work suggests that salivary CA125[24] and epidermal growth factor[25] levels have diagnostic value in ovarian cancer and breast cancer, respectively.

CONCLUDING REMARKS

Current efforts to elucidate the proteome for both WS and ductal saliva have progressed rapidly with advances in mass spectrometry and protein separation tools. A central repository is being established (www.hspp.ucla.edu) to consolidate the acquired proteomic data and link the identified proteins to public annotated protein databases. The integration of the large datasets from different laboratories is ongoing, and a comparative analysis of the salivary proteome with other body fluid proteomes is planned. Nevertheless, the characterization of the salivary proteome is far from complete as salivary proteins are often present in polymorphic isoforms and as unique splice variants with deletions, truncations, and posttranslational modifications as additional sources of complexity.

An initial iteration of the salivary proteome will be an important resource for researchers who are interested in salivary gland and oral biology. This catalog will also have great value for the field of saliva-based diagnostics. A comprehensive list of salivary proteins will make possible the identification of significant changes in saliva protein composition that are associated with disease processes. These alterations are potential diagnostic and/or prognostic indicators that could be used in a clinical context for noninvasive detection and monitoring of human diseases. Although, a handful of salivary disease biomarkers have been identified, the availability of a comprehensive catalog of proteins that comprise this body fluid should fuel efforts to discover many more molecules that can be used for this purpose.

Acknowledgments

This work was supported by the National Institute of Dental and Craniofacial Research (U01 DE 016274 to UCSF, U01 DE016267 to TSRI-UR, U01 DE016275 to UCLA-USC, and R03-DE017144 to UCLA).

REFERENCES

1. Mandel ID. The functions of saliva. J Dent Res 1987;66:623–7.
2. Tabak LA. A revolution in biomedical assessment: the development of salivary diagnostics. J Dent Ed 2001;65:1335–9.
3. Yao Y, Berg EA, Costello CE, Troxler RF, Oppenheim FG. Identification of protein components in human acquired enamel pellicle and whole saliva using novel proteomics approaches. J Biol Chem 2003;278:5300–308.
4. Wolters DA, Washburn MP, Yates JR, III. An automated multidimensional protein identification technology for shotgun proteomics. Anal Chem 2001;73:5683–90.
5. Xie H, Rhodus NL, Griffin RJ, Carlis JV, Griffin TJ. A catalogue of human saliva proteins identified by free flow electrophoresis-based peptide separation and tandem mass spectrometry. Mol Cell Proteomics 2005;4:1826–30.
6. Guo T, Rudnick PA, Wang W, Lee CS, DeVoe DL, Balgley BM. Characterization of the human salivary proteome by capillary isoelectric focusing/nanoreversed-phase liquid chromatography coupled with ESI-tandem MS. J Proteome Res 2006;5:1469–78.
7. Hu S, Loo JA, Wong DT. Human body fluid proteome analysis. Proteomics 2006;6:6326–53.
8. Kelleher NL. Top-down proteomics. Anal Chem 2004;76:197A–203A.
9. Cooper HJ, Håkansson K, Marshall AG. The role of electron capture dissociation in biomolecular analysis. Mass Spectrom Rev 2005;24:201–22.
10. Yang Z, Hancock WS, Chew TR, Bonilla L. A study of glycoproteins in human serum and plasma reference standards (HUPO) using multilectin affinity chromatography coupled with RPLC-MS/MS. Proteomics 2005;5:3353–66.
11. Zhang H, Li X-j, Martin DB, Aebersold R. Identification and quantification of N-linked glycoproteins using hydrazide chemistry, stable isotope labeling and mass spectrometry. Nature Biotechnol 2003;21:660–66.

12. Salomon AR, Ficarro SB, Brill LM, et al. Profiling of tyrosine phosphorylation pathways in human cells using mass spectrometry. Proc Natl Acad Sci USA 2003;100:443–8.
13. Pinkse MWH, Uitto PM, Hilhorst MJ, Ooms B, Heck AJR. Selective isolation at the femtomole level of phosphopeptides from proteolytic digests using 2D-nanoLC-ESI-MS/MS and titanium oxide precolumns. Anal Chem 2004;76:3935–43.
14. Hu S, Xie Y, Ramachandran P, et al. Large-scale identification of proteins in human salivary proteome by liquid chromatography/mass spectrometry and two-dimensional gel electrophoresis-mass spectrometry. Proteomics 2005;5:1714–28.
15. Huang C.-M. Comparative proteomic analysis of human whole saliva. Arch Oral Biol 2004;49:951–62.
16. Wilmarth PA, Riviere MA, Rustvold DL, Lauten JD, Madden TE, David LL. Two-dimensional liquid chromatography study of the human whole saliva proteome. J Proteome Res 2004;3:1017–23.
17. Neyraud E, Sayd T, Morzel M, Dransfield E. Proteomic analysis of human whole and parotid salivas following stimulation by different tastes. J Proteome Res 2006;5:2474–80.
18. Giusti L, Baldini C, Bazzichi L, et al. Proteome analysis of whole saliva: a new tool for rheumatic diseases—the example of Sjögren's syndrome. Proteomics 2007;7:1634–43.
19. Walz A, Stühler K, Wattenberg A, et al. Proteome analysis of glandular parotid and submandibular-sublingual saliva in comparison to whole human saliva by two-dimensional gel electrophoresis. Proteomics 2006;6:1631–9.
20. Ramachandran P, Boontheung P, Xie Y, Sondej M, Wong DT, Loo JA. Identification of N-linked glycoproteins in human saliva by glycoprotein capture and mass spectrometry. J Proteome Res 2006;5:1493–503.
21. Hu S, Wang J, Meijer J, et al. Salivary proteomic and genomic biomarkers for primary Sjögren's syndrome. Arthrit Rheum 2007;56:3588–600.
22. Nagler R, Bahar G, Shpitzer T, Feinmesser R. Concomitant analysis of salivary tumor markers—a new diagnostic tool for oral cancer. Clin Cancer Res 2006;12:3979–84.
23. Malamud D. Oral diagnostic testing for detecting human immunodeficiency virus-1 antibodies: a technology whose time has come. Am J Med 1997;102:9–14.
24. Chen DX, Schwartz PE, Li FQ. Saliva and serum CA 125 assays for detecting malignant ovarian tumors. Obstet Gynecol 1990;75:701–704.
25. Navarro MA, Mesía R, Díez-Gibert O, Rueda A, Ojeda B, Alonso MC. Epidermal growth factor in plasma and saliva of patients with active breast cancer and breast cancer patients in follow-up compared with healthy women. Breast Cancer Res Treat 1997;42:83–6.

12

Genomic targets in saliva

Bernhard G. Zimmermann, Zhanzhi Hu, and David T. Wong

GENOMIC CANCER BIOMARKERS IN SALIVA

Saliva is a convenient and noninvasive source of genomic DNA, but disease-related genetic information is also contained in the cellular component of oral fluid—which is usually collected as the pellet of an oral rinse. In the past decade, it has been shown that genetic alterations of nuclear and mitochondrial DNA (mtDNA) in the tumor tissue of oral cancer can also be found in the cell pellet. Unfortunately, the low level of target and the high normal background as well as the subtleness of the genetic changes and the heterogeneity of early events in cancer development have prevented the translation of these findings to the clinic. Elevated mtDNA was associated with head and neck squamous cell cancer (HNSCC), and with advanced stage disease while after treatment, mtDNA content was shown to decrease. However, it is also associated with smoking. Nonetheless, these efforts carry high potential for the noninvasive diagnosis.

All these genetic applications are based on the analysis of the cellular compartment of saliva. The cell-free phase of saliva has been presumed to be devoid of nucleic acids due to its hostile nucleolytic nature. Much to the contrary, we have shown that stable, cell-free nucleic acids exist in the supernatant of saliva. The existence of circulating DNA and RNA has been recognized for decades. Cell-free circulating DNA in plasma was first observed almost 60 years ago. Increased circulatory DNA levels were shown in plasma of cancer patients, and DNA derived from cancer patients displays tumor-specific characteristics. These include somatic mutations in tumor suppressor genes, microsatellite alterations, abnormal promoter methylation, and the presence of tumor-related viral DNA. Genetic alterations can successfully be identified in body fluids that drain from organs affected by tumors (Chapter 8). Thus, cell-free biomarkers derived from the tumor "travel" through the body and can be detected in blood and other body fluids. As studies of tumor-derived DNA detection in plasma of cancer patients were being pursued, "fetal" DNA was detected in the plasma of pregnant women.[1] In the following years, the presence of placenta and tumor-specific cell-free RNA in plasma were also demonstrated. These works increased the interest and efforts in the analysis of nucleic acids in body fluids for diagnostic purposes.

SALIVARY TRANSCRIPTOME

With the development of DNA microarrays and the completion of the human genome project, biomedical research has entered the postgenomic era. Technology advancement has allowed high-throughput studies at an unprecedented scale. With microarrays, the whole genome can be monitored, giving researchers the power to detect expression profile changes in a short time. Similarly, mass spectrometry has enabled detection of thousands of proteins from a single biological sample. This has promoted saliva-based diagnostic research to a new level. In 2004, a multi-institutional research consortium was initiated and funded by the National Institute of Dental and Craniofacial Research (NIDCR) to generate a complete catalog of all salivary secretory proteins (Human Salivary Proteome Project). The first salivary diagnostic alphabet is discussed in detailed in Chapter 11.

HUMAN SALIVARY mRNA: NOVEL CANCER BIOMARKER

In addition to all the previously known analytes, a stable, cell-free transcriptome was found to exist in saliva, and a group of "core" RNA species were consistently found in healthy saliva samples. This presented a second diagnostic alphabet in saliva and has opened the door to another chamber of saliva-based diagnostics—saliva transcriptome analyses. In an initial report, human interleukin 8 (IL-8) mRNA and protein were described.[2] The presence of cell-free human transcripts in saliva opens up new possibilities of noninvasive gene expression profiling. Since its discovery, the science behind saliva mRNA and the application of this analyte to identify molecular biomarkers has been actively pursued. Using the U133A high-density oligonucleotide microarray from Affymetrix global profiling of the salivary transcriptome led to the generation of a reference database of over 3,000 RNA species.[3] One hundred and eighty-five transcripts were denominated the "normal salivary core transcripts" (NSCT) as they were present in each saliva supernatant of the studied 10 healthy subjects. This work was followed up by a study to explore the translational utility of the salivary transcriptome: Saliva mRNA from patients with primary T1/T2 oral squamous cell carcinoma was compared to healthy subjects' profiles.[4] Real-time polymerase chain reaction (PCR) validation confirmed seven mRNAs that were at least 3.5-fold elevated in saliva from cancer patients. These salivary RNA biomarkers are transcripts of DUSP1, HA3, OAZ1, S100P, SAT, IL8, and IL1B. In this initial study, the combination of these biomarkers displayed a sensitivity and specificity of 91% in distinguishing patients from controls. Today, over 220 additional patients have been tested and the clinical accuracy holds up at >82% (Wang et al., in preparation). The clinical accuracy of the salivary oral cancer mRNA biomarkers is among the most discriminatory panels cancer biomarkers to date. It should be noted that the National Cancer Institute's Early Disease Detection Network (EDRN) has recently independently validated the salivary transcriptome biomarkers for oral cancer detection. The NCI/EDRN validation firmly established the scientific foundation and clinical diagnostic utility of the salivary transcriptome.

The presence of human mRNA in saliva may seem surprising. However, we have shown that salivary endogenous mRNA is protected from immediate degradation in a similar fashion as cell-free RNA in plasma.[5,6] The utilization of this related analyte has been widely accepted and recently peaked in the noninvasive determination of fetal aneuploidies from maternal plasma.[7] Contrarily, the authenticity of the salivary mRNA finding is often met with skepticism and has even been challenged by a group that was unable to reproduce the finding of mRNA in saliva supernatant and whole saliva.[8] However, the report gives rise to a number of technical reservations, and the inability to extract RNA even from the cell pellet "suggest a problem with their experimental technique that puts the validity of their conclusions about the nonpersistence of mRNA in the cell-free portion of saliva in doubt".[9] Meanwhile, a number of groups have been able to detect and quantify mRNA in saliva. In forensics, a molecular-based test allows the identification of body fluid stains, demonstrating the utility and validity of salivary mRNA testing. Based on panels of body fluid-specific transcripts, the distinction of stains originating from different body fluids such as blood, urine, semen, and saliva has been demonstrated for the purpose of identification.[10] Recently, even whole genome expression analysis was performed to identify stable, saliva-specific mRNAs.[11] Shaw and coworkers have identified a biomarker, amylase, which is highly correlated with sleep drive. Both salivary amylase activity and mRNA levels are also responsive to extended waking periods in humans.[12] These studies further support our work by showing that mRNA can be extracted from human saliva and used for molecular analysis.

Since the initial report we have accumulated an abundance of additional evidence, ranging from the characterization of salivary RNA,[5] to assessing salivary RNA integrity by cDNA library analysis,[13] to identifying and supporting the commercialization of the most effective stabilizer, RNAprotect® Saliva (QIAGEN).[14] A second commercial product Oragene-RNA was recently launched advocating saliva as a noninvasive source of human RNA (http://www.dnagenotek.com/products_oragerna.htm). Salivary cDNA library analysis showed that none of the 117 cloned mRNAs from saliva supernatant is from a pseudogene of contaminating genomic origin, disputing DNA as a source of templates giving rise to false-positive RNA signals.

ANALYSIS OF SALIVARY mRNA

Over the past 3 years, our group has been actively developing the application of patient-based transcriptome-wide technologies to identify RNA biomarkers in saliva. In the following we discuss concepts of saliva analysis that illustrate the analysis of salivary RNA and also the need for expanding the basic understanding of sample handling and analysis. Improvements are still necessary to harvest the full potential of genomic and transcriptomic information for diagnostic applications of the future.

We previously demonstrated that, despite rapid degradation of exogenous RNA, endogenous salivary RNA is protected from immediate degradation by association with macromolecules.[5] We have recently identified a common stabilization motif (AU rich element, ARE) in approximately 60% of salivary mRNA. We have further identified two ARE-binding proteins in saliva—AUF1 and HuF—that bind to ARE in salivary mRNA and may confer stability (Palanisamy V. et al., 2008). While salivary RNA is surprisingly stable, the accurate quantitative analysis warrants immediate sample processing or stabilization. Sample collection and processing on ice halt the "degeneration" of transcriptional patterns for some hours, and immediate freezing of the specimen is effective. However, this is not always possible in clinical or even home-based sampling. The identification of suitable stabilization reagents fitting the needs and constraints of the analytical goals is an important step toward practicability of molecular profiling. These enabling technologies are currently being actively pursued.

We compared the stability of RNA profiles from whole saliva at room temperature with three stabilizing reagents: Superase Inhibitor (Invitrogen), RNAlater (Ambion), or the RNAprotect Saliva reagent (RPS, QIAGEN).[14] Comparison between 0 and 7 days clearly showed that RNAlater, which is very successful in the stabilization of blood and tissue RNA, shows even greater discrepancy than unstabilized sample. Superase Inhibitor only displays a moderate stabilizing effect, while the overall expression profile is well preserved by the RPS reagent. Even storage of up to 1 week at room temperature did not affect the expression profile of 7 oral cancer markers compared to the fresh sample. Consequently, for the analysis of mRNA from whole saliva, RPS should be the preservation reagent of choice. However, for saliva supernatant preservation currently the best choice is Superase Inhibitor and immediate freezing.

RNA EXTRACTION

RNA extraction from saliva is relatively straightforward. Several commercial kits have been used successfully for the isolation of saliva RNA, employing protocols with minor modifications to allow a large sample volume. However, there are some limitations to the use of silica membranes for saliva. Due to the viscosity and nonhomogeneity of saliva, clogging of the filter may occur. Magnetic beads-based methods may prove suited to overcome this problem and offer a robust strategy for automated RNA extraction.

It should be noted that two commercially available RNA stabilization kits are specifically designed for saliva applications. QIAGEN's RNA Protect Saliva and DNA Genotek's Oragene-RNA are two prime examples of the rapid exploration by the commercial section of the clinical values and utilities of salivary transcriptome.

DNase TREATMENT

To avoid potential false positive results from genomic DNA (gDNA) contamination, it is imperative that quality control steps are built in the analysis. The use of DNase I treatment is very effective in removal of gDNA as illustrated in a control experiment (Fig. 12.1). DNAse I-treated RNA from seven saliva supernatant samples was treated with RNase cocktail and analyzed by

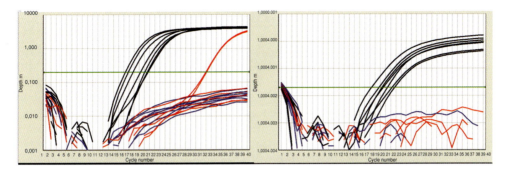

Figure 12.1 RNA was extracted from saliva and DNase I treated (seven samples). RNA was RT-PCR preamplified (*black*); RNA was RNase treated and RT-PCR preamplified (*red*). RNA was preamplified without RT (*blue*). Preamplification products were analyzed by TaqMan real-time PCR with intron spanning assays for IL8 and RPL37.

RT-PCR. While all untreated samples have detectable levels of both transcripts, the RNase digestion abolishes all signals except in two cases where the signal arises 15 cycles later, which is a reduction of template by a factor of 10,000. Concordantly, the controls without reverse transcription show no amplification. Thus, both controls show that the method detects and quantifies RNA and not genomic DNA.

QUANTITATIVE PCR ANALYSIS

Quantitative real-time PCR (qPCR) is currently the gold standard for mRNA quantification. It is perfectly suited for the analysis of samples with low concentration and even for fragmented RNA, as the method generally targets less than 150 nucleotide stretches, and the length can easily be reduced to 50. To ensure high sensitivity, reverse transcription should be carried out with target-specific primers.

One of the challenges of salivary research is that with traditional qPCR only a few targets can be analyzed before the sample is used up. To meet this problem, we have developed a new multiplex RT-PCR-based preamplification that allows the accurate quantification of over 50 targets from one reaction. The method yields unbiased quantitative results for target input ranges of six orders of magnitude (Hu et al., 2008). This novel method is tailored to the short nature of salivary RNA, and makes economical use of precious sample while increasing sensitivity by allowing high sample input and omitting a dilution effect prior to amplification. It offers great cost-effectiveness by reducing RT reactions per sample and allowing small qPCR volumes. In a proof of principle study, we demonstrated that the quantification in a PCR array with 30 nanoliter reaction volumes is possible on the BioTrove "Through Hole Array" which allows 3,072 parallel reactions, a new dimension in qPCR-based mRNA analysis.

MICROARRAY ANALYSIS: THE ALL EXON ARRAY

The main strategy to identify disease-associated mRNAs in saliva is through microarray analysis. For whole saliva, 3′ based arrays employing poly dT priming and 2 rounds of IVT (in vitro transcription) amplification is successful. While this approach also works for saliva supernatant RNA, a large amount of information may be missed as approximately 50% of salivary RNAs are fragmented and do consequently not carry a poly-A tail. Random priming approaches however result in an additional shortening of the fragments. We have recently made a significant advancement in saliva transcriptome diagnostics by achieving the ability to linearly amplify and recover all salivary RNA fragment and profile on the new Affymetrix all exon array (AEA). This novel approach allows the investigation of the whole salivary transcriptome with a resolution down to individual exons. We have defined the salivary exon core transcriptome (SECT), which contains 1,370 probe sets representing 851 unique genes that are present in over 85% of the tested saliva samples (Hu et al., 2008). Preliminary data are consistent with our previous findings and do expand the number of sequences and genes detected. Initial results with specimen from oral and pancreatic cancer raise the hope that the increased resolution will lead to the discovery of highly discriminatory disease markers for systemic diseases.

OUTLOOK

The demonstration of the clinical utilities of the salivary transcriptome will be a defining moment for salivary diagnostics: recognition of the full potential of saliva analysis will promote the establishment of extensive saliva collections in addition to the traditional specimen.

We aim to expand the diagnostic toolbox of oral fluid-based diagnostics by developing a second salivary diagnostic alphabet, the salivary transcriptome. With the salivary proteome and transcriptome diagnostics alphabets, information related to oral and systemic diseases that come in many forms can be envisioned to be harnessed from a single drop of saliva. Technologies are now available to enable the harnessing of highly discriminatory salivary proteomic and genomic biomarkers for early detection of disease, treatment monitoring, and evaluation of therapeutic efficacies. The pharmacogenomics and pharmacoproteomics of saliva will allow clinical utilities for personalized medicine. Enormous opportunities lie ahead and our intent is to establish the rationale, methodology, and targets to harness this potential for the improvement of healthcare.

Acknowledgments

Supported by PHS grants RO1 DE017170 and R21 CA126733.

REFERENCES

1. Lo YM, Corbetta N, Chamberlain PF, et al. Presence of fetal DNA in maternal plasma and serum. Lancet 1997;350:485–7.
2. St John MA, Li Y, Zhou X, et al. Interleukin 6 and interleukin 8 as potential biomarkers for oral cavity and oropharyngeal squamous cell carcinoma. Arch Otolaryngol Head Neck Surg 2004;130:929–35.
3. Li Y, Zhou X, St John MA, Wong DT. RNA profiling of cell-free saliva using microarray technology. J Dent Res 2004;83:199–203.
4. Li Y, St John MA, Zhou X, et al. Salivary transcriptome diagnostics for oral cancer detection. Clin Cancer Res 2004;10:8442–50.
5. Park NJ, Li Y, Yu T, et al. Characterization of RNA in saliva. Clin Chem 2006;52:988–94.
6. Ng EKO, Tsui NBY, Lau TK, et al. mRNA of placental origin is readily detectable in maternal plasma. PNAS 2003;100:4748–53.
7. Lo YM, Tsui NB, Chiu RW, et al. Plasma placental RNA allelic ratio permits noninvasive prenatal chromosomal aneuploidy detection. Nat Med 2007;13:218–23.
8. Kumar SV, Hurteau GJ, Spivack SD. Validity of messenger RNA expression analyses of human saliva. Clin Cancer Res 2006;12:5033–9.
9. Ballantyne, J. Validity of messenger RNA expression analyses of human saliva. Clin Cancer Res 2007;13:1350.
10. Juusola J, Ballantyne J. Messenger RNA profiling: a prototype method to supplant conventional methods for body fluid identification. Forensic Sci Int 2003;135:85–96.
11. Zubakov D, Hanekamp E, Kokshoorn M, van Ijcken W, Kayser M. Stable RNA markers for identification of blood and saliva stains revealed from whole genome expression analysis of time-wise degraded samples. Int J Legal Med 2008;122:135–42.
12. Seugnet L, Boero J, Gottschalk L, Duntley SP, Shaw PJ. Identification of a biomarker for sleep drive in flies and humans. PNAS 2006;103:19913–18.
13. Park NJ, Zhou X, Yu T, et al. Characterization of salivary RNA by cDNA library analysis. Arch Oral Biol 2007;52:30–35.
14. Park NJ, Yu T, Nabili V, et al. RNAprotect saliva: an optimal room-temperature stabilization reagent for the salivary transcriptome. Clin Chem 2006;52:2303–304.

13

Point-of-care diagnostics for infectious diseases

Paul L.A.M. Corstjens and Daniel Malamud

INTRODUCTION

Point-of-care (POC) diagnostics represent a rapidly growing industry. As the healthcare system becomes more managed and more expensive, any advance that leads to simplification and decreased costs is well received. POC testing removes several steps from the process and thus reduces cost. Oral-based POC diagnosis has the added advantages of lesser invasiveness and, therefore, increased acceptance, and since a phlebotomist is not required, a further decrease in cost. Infectious diseases are particularly applicable to oral-based POC. In most cases, one only requires a qualitative result; the individual either has the disease/infection or does not. It is also possible to carry out quantitative POC testing, for example, to determine bacterial or viral load. However, it is often more important to have a rapid yes/no result so that appropriate therapy can be administered promptly. Thus, distinguishing on-site if the patient is infected with a bacterial or viral pathogen can lead to prompt administration of antibiotics, if appropriate, or prevent unnecessary drugs if the disease is viral.

In this paper, we review the literature and provide an overview of infectious diseases and immunity detected using oral fluids (saliva samples).

INFECTIOUS DISEASES, CURRENT APPROACHES FOR DIAGNOSIS

An infectious disease results from the action of a pathogenic agent present in a host organism. The pathogenic agent may be a microorganism or proteinous infectious particles without nucleic acid such as prions. We distinguish primary and opportunistic pathogens; primary pathogens cause a disease in an otherwise healthy individual, whereas opportunistic pathogens typically cause a disease in immunocompromised patients.

Communicable infectious diseases caused by primary pathogens are important since infection easily spreads from person to person. This can transpire directly by respiratory transmission (as in the case of tuberculosis and measles) or by sexual or mucosal contact (e.g., human immunodeficiency and hepatitis virus infections). Another form of transmission transpires indirectly by means of insect vectors. Well-known examples include the female mosquitoes carrying protozoan *Plasmodium* species that cause malaria and ticks carrying *Borrelia burgdorferi* bacteria that cause Lyme disease.

New communicable infectious diseases are identified regularly; two recent examples are severe acute respiratory syndrome (SARS) caused by coronavirus and avian flu caused by influenza A virus subtype H5N1. The new infectious diseases are of major concern since their emergence often leads to high mortality rates, for example, 10 and 60% mortality for SARS and H5N1, respectively. Also of concern is the reemergence and spread of bacterial infections by strains that have developed multiple drug resistance. Two examples are multidrug-resistant tuberculosis (MRTB) and methicillin-resistant *Staphylococcus aureus* (MRSA); in both cases multidrug resistance is linked to increased mortality.

The key to efficacious treatment of infectious diseases is early and accurate identification of the infectious agent. While this might sound like a simple task, in many cases the clinical signs and symptoms are insufficient to identify the correct diagnostic test. For example, a fever, sore throat, and fatigue might suggest a test for a streptococcal infection, but the patient's history might not suggest a test for viral infectious mononucleosis. Moreover, while infectious diseases may be caused by distinct bacterial, viral, fungal, or protozoan agents, often there are secondary infections and/or immune suppression that further complicate appropriate diagnosis.

A major issue is to decide what type of specimen to collect for testing. For many pathogens the obvious choice is a blood sample; for local infections (surface lesions or localized infections) a sample may be taken from the site of the infection. Typically, an oral swab is used to confirm a streptococcal infection. In the case of tuberculosis (TB) a sputum sample is indicated, while for a suspected kidney or bladder infection, urine may be the sample of choice. The type of sample collected is also influenced by the site and available medical staff. With respect to future home, on-site, and POC test applications, saliva as a diagnostic sample is an excellent alternative to a blood specimen. Moreover, saliva collection and analysis may provide a cost-effective approach for large populations screening for epidemiological testing or to monitor immunity to common viral infections.[1-3]

The use of saliva as a diagnostic sample in laboratory tests has recently been reviewed.[4] As with other types of samples, salivary tests may be carried out at POC (e.g., the physician office) or the collected saliva may be sent to a centralized testing facility. When developing any diagnostic test, there are a series of standard issues including sensitivity, specificity, reproducibility, cost, and sample preparation. The ideal test would have 100% sensitivity and 100% specificity, yielding zero false negatives and zero false positives. This is rarely, if ever, seen.

The primary value of oral fluid testing is the noninvasive nature of the procedure; although obtaining glandular duct saliva is somewhat more complicated than analyzing whole saliva or mucosal transudates. Advantages include home testing or collection at nontraditional settings (dental office, nursing home, remote geographical locations) and for patients with fear of venipuncture, or for the elderly and pediatric populations.

Rapid direct detection and identification of the infectious microorganism by molecular methods is not yet widely implemented in hospital and medical laboratories. Therapy in most of the cases is initiated immediately, even before blood sample results are available. If the identity of the bacterial pathogen is unknown, wide-spectrum antibiotics are applied. In resource-poor countries where certain infections are endemic, medication is often provided without concomitant laboratory diagnosis. This approach, especially when it concerns prescription of antibiotics, may eventually accelerate the emergence of multidrug-resistant microorganisms. In the ideal situation the physician would have access to a POC device that permitted direct testing of a specimen for common diseases. With infectious diseases, the device would allow the unambiguous identification of the organism causing the infection so that specific medication can be offered.

INFECTIONS DETECTABLE UTILIZING ORAL FLUIDS

Oral fluid is regarded as a mirror of blood and as such offers a specimen for diagnostic purposes.[5] The presence of molecular markers (human antibodies and pathogen-derived analytes including nucleic acids) in oral fluid has been demonstrated for many infectious diseases.

A selection of references to the indirect and direct detection of bacterial, viral, and other pathogens in oral samples is presented in Tables 13.1–13.3. The list includes studies describing detection of antibodies upon immunization. Multiple references and evaluation studies from the same research group are omitted unless they detect different pathogens or utilize different technologies. References to sputum, dental/denture plaque, pharyngeal throat swabs, or nasopharyngeal samples were not included. Most references describe clinical studies; case studies were included when they described the development of new assays.

Bacterial infections

Over 500 bacterial species are present in the mouth; however, most of these are commensal and not pathogenic. Isolation of periodontal and cariogenic bacteria from various types of oral samples has been carried out by cultivation and their identity confirmed by molecular methods. However, it is doubtful that viable primary pathogenic bacteria, other than the periodontophatic and cariogenic bacteria or organisms causing upper, lower, or parenchymal respiratory diseases, can be routinely detected in oral samples using culture methods. For instance, a 98% detection rate of *Mycobacterium tuberculosis* was obtained by polymerase chain reaction (PCR) using mixed saliva, in contrast to a 17.3%

Table 13.1 Examples in context of bacterial infectious diseases using saliva samples.

Bacterium	Antibody	Antigen	DNA
Bordetella pertussis	Granström, G. 1988; Litt, D. 2006; Zackrisson, G. 1990		
Campylobacter jejuni	Cawthraw, S. 2002		
Clostridium tetani[a]	Cardinale, F. 2001; Engström, P. 2002; Layward, L. 1995; Lue, C. 1994		
Escherichia coli O157	Ludwig, K. 2002		
Helicobacter pylori	Christie, J. 1996; Fallone, C. 1996; Gilger, M. 2002; Hooshmand, B. 2004; Marshall, B. 1999; Loeb, M. 1997; Luzza, F. 2000; Pellicano, R. 2001; Simor, A. 1996; Wienholt, M. 1993.		Basso, D. 1996; Bonamio, M. 2004; Hammar, M. 1992; Tiwari, S. 2005
Leptospira species	da Silva, M. 1992		
Moraxella catarrhalis	Stutzmann, M. 2003		Eguchi, J. 2003; Lee, S. 2004
Mycobacterium tuberculosis	Araujo, Z. 2004; de Larrea, C. 2006		
Porphyromonas gingivalis[b]	Hägewald, S. 2003		Beikler, T. 2006; Iwai, T. 2005; Mager, D. 2005; Umeda, M. 1998
Salmonella thyphi	Herath, H. 2003		
Shigella species[c]	Khazenson, L. 1981; Salamotova, S. 1993; Schultsz, C. 1992		
Streptococcus species[d]			Hoshino, T. 2004; Mager, D. 2005; Napimoga 2004
Streptococcus pneumoniae[e]	Huo, Z. 2004; Nurkka, A. 2005; Zhang, Q. 2006	Krook, A. 1986	
Treponema pallidum	Baguley, S. 2005; Maple, P. 2006		Palmer, H. 2003[f]

[a] Detection of salivary antibodies upon immunization with inactivated tetanus toxoid isolated from *Clostridium tetani*.

[b] Including other (not specified in the table) oral/periodontophatic bacteria: *Actinobacillus actinomycetemcomitans*, *Bacteroides forsythus*, *Campylobacter rectus*, *Capnocytophaga gingivalis*, *Eikenella corrodens*, *Prevotella intermedia*, *Prevotella melaninogenica*, *Prevotella nigrescens*, *Streptococcus mitis*, *Tannerella forsythensis*, and *Treponema denticola*. Does not include the numerous references in which detection was performed on subgingival plaque samples only.

[c] Including *Shigella dysenteriae*, *Shigella flexneri*, and *Shigella sonnei*.

[d] Not including *Streptococcus pneumoniae*, but including other species from mutans, mitis, and salivarius group streptococci: *Streptococcus gordonii*, *Streptococcus mutans*, *Streptococcus oralis*, *Streptococcus salivarius*, *Streptococcus sanguinis*, and *Streptococcus sobrinus*.

[e] Antigen detection based on the presence of pneumococcal C polysaccharide.

[f] Sampling: swabs of oral ulcers suspected to be syphilitic in origin.

139

detection rate by cultivation.[6] Only when acute infection with high bacterial loads occurs, will the pathogenic organism appear in the oral cavity.

Helicobacter pylori is a major cause of peptic ulcers and is currently regarded as an early risk factor for gastric carcinoma and the mucosa-associated lymphoid tissue lymphoma. It is theorized to be fecal-oral; however, few studies report cultivation of *H. pylori* from oral samples or fecal samples.[7] The gold standard to indicate active infection is still based on the collection of gastric mucosal biopsy for cultivation. However, detection of *H. pylori*-specific rDNA sequences by PCR of saliva samples of symptomatic patients indicated that this is a reliable specimen to indicate active infection.[8,9]

Results with *M. tuberculosis* and *H. pylori* demonstrate that although viable bacteria may not be detectable in oral fluid, saliva still contains pathogen-derived analytes. In these two examples, pathogen DNA was analyzed, but other markers as 16S rRNA sequences[10] could be targeted as well. A non-nucleic acid example is the detection of *Streptococcus pneumoniae* in patients with pneumonia.[11] *S. pneumoniae* infection was detected by screening for the presence of a pneumococcal C polysaccharide in saliva.

Viral infections

Worldwide, fatalities from most infectious diseases have not significantly increased in the past two decades. This is due to improved medical care, new vaccines, vaccination policies, development of novel drugs, and a spectacular increase in antibiotic prescription for bacterial infections. If the same resources applied in the Western world become available in developing countries, the number of infectious disease-related deaths will significantly decrease.

Besides the occurrence of multidrug-resistant microorganisms (MRTB and MRSA), the new and reemerging viral infections are a current concern. For instance, the number of deaths related to HIV infection increased since 1993 from 0.7 million to 2.8 million in 2002 (World Health Organization report 2004). Newly emerging diseases primarily result from new or modified viral strains. These strains are often insensitive to existing antiviral drugs.

Literature shows that the direct detection and identification of many viruses in saliva by PCR could become a standard method. Numerous clinical and/or validation studies have been reported, and a selection is shown in Table 13.2. Besides targeting the genome, presence of a virus can be measured by detecting genes transcribed during the productive phase of the infection.[12]

RNA viruses including dengue, hepatitis C (HCV), and HIV may be more difficult to detect in saliva as their single-stranded RNA genome is orders of magnitude less stable than a double-stranded DNA genome. Sampling and sample handling in these situations are crucial. Literature shows that HCV and HIV saliva studies are well represented and standard detection methods have been developed. The presence and frequency of infectious HIV particles in saliva is still controversial.[13–15] However, detection of HIV RNA was clearly demonstrated in several studies, although viral load values in saliva can be

Table 13.2 Examples in context of viral infectious diseases using saliva samples.

Virus	Antibody	Antigen	Nucleic acid
Cytomegalovirus[a]	Zhang, C. 2006		Blackbourn, D. 1998; Idesawa, M. 2004; Lucht, E. 1993; Miller, C. 2005; Saygun, I. 2005; Yamamoto, A. 2006
Dengue virus	Balmaseda, A. 2003; Cuzzubbo, A. 1998; de Oliveira, S. 1999; Vázquez, S. 2007		
Ebola virus[b]		Formenty, P. 2006	Formenty, P. 2006
Epstein-Barr virus[a]	Sheppard, C. 2001; Vyse, A. 1997		Blackbourn, D. 1998; Idesawa, M. 2004; Miller, C. 2005; Saygun, I. 2005
Hepatitis A virus	Amado, L. 2006; Morris-Cunnington, M. 2004; Ochino, J. 2007; Parry, J. 1989; Skidmore, S. 2001; Thieme, T. 1992		Mackiewicz, V. 2004
Hepatitis B virus[c]	Amado, L. 2006; Farghaly, A. 1998; Fisker, N. 2002; Parry, J. 1989	Chaita, T. 1995; Farghaly, A. 1998; Hutse. V. 2005; Noppornpanth, S. 2000; Richards, A. 1996; Thieme, T. 1992	Kidd-Ljunggren, K. 2006; Noppornpanth, S. 2000; van der Eijk, A. 2004
Hepatitis C virus	Amado, L. 2006; Bélec, L. 2003; de Cock, L. 2005; El-Medany, O. 1999; Farghaly, A. 1998; Judd, A. 2003; Maticic, M. 2003; Thieme, T. 1992; Zmuda, J. 2001		Bélec, L. 2003; Chen, M. 1995; Eirea, M. 2005; Farghaly, A. 1998; Rey, D. 2001; Roy, K. 1998; Wang, C. 2006
Hepatitis G virus[d] (GB virus C)			Bourlet, T. 2002; Eugenia, Q. 2001; Yan, J. 2002
Herpes simplex virus[a,e]	Rune, S. 1984; Spicher, V. 2001; Välimaa, H. 2002		da Silva, L. 2005; Furuta, Y. 1998; Kaufman, H. 2005; Miller, C. 2005
Human herpesvirus (HHV-6, -7, or -8)[a]			Blackbourn, D. 1998; Casper, C. 2007; Gautheret, A. 1995; Miller, C. 2005; Pereira, C. 2004; Ramsay, M. 2002; Taylor, M. 2004; Zerr, D. 2005
Human immunodeficiency virus[f,g]	Archibald, D. 1986; Chohan, B. 2001; Granade, T. 1995; Kakizawa, J. 1996; Maticic, M. 2000; Matsuda, S. 1993; O'Connell, R. 2003; O'Shea, S. 1990; Parry, J. 1987; Yasuda, S. 1998	Katz, D. 1994; O'Shea, S. 1990	Bourlet, T. 2001; Freel, S. 2003; Goto, Y. 1991; Kakizawa, J. 1996; Lucht, E. 1993; Liuzzi, G. 1994/2002; Maticic, M. 2000; O'Shea, S. 1990; Qureshi, M. 1997; Shugars, D. 1999; Spear, G. 2005; Yagyu, F. 2002
Human papillomavirus	Buchinsky, F. 2006; Cameron, J. 2003; Gonçalves, A. 2006; Marais, D. 2006		Cameron, J. 2003; Gonçalves, A. 2006; Marais, D. 2006; Zhao, M. 2005
Human parvovirus B19	Cubel, R. 1996; Rice, P. 1996		

(Continued)

Table 13.2 *(cont.)*

Virus	Antibody	Antigen	Nucleic acid
Influenza virus	Brokstad, K. 2002; el-Madhun, A. 1998		
Measles virus	Friedman, M. 1982; Gill, J. 2002; Helfand, R. 1999; Kremer, J. 2005; Nigatu, W. 1999/2001; Perry, K. 1993; Samuel, D. 2003; Thieme, T. 1992		Chibo, D. 2005; Nigatu, W. 2006; Oliveira, S. 2003
Mumps virus	Friedman, M. 1982; Jin, L. 2004; Perry, K. 1993; Thieme, T. 1992; Warrener, L. 2006		Jin, L. 2004; Sanz, J. 2006
Norwalk virus	Moe, C. 2004		
Poliovirus	Abrahamsson, J. 1999; Cardinale, F. 2001; Hanslon, L. 1984; Herremans, T. 1999; Ivanov, A. 2005; Smith, D. 1987; Sirisinha, S. 1970		
Rabies virus[h]		Madhusudana, S. 2004	Crepin, P. 1998; Nagaraj, T. 2006; Smith, J. 2003; Wacharapluesadee, S. 2001
Rotavirus	Coulson, B. 1989; Friedman, M. 1996; Jayashree, S. 1988; Ramachandran, M. 1998; Ward, R. 1992		
Rubella virus	Gill, J. 2002; Morris, M. 2002; Nokes, D. 1998; Ramsay, M. 2002; Thieme, T. 1992; Vijaylakshmi, P. 2006		Vyse, A. 2002
SARS coronavirus[i]			Drosten, C. 2004; Wang, W. 2004
Torque teno virus[j]			Deng, X. 2000; Goto, K. 2000; Inami, T. 2000; Kasirga, E. 2005; Matsubara, H. 2000; Ross, R. 1999; Rotundo, R. 2004; Yan, J. 2002
Varicella-Zoster virus[a]	Talukder, Y. 2005; Terada, K. 2002		Mehta, S. 2004; Ohtani, F. 2006; Yamakawa, K. 2007

[a] Human herpesvirus (HHV) types: Cytomegalovirus is HHV-5; Epstein-Barr is HHV-4; Herpes simplex virus-1 and virus-2, respectively, HHV-1 and HHV-2; Varicella-Zoster virus is HHV-3; HHV-6 and HHV-7 are used when referring to roseolovirus; and HHV-8 is a rhadinovirus type.

[b] Antigen detection with a polyvalent hyperimmune rabbit serum to virus subtypes isolated/identified during outbreaks of Ebola hemorrhagic fever.

[c] Antigen detection based on the presence of hepatitis B surface antigen (HBsAg).

[d] A currently more preferred name for hepatitis G virus (HGV) is GB virus C (GBV-C). The virus does not cause hepatitis; whether it causes a specific disease is uncertain.

[e] Including type-1 and type-2 human simplex virus.

[f] Antigen detection based on the presence of HIV p24 core protein.

[g] Besides detection of genomic RNA sequences, some also report detection of proviral DNA sequences.

[h] Antigen detection based on the presence of rabies nucleoprotein.

[i] SARS is the "severe acute respiratory syndrome."

[j] Torque teno virus (TTV) is also referred to as "transfusion-transmitted virus." The virus is associated with blood transfusions and hepatitis, but so far has no established etiological role in hepatitis.

2–3 orders of magnitude lower than blood.[16–18] For HCV, lower RNA values in saliva as compared to serum are also reported, but differences are not as large as observed for HIV.[19] In a few cases, hypersecretion of HIV RNA in nonblood compartments was reported with higher viral loads for saliva than blood levels.[20] However, the correlation between saliva and blood viral load is not always clear, which in part may be a consequence of the presence of salivary PCR inhibitors.[21] Although oral transmission of HIV is rare, it cannot be excluded; secondary factors including gingivitis and periodontitis could increase the risk of transmission.

As there is no vaccination against HIV, detection of antibodies against specific HIV antigens is sufficient to conclude that the individual is infected and most likely is contagious. Currently, fourth-generation HIV screening assays are available that combine antibody detection and p24 detection to identify viral infection within the seroconversion window.[22] Viral load determination, by RNA detection or, to a lesser extent, using p24 antigen detection, is mainly used to monitor the response to drug therapy.

A different situation exists with Ebola infection. Infection must be diagnosed by direct detection of the virus (using antigen or RNA detection) as mortality rate is 80% with most fatal cases being seronegative.[23] For dengue infection, the presence of antibodies to dengue derived from a primary infection with one of four different strains is a potential risk marker. In those cases, secondary infection with a different dengue serotype may lead to a hemorrhagic fever or dengue shock syndrome (see reference 24).

Other infections

While most pathogens are viral or bacterial, multicellular parasites including *Candida*, other fungi, and metazoans can also cause infection. A fourth group of pathogens are the protozoa. *Plasmodium* species are transmitted by mosquitoes and cause malaria in humans. Another example involves the microsporidia *Enterocytozoon bieneusi* and *Septata intestinalis* recognized as pathogens primarily in immunocompromised and AIDS individuals. The sporozoa, especially *Toxoplasma gondii*, cause an opportunistic infection in immunocompromised patients and is a risk factor in pregnancy, as congenital toxoplasmosis can seriously affect the fetus.

Most multicellular parasites and protozoa will not directly affect the respiratory tract or the oral cavity. Exceptions may be blood-borne pathogens that can enter the oral cavity through bleeding gums. A multicellular parasite that does occur in the mouth is *Candida*. *Candida albicans* is typically found on skin and mucous membranes. It is not a primary pathogen, but it can lead to oropharyngeal candidiasis when the environment in the oral cavity becomes unbalanced, as a consequence of another infection, a compromised immune system, or long-term antibiotic use. Table 13.3 shows an overview of some of the results on infections from nonbacterial and nonviral pathogenic microorganisms that have been analyzed in oral fluid.

Table 13.3 Examples in context of nonbacterial and nonviral infectious diseases using saliva samples.

Other pathogens	Antibody	Antigen	Nucleic acid
Candida albicans	Jeganathan, S, 1987; Millon, L. 2001		
Entamoeba histolytica[a]	Abd-Alla, M. 2000; Aceti, A. 1991; del Muro, R. 1990; El-Hamshary, E. 2004; Punthuprapasa, P. 2001	Abd-Alla, M. 2000	
Naegleria fowleri	Rivera-Aguilar, V. 2000		
Schistosomas species[b]	Santos, M. 2000; Wang, Z. 2002		
Taenia solium	Acosta, E. 1990; Bueno, E. 2000; Feldman, M. 1990		
Toxoplasma gondii	Hajeer, A. 1994; Loyola, A. 1997		

[a] Antigen detection based on the presence of a specific galactose-inhibitable lectin.
[b] Including *Schistosmas japonica* and *Schistosomas mansoni*.

INDIRECT OR DIRECT DETECTION OF PATHOGENS

The humoral immune response can be a marker of past infection, and the prevalence of pathogen-specific IgG can be used as an indication of the level of immunity in a population. On the other hand, the presence of specific IgG can also reflect persistent infection. In some cases active infection can be evaluated by determining the ratio between IgM and IgG. For instance, in patients with acute pneumococcal infection, the IgG concentration was significantly lower than in healthy controls, whereas the IgM concentration in the infected individuals was significantly higher.[25] Salivary IgA has also been proposed for early diagnosis, for example, typhoid fever.[26] IgG and IgM detected in saliva are derived from blood via the gingival crevicular fluid whereas IgA is found in mucosal areas. IgA prevents colonization of mucosa, whereas IgM is responsible for the early stages of cell-mediated immunity before there is sufficient IgG.

The main problem in using antibodies for detecting acute and active infections is the lack of antibody data from individuals before infection. Large variations in levels of specific immunoglobulins between individuals make it difficult to use antibody screening as a general diagnostic tool. The detection of antibodies is sufficient to demonstrate infection only for infections for which no immunization is available, such as HIV and human T-lymphotropic virus (HTLV). Detection of HIV and HTLV antibodies therefore is used for screening of blood donations.

Other antibody tests that are still used in screening of the US blood supply are for HBV, HCV, and syphilis. However, to further reduce the chance of transmission by blood donations, nucleic acid testing (NAT) is also implemented. NAT is used because it allows detection of an infection before seroconversion. It is currently applied to detect active infections of HIV, HCV, and West Nile virus.[27] Active hepatitis B virus (HBV) infection is tested by screening for a specific antigen (hepatitis B surface antigen). Obviously, the detection of antibodies is not always useful to detect acute or active infection. Moreover, antibody assays are not applicable to immunodeficient patients.

Diagnostic tests that simultaneously detect host-derived antibodies and pathogen-derived antigens and nucleic acids are valuable not only because they could identify active infection but also because they can track disease progression. A schematic of such a device is shown in Figure 13.1.[28] The modular device divides a single saliva sample into separate pathways that can detect multiple targets. One pathway is for detecting antibodies, a second channel detects proteinous or polysaccharide antigens, whereas the third and fourth channels are for the detection of nucleic acids (RNA or DNA). The antibody pathway does not require sample processing, whereas the antigen and nucleic acid pathways do require processing of varying complexity. Note again that each pathway can handle multiple targets, various antibodies, antigens, and nucleic acid targets that can be simultaneously detected. To validate this microfluidic device for saliva testing, HIV-specific assays have been developed. The HIV assay includes antibody detection; lysis and p24 antigen detection; lysis, DNA purification and PCR amplification of proviral DNA; and RNA isolation and RT-PCR amplification of HIV RNA. Primary acute infection with HIV would be unequivocally demonstrated when data indicate p24, HIV DNA and RNA, but no HIV antibodies. After seroconversion antibodies will be detectable, but the p24 signal is decreased or may even be absent due to the formation of immune complexes with human antibodies, whereas HIV DNA and RNA are still detectable. The correlation between HIV DNA (proviral copies of HIV integrated in the human genome) and HIV RNA may be an indicator of disease progression.

What is unique in this device is that the pathways follow a generic approach such that the assay-specific part is only determined by the lateral flow (LF)-based capture and the pathogen-specific probes in the nucleic acid paths. As demonstrated recently,[29] the antibody path allows convenient multiplexed detection of antibodies against multiple pathogens. Moreover, multiplexing of different types of biomolecules also addresses interference issues that may occur in various kinds of immunoassays.

CONCLUDING REMARKS

The development and application of rapid POC devices for detection of infectious diseases using saliva has already proved its benefit in HIV testing. Currently, only POC devices detecting the presence of human antibodies against the pathogen are available. As soon as saliva-based POC devices allowing the direct detection/identification of the pathogen causing the infection become available, POC will replace the current hospital/laboratory testing. Increased POC testing may result in fewer patients being referred for more elaborate

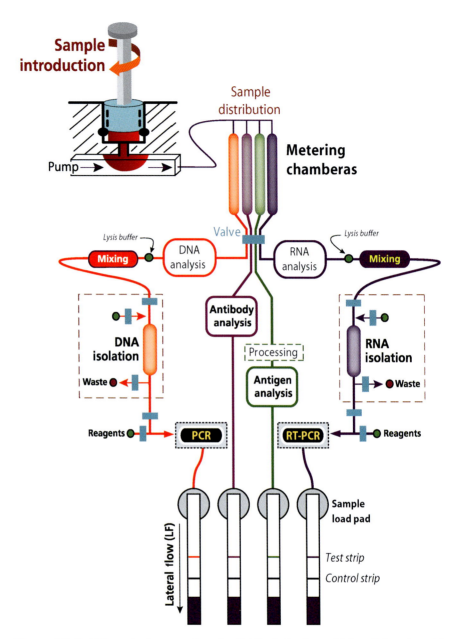

Figure 13.1 Schematic diagram of a microfluidic device for multiplexed detection of infectious disease pathogens. (From top to bottom) A saliva collection device is inserted in the microfluidic device, and saliva from the absorbent pad is pumped into the microfluidic channels. The saliva specimen is divided over four different metering chambers connected to four different paths for antibody, antigen, RNA, and DNA targets, respectively. Each path includes a target type-specific processing. The nucleic acid paths include amplification steps that utilize target-specific probes. Detection of the targets utilizes (generic) reporter conjugates that are deposited at target-specific capture sites on the lateral flow strips. Lateral flow strips can have either one or multiple specific capture zones.

testing. An example is the POC testing for active *H. pylori* infection, which could reduce the number of patients referred for endoscopy.

When developing widely applicable saliva-based POC devices for infectious diseases (1) the assays should be inexpensive; (2) test devices should be disposable; (3) test results need to be rapidly available; and (4) assays should accommodate the identification of pathogens responsible for the most common infections. This might include the combination of testing for antibodies against HIV and other common HIV-associated opportunistic pathogens. It is obvious that for bedside testing at the patients home, handheld devices are convenient. But the large majority of individuals will receive POC testing at the office of a general practitioner where small portable bench top devices are acceptable and recommended if their use increases sensitivity.

Acknowledgments

Dr Karoly Szuhai (MD, PhD; Leiden University Medical Center) is acknowledged for pertinent and critical remarks during the preparation of this manuscript. Claudia de Dood (Leiden University Medical Center) is acknowledged for her help with the literature references. Dr William R. Abrams (New York University College of Dentistry) is acknowledged for creating Figure 13.1. Preparation of this manuscript was supported by NIH grants UO1-DE-0114964, UO1-DE-017855, and the New York State Office of Science Technology and Academic Research (NTSTAR).

REFERENCES

1. Kaufman E, Lamster IB. The diagnostic applications of saliva—a review. Crit Rev Oral Biol Med 2002;13(2):197–212.
2. Morris-Cunnington MC, Edmunds WJ, Miller E, Brown DW. A novel method of oral fluid collection to monitor immunity to common viral infections. Epidemiol Infect 2004;132(1):35–42.
3. O'Connell T, Thornton L, O'Flanagan D, et al. Oral fluid collection by post for viral antibody testing. Int J Epidemiol 2001;30(2):298–301.
4. Malamud D, Sam Niedbala R. (eds) *Oral-Based Diagnostics*, 1st edn. Boston, MA: Blackwell Publishing; 2007.
5. van Nieuw Amerongen A, Ligtenberg AJ, Veerman EC. Implications for diagnostics in the biochemistry and physiology of saliva. Ann N Y Acad Sci 2007;1098:1–6.
6. Eguchi J, Ishihara K, Watanabe A, Fukumoto Y, Okuda K. PCR method is essential for detecting *Mycobacterium tuberculosis* in oral cavity samples. Oral Microbiol Immunol 2003;18(3):156–9.
7. Shames B, Krajden S, Fuksa M, Babida C, Penner JL. Evidence for the occurrence of the same strain of *Campylobacter pylori* in the stomach and dental plaque. J Clin Microbiol 1989;27(12):2849–50.
8. Tiwari SK, Khan AA, Ahmed KS, et al. Rapid diagnosis of *Helicobacter pylori* infection in dyspeptic patients using salivary secretion: a non-invasive approach. Singapore Med J 2005;46(5):224–8.

9. Ahmed KS, Khan AA, Ahmed I, et al. Prevalence study to elucidate the transmission pathways of *Helicobacter pylori* at oral and gastroduodenal sites of a South Indian population. Singapore Med J 2006;47(4):291–6.

10. Granstrom G, Askelof P, Granstrom M. Specific immunoglobulin A to *Bordetella pertussis* antigens in mucosal secretion for rapid diagnosis of whooping cough. J Clin Microbiol 1988;26(5):869–74.

11. Krook A, Fredlund H, Holmberg H. Diagnosis of pneumococcal pneumonia by detection of antigen in saliva. Eur J Clin Microbiol 1986;5(6):639–42.

12. Slots J, Nowzari H, Sabeti M. Cytomegalovirus infection in symptomatic periapical pathosis. Int Endod J 2004;37(8):519–24.

13. Baron S, Poast J, Cloyd MW. Why is HIV rarely transmitted by oral secretions? Saliva can disrupt orally shed, infected leukocytes. Arch Intern Med 1999;159(3):303–10.

14. Campo J, Perea MA, del RJ, Cano J, Hernando V, Bascones A. Oral transmission of HIV, reality or fiction? An update. Oral Dis 2006;12(3):219–28.

15. Shugars DC, Alexander AL, Fu K, Freel SA. Endogenous salivary inhibitors of human immunodeficiency virus. Arch Oral Biol 1999;44(6):445–53.

16. Liuzzi G, Chirianni A, Clementi M, Zaccarelli M, Antinori A, Piazza M. Reduction of HIV-1 viral load in saliva by indinavir-containing antiretroviral regimen. Aids 2002;16(3):503–504.

17. Freel SA, Fiscus SA, Pilcher CD, et al. Envelope diversity, coreceptor usage and syncytium-inducing phenotype of HIV-1 variants in saliva and blood during primary infection. Aids 2003;17(14):2025–33.

18. Bourlet T, Cazorla C, Berthelot P, et al. Compartmentalization of HIV-1 according to antiretroviral therapy: viral loads are correlated in blood and semen but poorly in blood and saliva. Aids 2001;15(2):284–5.

19. Rey D, Fritsch S, Schmitt C, Meyer P, Lang JM, Stoll-Keller F. Quantitation of hepatitis C virus RNA in saliva and serum of patients coinfected with HCV and human immunodeficiency virus. J Med Virol 2001;63(2):117–19.

20. Shugars DC, Patton LL, Freel SA, et al. Hyper-excretion of human immunodeficiency virus type 1 RNA in saliva. J Dent Res 2001;80(2):414–20.

21. Ochert AS, Boulter AW, Birnbaum W, Johnson NW, Teo CG. Inhibitory effect of salivary fluids on PCR: potency and removal. PCR Methods Appl 1994;3(6):365–8.

22. Ly TD, Ebel A, Faucher V, Fihman V, Laperche S. Could the new HIV combined p24 antigen and antibody assays replace p24 antigen specific assays? J Virol Methods 2007;143(1):86–94.

23. Ksiazek TG, Rollin PE, Williams AJ, et al. Clinical virology of Ebola hemorrhagic fever (EHF): virus, virus antigen, and IgG and IgM antibody findings among EHF patients in Kikwit, Democratic Republic of the Congo, 1995. J Infect Dis 1999;179(Suppl 1):S177–87.

24. Cuzzubbo AJ, Vaughn DW, Nisalak A, Suntayakorn S, Aaskov J, Devine PL. Detection of specific antibodies in saliva during dengue infection. J Clin Microbiol 1998;36(12):3737–9.

25. Huo Z, Spencer O, Miles J, et al. Antibody response to pneumolysin and to pneumococcal capsular polysaccharide in healthy individuals and *Streptococcus pneumoniae* infected patients. Vaccine 2004;22(9–10):1157–61.

26. Herath HM. Early diagnosis of typhoid fever by the detection of salivary IgA. J Clin Pathol 2003;56(9):694–8.
27. American Red Cross Blood Services (Penn Jersey Region). *Blood Testing*. Available at: http://www.pleasegiveblood.org/blood-facts/blood-testing.html (accessed May 5, 2007).
28. Malamud D, Bau H, Niedbala S, Corstjens P. Point detection of pathogens in oral samples. Adv Dent Res 2005;18(1):12–16.
29. Corstjens PLAM, Chen Z, Zuiderwijk M, et al. Rapid assay format for multiplex detection of humoral immune responses to infectious disease pathogens (HIV, HCV, and TB). Ann N Y Acad Sci 2007;1098:437–45.

Dental caries risk assessment

Paul C. Denny and Patricia A. Denny

14

INTRODUCTION

A risk assessment for dental caries is accomplished with host factors that correlate with caries history in young adults, and are then used to predict individual risk levels that are tooth group specific in children. The host factors are oligosaccharides present on salivary glycoproteins. This test (CARE Test[TM] is the registered trademark of Proactive Oral Solutions, Inc.; the commercial test is in mid-phase development) is believed to be centered on the specific classes of oligosaccharides that either facilitate bacterial attachment and colonization at the surface of teeth or protect against colonization by promoting agglutination and removal of free bacteria (CARE Test[TM]). The ratio of the two classes of oligosaccharides is very strongly correlated with the numerical range of DFT (decayed and filled teeth) observed in a young adult population.

The value of saliva to the health and comfort of oral tissues is indisputable. In most cases, the function of specific components in saliva has been conjectured from their activities after isolation and purification.[1]

Many proteins in saliva are glycosylated,[2] and as a class, these glycoproteins have received considerable attention regarding their functional significance. Mucins and agglutinins are standouts in this group. Agglutinins interact with a variety of bacteria, forming aggregates, thereby preventing attachment to oral tissues and facilitating bacterial clearance from the oral cavity.[3] Mucins also possess this capacity, but in addition, form coatings that both lubricate and protect soft and hard tissues in the oral cavity.[4]

A long-recognized value of the oligosaccharides of salivary proteins is that they are blood-type specific, sharing identity with the blood types routinely found on red blood cells. Mucins and other salivary glycoproteins are the carriers of these blood-type oligosaccharides,[5] which like any blood type, may be broadly represented in one individual or nearly nonexistent in another. Several of the oligosaccharide motifs represented on salivary glycoproteins have a concentration range between individuals that exceeds 1,000-fold.[6] Individual differences in amounts of some of these oligosaccharides have been correlated with the number of dental caries in young adults, leading to development of a test, believed to predict caries susceptibility in children.[6,7] This approach of focusing on host factors as predictors of caries susceptibility and ultimately participants in the cariogenic process, while novel, is not unexpected. A variety of host factors with this potential have been identified.[8] However, in a survey of more than 30 clinical studies of models for predicting caries risk, past caries history was the most frequent and reliable indicator of risk of future with caries. Bacterial titers in saliva contribute to the accuracy of their predictability.[9] An inherent problem with these models is that failure to prevent all caries is precluded. Thus, to predict the risk before the onset of any disease is the most desirable.

MATERIALS AND METHODS

Subjects

The young adults accrued for this study were volunteer students from the Dental and Dental Hygiene programs at the University of Southern California, School of Dentistry and represented the reference group for development of the caries susceptibility algorithm. The subjects ranged in age from 24 to 35-year old. This age range represented a stable statistical endpoint for first-time caries acquisition as judged by a lack of significant correlation of their ages with caries history. The subjects included a variety of races and ethnicities. Although detailed medical histories were taken, the only exclusions from algorithm development were if dental sealants had been applied during childhood, or if the subject had taken a medication with known saliva altering properties within the last 24 h. Children, 7–10-years old, were selected because they represent an endpoint for the caries history of their deciduous teeth (decayed and filled surfaces, DFS) and also because an early record of caries in their permanent teeth is already evident. The children were equal in numbers of Asian and Hispanic.

Saliva collection

Resting whole saliva was collected by drooling. All dental examinations were visual and followed the saliva collection. For many of the children and young adults, annual dental examinations were made, spanning 4 and 5 years, and saliva samples were collected and archived at $-80°C$.

Oligosaccharide quantitation

Various species of oligosaccharides were quantitated using dot blot technology. Dried spots of whole saliva were probed with commercially available lectins. The amount of lectin binding was proportional to the amount of a particular oligosaccharide motif that is present in the spot of saliva. The bound lectin was then visualized and quantitated relative to the blood glycoprotein, glycophorin, using a streptavidin-alkaline phosphatase-based reporter system. Lectin combinations used in the test are proprietary.

Mathematical procedures

Linear regression has been reported to be one of best approaches for evaluating correlation of caries risk factors.[9] All results presented here have been achieved by multiple linear regression analyses. However, development of the most recent algorithms involved a combination of multiple linear regression and neural net mathematics. SigmaStat™(SPSS, Inc.) was the primary statistical program used for multiple linear regression, significance, and coefficient of determination (R^2). AI Trilogy™ (Ward Systems Group, Inc.) was used for the neural net mathematics.

The final embodiment of the test device is still in development, and thus, not available for presentation. However, we envision that the test will be able to be administered and evaluated chair side.

RESULTS

The caries risk test evolved from a relationship observed between the MUC7 mucin (MG2) concentration in saliva and caries history (decayed and filled teeth, DFT) in young Caucasian adults.[10] Analysis of the mucin assay system indicated that a negative correlation between this mucin and caries history was actually based on the amount of the sugar, sialic acid, that was bound to the mucin.[11] Sialic acid on mucins had already been shown to be a ligand for the surface adhesins (lectins) of several types of oral bacteria, which can lead to mucin-mediated agglutination and removal from the oral cavity.[12] This association with a likely deterrent of cariogenesis, prompted evaluation of lectins as possible reagents for assessing the relationship between individual patterns of oligosaccharides and caries susceptibility.

The test uses a battery of lectins, some of which target oligosaccharides that are positively correlated with caries history in young adults, while other lectins target oligosaccharides that are negatively correlated. An individual's ratio of these two groups of oligosaccharides correlates with caries history.

Figure 14.1a portrays the strength of the relationship between the oligosaccharide patterns of the salivary glycoproteins of young adults and their caries history, which is organized according to affected tooth groups. The tooth group test output metric has value when applied to children before caries occur, because it provides the rationale for an individualized, targeted program of prevention. The exact mathematical values from the test algorithm are shown in Figure 14.1a; whereas in practice, the test results are rounded to the nearest whole number, yielding an R^2 of 1.00 with sensitivity and specificity of 100% for this phase of test development.

The sensitivity and specificity of the predictive value of the test is still under study. When the algorithm developed in the adult reference group is applied to children, the risk levels are clear and unambiguous (Fig. 14.1b). Over a period of 3 or 4 years, on going studies indicate that these children continue to exhibit caries patterns consistent with their tested risk category. Furthermore, these children also continue to test to the same risk level on an annual repeat basis (not shown).

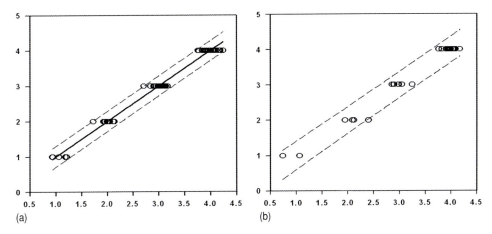

Figure 14.1 (a) Prediction of susceptibility levels in children: test development. Demonstration of algorithm-relating quantitated oligosaccharides in resting saliva to susceptibility levels based on the accumulated pattern of caries disease in adults 24–35-years old. Level 4 exhibits a pattern of caries in molars and premolars. Level 3 is equivalent to caries only in molars. Level 2 has caries in no more than two teeth either in the molars or in combination with a P2 premolar and do not usually appear before age 15. Level 1 is devoid of caries. Regression line of formula (solid line); bracket for the 98% confidence interval of prediction (dashed lines). $N = 71$ subjects; coefficient of determination $(R^2) = 0.985$; significance, $p = <0.0001$. (b) Prediction of susceptibility levels in children: test application. Performance of algorithm, demonstrated in (a), when applied to the saliva of children 7–10-years old. The algorithm formula delivers unambiguous susceptibility levels, based on patterns of caries disease, which are projected to occur by 24-years old if preventive measures are not instituted. 98% confidence interval of prediction (dashed lines). $N = 27$ subjects.

An example of a targeted preventive treatment plan for a child that falls into the highest susceptibility level would be to preemptively seal 14 of their molars and premolars. Observations in adults indicate that caries in the lower P1 premolars is relatively rare, and thus, application of sealant is not expedient. The preventive treatment for level 3 would require only the molars be sealed. We would not recommend sealants for level 2, except perhaps in the later teen years and then only on those teeth that show early signs of cavitation. Level 1 would require no sealants. The results of the test and suggested patterns of sealant application in no way substitute for continuing good oral health and nutrition practices, regular dental visits, and the use of fluoride treatments, especially to prevent smooth surface lesions. The test is complementary to these copreventives and together provides a strategy for near-complete prevention of caries.

DISCUSSION

Dental caries is an infectious disease that, in many ways, resembles other infectious diseases.[13] To initiate the process, most pathogens utilize their surface lectins to bind to specific host oligosaccharides. These oligosaccharides protrude from the cell membranes of the target tissues. For teeth, the host oligosaccharides are components of the saliva-based pellicle coating, and pathogen binding is the step that precedes formation of the cariogenic plaque biofilm.

Most of the target epithelia of the gastrointestinal and respiratory tracts is blanketed with a mucus coating. Pathogens specific for these sites have devised strategies for penetrating or living in the mucus of these tissues as a prelude to attaching to the underlying epithelia. The relationship between mucins and pathogens in the oral cavity appears to be manifested differently. The large gel-forming mucins, such as MUC5B (MG1), are components of the tooth pellicle and contribute lubricity to the coating. By contrast, the smaller mucin MUC7 seems to be primarily involved in management of the microbiota of the oral cavity. The ability of MUC7 mucin to interact with and agglutinate bacteria is dependent on the type of oligosaccharides in the mucin glycoprofile.[12]

As noted earlier, when comparing the dot blot patterns, individual oligosaccharides appear to vary independently with regard to the total amount in saliva. This variation may also be true for different oligosaccharide motifs on the same molecule. MUC7 mucin can carry two different oligosaccharide motifs that bind to human neutrophils on one hand and a variety of oral bacteria on the other.[14,15] In a functional sense, this raises the possibility that the mucin may facilitate opsonization by forming coaggregates of neutrophils and bacteria. Reduced levels of 1 or both oligosaccharides could dramatically alter the functionality of the mucin and thereby result in health-related consequences.

In view of the potential for functional variability due to differences in oligosaccharide patterns on salivary glycoproteins, a model for the caries susceptibility test is proposed that attempts to incorporate fundamental features of the caries test into a context of functional elements of saliva. This model suggests that the oligosaccharide group that is positively correlated with caries history is associated primarily with glycoproteins that contribute to pellicle formation. Alternatively, oligosaccharides that are negatively correlated with caries history would be associated with salivary glycoproteins that function to agglutinate oral bacteria. The ratio of these two groups of oligosaccharides provides the best correlation with caries history and is the best predictor of risk of future caries in children.

Acknowledgments

This project is supported by NIDCR STTR Phase I and Phase II grants, 2 R42 DE014650, "Saliva Test for Caries Risk" to Proactive Oral Solutions, Inc. (P. C. Denny, PI). Clinical studies are performed under subcontract to USC School of Dentistry (J. M. Galligan, PI)

REFERENCES

1. Lamkin MS, Oppenheim FG. Structural features of salivary function. Crit Rev Oral Biol Med 1993;4:251–9.

2. Sondej MA, Denny PA, Xie Y, et al. Glycoprofiling of the human salivary proteome. In: *Proceedings of the 54th ASMS Conference of Mass Spectrometry and Allied Topics*, Seattle, WA, May 28–June 1, 2006.

3. Ligtenberg AJ, Veerman EC, Nieuw Amerongen AV. A role for Lewis a antigens on salivary agglutinin in binding to *Streptococcus mutans*. Antonie van Leeuwenhoek 2000;77:21–30.

4. Nieuw Amerongen AV, Bolscher JGM, Veerman ECI. Salivary mucins: protective functions in relation to their diversity. Glycobiology 1995;5:733–40.

5. Prakobphol A, Leffler H, Fisher SJ. The high-molecular-weight human mucin is the primary salivary carrier of ABH, Le[a], and Le[b] blood group antigens. Crit Rev Oral Biol Med 1993;4:325–33.

6. Denny PC, Denny PA, Takashima J, Si Y, Navazesh M, Galligan, JM. A novel saliva test for caries risk assessment. CDA J 2006;34:287–94.

7. Denny PC, Denny PA, Takashima J, Galligan J, Navazesh M. A novel caries risk test. Ann NY Acad Sci 2007;1098:204–15.

8. Anderson M. Risk assessment and epidemiology of dental caries: review of the literature. Pediat Dent 2002;24:377–85.

9. Powell LV. Caries prediction: a review of the literature. Community Dent Oral Epidemiol 1998;26:361–71.

10. Denny PC, Denny PA, Navazesh M. Correlation of saliva mucin concentrations with caries history in Caucasian young adults. J Dent Res 2003;82(Special Issue B):250.

11. Baughan LW, Robertello FJ, Sarrett DC, Denny PA, Denny PC. Salivary mucin as related to oral *Streptococcus mutans* in the elderly. Oral Micro Immunol 2000;15:10–14.

12. Murray PA, Levine MJ, Reddy MS, Tabak LA, Bergey EJ. Preparation of a sialic acid-binding protein from *Streptococcus mitis* KS32AR. Infect Immun 1986;53:359–65.

13. Sharon N. Carbohydrate-lectin interactions in infectious disease. Adv Exp Med Biol 1996;408:1–8.

14. Prakobphol A, Thomsson KA, Hansson GC, et al. Human low-molecular-weight salivary mucin expresses the sialyl Lewis[x] determinant and has L-selectin ligand activity. Biochemistry 1998;37:4916–27.

15. Prakobphol A, Tangemann K, Rosen SD, Hoover CI, Leffler H, Fisher SJ. Separate oligosaccharide determinants mediate interactions of the low-molecular-weight salivary mucin with neutrophils and bacteria. Biochemistry 1999;38:6817–25.

15

Periodontal disease

Christoph A. Ramseier, Thiago Morelli, Janet S. Kinney,
Meghan Dubois, Lindsay Rayburn,
and William V. Giannobile

INTRODUCTION

Periodontal disease—background

Chronic diseases of the oral cavity include dental decay and periodontal disease, the former being a destruction of the hard tissue of the teeth, while the latter is a group of inflammatory conditions affecting the supporting structures of the dentition.[1] The impact of the dental biofilm on the etiology of periodontal diseases has been well studied. However, it is the paradoxical impact of the susceptible host's inflammatory response to the microbial challenge that ultimately leads to the destruction of periodontal structures and subsequent tooth loss.[2]

Periodontal diseases are further divided into reversible and nonreversible categories. Gingivitis is a reversible inflammatory reaction of the marginal gingiva to dental biofilms. Gingivitis is characterized by an increase in gingival blood flow, enhanced vascular permeability, and influx of cells (polymorphonuclear leukocytes (PMN) and monocyte-macrophages) from the peripheral blood into the periodontal connective tissue. Therefore, clinical soft tissue alterations during the state of gingivitis include redness, edema, and maybe bleeding, or tenderness.

Periodontitis, the destructive category of periodontal disease, is a chronic nonreversible inflammatory state of the supporting structures (Fig. 15.1). After its initiation, the disease progresses with the loss of collagen fibers and attachment to the root surface, apical migration of the pocket epithelium, formation of deepened periodontal pockets, and the resorption of alveolar bone. If left untreated, the disease continues with progressive alveolar bone destruction, leading to increased tooth mobility and subsequent tooth loss.[3]

Chronic periodontitis is the most prevalent form of destructive periodontal disease. From 1988 to 1994, approximately half of US adults (30 years and older) had chronic periodontitis. Further breakdown of these findings indicate that 31% of the US population exhibit mild forms of the disease, 13% display moderate severity, and 4% suffer advanced disease.[4]

Regarding the microbiological challenge aforementioned, an estimate of more than 600 different bacteria are capable of colonizing the human mouth

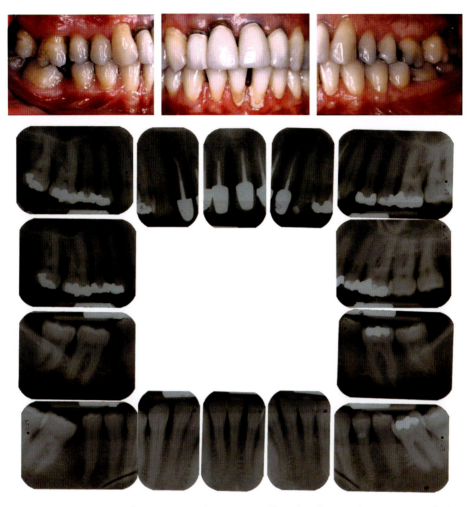

Figure 15.1 Female patient aged 38 years afflicted with periodontitis. Intraoral photographs and radiographs depict gingival tissue loss, plaque biofilm, and radiographic bone loss due to multiple local and systemic risk factors of disease.

with any individual typically harboring 150–200 varying species. Inherent virulence factors of these pathogenic species enable the bacteria to (1) colonize on the tooth and in the gingival sulcus and (2) cause tissue damage to the periodontal tissue by producing potent substances that subsequently trigger the host innate inflammatory response.[5]

Early disease detection and evaluation of periodontal therapy

A periodontal diagnostic tool, in general, provides pertinent information for differential diagnosis, localization of disease, and severity of infection. It serves as a basis for treatment planning and provides means for assessing the effectiveness of periodontal therapy. Current clinical diagnostic parameters that were introduced more than half a century ago continue to function as the basic model for periodontal diagnosis in clinical practice today. They include various parameters such as probing pocket depths, bleeding on probing, clinical attachment levels, plaque index, and radiographs quantifying alveolar bone levels.[6] Albeit easy to use, cost-effective, and relatively noninvasive, clinical attachment loss evaluation by the periodontal probe measures damage from past episodes of destruction and requires a 2- to 3-mm threshold change before a site with significant breakdown can be identified. Furthermore, the use of subtraction radiography offers means to detect minute changes in alveolar bone calcium content. These measures, however, are rarely seen in dental clinical practice today. Moreover, they lack the capacity to identify highly susceptible patients who are at risk for future breakdown.[7]

Need for a periodontal diagnostic indicator

The diagnosis of active phases of periodontal disease and the identification of patients at risk for active disease represents challenges for clinical investigators and practitioners. Researchers are confronted with the need for an innovative diagnostic test that focuses on the early recognition of the microbial challenge to the host. Optimal innovative approaches would correctly determine the presence of current disease activity, predict sites vulnerable for future breakdown, and assess the response to periodontal interventions. A new paradigm for periodontal diagnosis would ultimately affect improved clinical management of periodontal patients.

Researchers involved in periodontal disease diagnostics are currently investigating the possible use of oral fluids such as saliva for disease diagnosis.[8] Professionals in seemingly unrelated arenas such as the insurance industry, Environmental Protection Agency, and Homeland Security are interested in the possibility of oral fluid use as well for rapid screening of oral and systemic health status.

MARKERS OF PERIODONTAL DISEASE FROM SECRETED SALIVA

Secretions from the major salivary glands (parotid, submandibular, and sublingual), which have a large number of proteins and peptides, are responsible for maintenance of oral cavity integrity (Table 15.1). Also, because of its importance in oral biofilm formation and host defense, secreted saliva may have a significant role in the establishment and progression of periodontal disease.

Markers affecting the dental biofilm

Specific markers

Immunoglobulins (Ig) are important specific defense factors of saliva. Of the different classes of immunoglobulins, IgA, IgG, and IgM influence the oral

Table 15.1 Major salivary gland secretion mediators associated with periodontal diseases.

Marker	Relationship to periodontal disease	Type of periodontal disease
Specific		
Immunoglobulins (IgA, IgM, IgG)	Interfere in the adherence and bacterial metabolism/↑ concentration in saliva of periodontal patients	Chronic and aggressive
Nonspecific		
Mucins	Interfere in the colonization of *A. actinomycetemcomitans*	Aggressive
Lysozyme	Regulates plaque biofilm accumulation	Chronic
Lactoferrin	Inhibits microbial growth/↑ correlation with *A. actinomycetemcomitans*	Aggressive
Histatin	Neutralizes LPS and enzymes known to affect the periodontium	Chronic and aggressive
Peroxidase	Interferes in plaque accumulation/↑ correlation with periodontal patients	Chronic
Systemic		
CRP	↑Concentration found in serum and saliva of periodontal patients	Chronic and aggressive

microbiota by interfering in the adherence of bacteria or by inhibiting bacterial metabolism, IgA being the predominant immunoglobulin. Patients with periodontal disease are shown to have higher salivary concentrations of IgA, IgG, and IgM specific to periodontal pathogens as compared to healthy patients.[9] Additionally, levels of these immunoglobulins in saliva are greatly reduced after periodontal treatment.[10] As a consequence, the screening of saliva, especially for IgA antibodies, has been previously discussed as a useful, noninvasive technique to identify individuals with potential to develop periodontal disease or those who are currently responding to a periopathogenic infection.[11]

Nonspecific markers

Mucins are glycoproteins produced by submandibular and sublingual salivary glands and numerous minor salivary glands. The physiological functions of the mucins (MG1 and MG2) are cytoprotection, lubrification, protection against dehydration, and maintenance of viscoelasticity in secretions. MG2 mucin affects the aggregation and adherence of bacteria and is known to interact with *Aggregatibacter actinomycetemcomitans* and the decline of MG2 concentration in saliva may increase colonization of this periopathogen.[12]

Lysozyme is an antimicrobial enzyme able to cleave chemical bonds in the bacterial cell wall. It can lyse some bacterial species by hydrolyzing glycosidic linkages in the cell wall peptidoglycan. It may also cause lyses of bacterial cells by interacting with monovalent anions and with proteases found in saliva. This combination leads to destabilization of the cell membrane likely due to activation and deregulation of endogenous bacterial autolysins. Patients with low levels of lysozyme in saliva are more susceptible to plaque accumulation, which is considered a risk factor for periodontal disease.[13]

Lactoferrin is an iron-binding glycoprotein produced by salivary glands, which inhibits microbial growth by sequestering iron from the environment, and thus depriving bacteria of this essential element. This glycoprotein is strongly upregulated in mucosal secretions during gingival inflammation and is detected in high concentration in saliva of patients with periodontal disease as compared to healthy patients.[14]

Histatin is a salivary protein with antimicrobial properties secreted in parotid and submandibular glands. It neutralizes the endotoxic lipopolysaccharide located in the membrane of gram-negative bacteria. Histatin is also an inhibitor of host and bacterial enzymes involved in the destruction of the periodontium. In addition to its antimicrobial activities, histatin is involved in the inhibition of the release of histamine from mast cells, affecting its role in oral inflammation.[15,16]

Peroxidase is a salivary enzyme produced by acinar cells in salivary glands. This enzyme removes toxic hydrogen peroxide produced by oral microorganisms and reduces acid production in dental biofilm, decreasing plaque accumulation and establishment of gingivitis and caries. Patients with periodontal disease have demonstrated high levels of this enzyme in saliva.[17]

Systemic markers related to periodontal infection

C-reactive protein (CRP) is a systemic marker released during the acute phase of an inflammatory response. CRP is produced by the liver and is stimulated by circulating cytokines, such as TNF-α and IL-1, affected by periodontal inflammation. Circulating CRP may reach saliva via gingival crevicular fluid (GCF) or the salivary glands (Fig. 15.2). Chronic and aggressive periodontal diseases have been associated with high levels of CRP in addition to other inflammatory biomarkers.[18] Studies have demonstrated that periodontal patients display elevated concentrations of serum CRP as compared to healthy individuals.[19] CRP has recently been measurable in saliva from periodontal patients using a "lab-on-a-chip" method.[20]

MARKERS OF PERIODONTAL DISEASE FROM WHOLE SALIVA

Significance of gingival crevicular fluid

Easily collected and containing local and systemic-derived biomarkers of periodontal disease, oral fluids may offer the basis for patient-specific diagnostic tests for periodontal disease (Fig. 15.3). GCF is both a physiological fluid as well as an inflammatory exudate originating from the gingival plexus of blood vessels in the gingival corium, subjacent to the epithelium lining of the

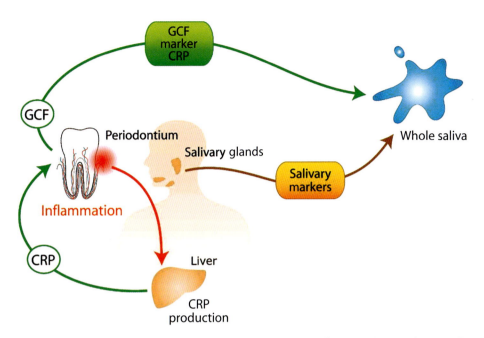

Figure 15.2 Schematic overview of the stimulation of CRP in the liver by periodontal pathogens and its subsequent release into GCF and whole saliva, respectively.

dentogingival space. As GCF traverses through inflamed periodontal tissues en route to the sulcus, biological molecular markers are gathered from the surrounding site and subsequently deluded into whole saliva. GCF sampling methods have been shown to accurately capture inflammatory and connective tissue breakdown mediators. More than 90 different components in GCF have been evaluated to date for periodontal diagnosis.[21] Of the numerous constituents in GCF, however, the vast majority constitute soft tissues inflammatory events, while only a few are regarded as specific biomarkers of alveolar bone destruction.[22]

Markers of periodontal soft tissue inflammation

During the initiation of an inflammatory response in the periodontal connective tissue, numerous cytokines such as PGE_2, IL-1β, IL-6, or TNF-α are released from cells of the junctional epithelia, connective tissue fibroblasts, macrophages, and PMNs (Fig. 15.4). Subsequently, a number of enzymes such as MMP-8, MMP-9, or MMP-13 are produced by PMNs and osteoclasts, leading to the degradation of connective tissue collagen and alveolar bone. During the inflammatory process, intercellular products are created and migrate toward the gingival sulcus or periodontal pocket.

Prostaglandins are arachidonic acid metabolites composed of ten classes, of which D, E, F, G, H, and I are of main importance. Of this group, PGE_2 is one of the most extensively studied mediators of periodontal disease activity. During the host's innate defense response to bacterial lipopolysaccharide, monocytes,

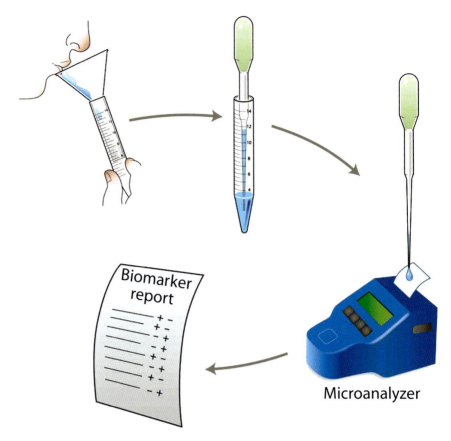

Figure 15.3 Strategy for oral fluid sampling and analysis with a rapid point-of-care, or lab-on-a-chip device for the generation of a periodontal disease biomarker report.

PMNs, macrophages, and other cells release IL-1, TNF, and PGE_2. PGE_2 acts as a potent vasodilator and increases capillary permeability, which elicit clinical signs of redness and edema. PGE_2 also stimulates fibroblasts and osteoclasts to increase production of matrix metalloproteinases (MMPs).[23]

Markers of alveolar bone loss

Many different biomarkers associated with bone formation, resorption, and turnover have been evaluated in GCF and saliva such as alkaline phosphatase, osteocalcin, osteonectin, and collagen telopeptidases, reviewed in reference 22. These mediators are associated with local bone metabolism (in the case of periodontitis) as well as systemic conditions (such as osteoporosis or metastatic bone cancers).

MMPs are host proteinases responsible for both tissue degradation and re-modeling. During progressive periodontal breakdown, gingival and periodontal ligament collagens are cleaved by host cell-derived interstitial collagenases. Matrix metalloproteinase-8 (MMP-8) is the most prevalent MMP found in

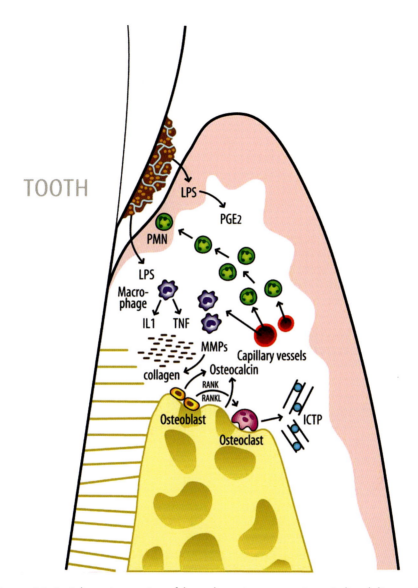

Figure 15.4 Schematic overview of the pathogenic processes in periodontal disease. Initial events are triggered by lipopolysaccharide (LPS) from gram-negative plaque biofilms on the tooth root surfaces. As a first line of defense, polymorphonuclear leukocytes (PMNs) are recruited to the site. Monocytes and activated macrophages respond to endotoxin by releasing cytokines (tumor necrosis factor alpha, TNF-α, and interleukin 1 beta, IL-1β), which stimulate further tissue destruction. Matrix metalloproteinases (MMPs), powerful collagen-destroying enzymes, are produced by fibroblasts and PMNs. TNF-α, IL-1β, and receptor activator of NF-$\kappa\beta$ ligand (RANKL) are elevated in active sites and mediate osteoclastogenesis and bone breakdown. Bone-specific markers such as pyridinoline cross-linked carboxyterminal telopeptide of type I collagen (ICTP) are released into the surrounding area and transported by way of gingival crevicular fluid (GCF) into the pocket and serve as potential biomarkers for periodontal disease detection.

diseased periodontal tissue and GCF. Elevated MMP-8 levels in active disease progression were observed in a longitudinal study using patients with gingivitis, nonprogressive and progressive periodontitis.[24,25] Recently, MMP-8 was demonstrated to be highly elevated in saliva from patients with periodontal disease using a rapid point-of-care microfluidic device.[26] MMP-8 is also elevated in peri-implant sulcular fluid from peri-implantitis lesions.[27] Collectively, these results offer optimistic hope for the use of MMP-8 as a biomarker for the active phase of peri-implant disease. Longitudinal studies are required to evaluate MMP-8 either alone or in conjunction with other molecular biomarkers to predict the risk of future disease occurrence and monitor treatment interventions.

Gelatinase (MMP-9), another member of the collagenase family, is produced by neutrophils and degrades collagen intercellular ground substance. In a longitudinal study, patients were asked to rinse and expectorate, providing subject-based instead of site-based GCF samples.[28] When analyzed, a twofold increase in mean MMP-9 levels was reported in patients with progressive attachment loss. Given these results, future use of MMP-9 in oral fluid diagnostics may serve as a guide in periodontal treatment monitoring.

Collagenase-3, referred to as matrix metalloproteinase 13 (MMP-13), is another collagenolytic matrix metalloproteinase with an exceptionally wide substrate specificity. MMP-13 has also been implicated to peri-implantitis. It was concluded that elevated levels of both MMP-13 and MMP-8 correlated with irreversible perio-implant vertical bone loss around loosening dental implants.[29] In the future, MMP-13 may be useful for diagnosing and monitoring the course of periodontal disease as well as tracking the efficacy of therapy.[30]

Given the specificity and sensitivity for bone resorption, pyridinoline cross-links, such as pyridinoline cross-linked carboxyterminal telopeptide of type I collagen (ICTP), represent a potentially valuable diagnostic aid for periodontal disease. Several investigations have explored the ability of pyridinoline cross-links to detect bone resorption in periodontitis, peri-implantitis as well as in response to periodontal therapy.[31–33] In brief, these studies assessing the role of GCF ICTP levels as a diagnostic marker of periodontal disease activity have produced promising results to date. ICTP has been shown to be a promising predictor of both future alveolar bone loss and attachment loss. Furthermore, ICTP was strongly correlated with clinical parameters and putative periodontal pathogens, and demonstrated significant reductions after periodontal therapy. Controlled human longitudinal trials are needed to fully establish the role of salivary ICTP as a predictor of periodontal tissue destruction, disease activity, and response to therapy in periodontal patients.

Elevated serum osteocalcin levels have been found during periods of rapid bone turnover such as osteoporosis, multiple myeloma, and fracture repair. Therefore, studies have investigated the relationship between GCF osteocalcin levels and periodontal disease. When a combination of the biochemical markers such as osteocalcin, collagenase, PGE_2, α-2 macroglobulin, elastase, and alkaline phosphatase was evaluated, increased diagnostic sensitivity and specificity values of 80 and 91%, respectively, were reported.[34]

Osteopontin (OPN) is a single-chain polypeptide having a molecular weight of approximately 32,600. In bone matrix, OPN is highly concentrated at sites where osteoclasts are attached to the underlying mineral surface, that is, the clear zone attachment areas of the plasma membrane. Results from periodontal studies indicated that OPN concentrations in GCF increased proportionally with the progression of disease; and when nonsurgical periodontal treatment was provided, GCF OPN levels were significantly reduced. Although additional long-term prospective studies are needed, at this point OPN appears to hold promise as a possible salivary biomarker of periodontal disease progression.[35]

CLINICAL APPLICATIONS

Rapid point-of-care diagnostics for periodontal disease

Periodontal surveillance and disease diagnosis will greatly advance over the coming years via the use of rapid point-of-care (POC) oral diagnostics. The drug discovery process has been an excellent catalyst to link together novel therapeutics to emerging diagnostic disease biomarkers. This connection in biomedicine has led to the development of prototype rapid, accurate, and "real-time" assessment of multiple diseases, including periodontal disease. Novel technologies such as lab-on-a-chip and microfluidic devices offer potential to manage complex oral fluids like saliva and GCF to provide a determination of a patient's periodontal disease risk profile, current disease "activity," and response to therapeutic interventions. This approach should accelerate clinical decision making and monitoring of episodic disease progression in a chronic infectious disease such as periodontitis.[36]

The use of optimized POC devices for periodontal surveillance will likely require less training and fewer resources than current diagnostic tests; could lead to better utilization of skilled clinicians for simpler and less intensive treatment; and result in a more cost-effective healthcare delivery. The portable, easy-to-use diagnostic tools will allow patients to be screened for periodontal disease in settings other than the dental practice, such as at a physician's office or in the home, allowing patients to be directed for treatment. Periodontal oral diagnostic devices will also enable screening of large populations, especially the underserved communities and resource-poor areas, around the globe more quickly and effectively than current inefficient screening approaches. The potential to sample various populations will help better identify at-risk groups and increase access to treatment for those most at need, improving public health.[37]

While the future of periodontal disease diagnosis using salivary diagnostics looks promising, significant obstacles lay ahead before these approaches will be widely available in the clinical setting. Validation of novel periodontal diagnostics will need to be benchmarked with existing "gold standards" of disease such as alveolar bone levels and clinical attachment levels in large patient populations. Acceptance by dentists and treatment clinicians is also necessary and may prove difficult. The dental community is not familiar with mass screening of populations for oral and systemic diseases. If more efficient periodontal therapy can be delivered, clinicians will be more likely to utilize new diagnostic approaches. A greater emphasis must be placed on clinician education in diagnostics, disease risk, and disease prevention through the public health sector before diagnostics will be integrated into routine clinical periodontal practice.[38]

Although many challenges lay ahead, the use of saliva-based oral fluid diagnostics appears promising for future application to diagnose and prognosticate periodontal treatment outcomes.

Acknowledgments

The authors appreciate Mr. Chris Jung for preparation of the figures. This work was supported by NIH/NIDCR grant U01-DE14961 and NCRR grant M01-RR000042 to William V. Giannobile, 5 T32 RR023257 to Meghan Dubois and Lindsay Rayburn, and research scholarship from the Swiss Society of Periodontology (SSP) to Christoph A. Ramseier.

REFERENCES

1. Armitage GC. Development of a classification system for periodontal diseases and conditions. Ann Periodontol 1999;4(1):1–6.
2. Page RC, Kornman KS. The pathogenesis of human periodontitis: an introduction. Periodontology 2000 1997;14:9–11.
3. Offenbacher S. Periodontal diseases: pathogenesis. Ann Periodontol 1996;1(1):821–78.
4. Albandar JM, Brunelle JA, Kingman A. Destructive periodontal disease in adults 30 years of age and older in the United States, 1988–1994. J Periodontol 1999;70(1):13–29.
5. Listgarten MA. Structure of surface coatings on teeth. A review. J Periodontol 1976;47(3):139–47.
6. Armitage GC. The complete periodontal examination. Periodontology 2000 2004;34:22–33.
7. Goodson JM. Diagnosis of periodontitis by physical measurement: interpretation from episodic disease hypothesis. J Periodontol 1992;63(4 Suppl):373–82.
8. Malamud D. Salivary diagnostics: the future is now. J Am Dent Assoc 2006;137(3):284–6.
9. Seemann R, Hagewald SJ, Sztankay V, Drews J, Bizhang M, Kage A. Levels of parotid and submandibular/sublingual salivary immunoglobulin A in response to experimental gingivitis in humans. Clin Oral Investig 2004;8(4):233–7.
10. Reiff RL. Serum and salivary IgG and IgA response to initial preparation therapy. J Periodontol 1984;55(5):299–305.
11. Mandel ID. Markers of periodontal disease susceptibility and activity derived from saliva. In: Johnson NW, ed., *Periodontal Diseases—Markers of Disease Susceptibility and Activity*. Cambridge, NY: Cambridge University Press; 1991:228–53.

12. Groenink J, Ligtenberg AJ, Veerman EC, Bolscher JG, Nieuw Ameron-gen AV. Interaction of the salivary low-molecular-weight mucin (MG2) with *Actinobacillus actinomycetemcomitans*. Antonie Van Leeuwenhoek 1996;70(1):79–87.
13. Jalil RA, Ashley FP, Wilson RF. The relationship between 48-h dental plaque accumulation in young human adults and the concentrations of hypothiocyanite, "free" and "total" lysozyme, lactoferrin and secretory immunoglobulin A in saliva. Arch Oral Biol 1992;37(1):23–8.
14. Groenink J, Walgreen-Weterings E, Nazmi K, et al. Salivary lactoferrin and low-Mr mucin MG2 in *Actinobacillus actinomycetemcomitans*-associated periodontitis. J Clin Periodontol 1999;26(5):269–75.
15. Gusman H, Travis J, Helmerhorst EJ, Potempa J, Troxler RF, Oppenheim FG. Salivary histatin 5 is an inhibitor of both host and bacterial enzymes implicated in periodontal disease. Infect Immun 2001;69(3):1402–408.
16. Helmerhorst EJ, Oppenheim FG. Saliva: a dynamic proteome. J Dent Res 2007;86(8):680–93.
17. Guven Y, Satman I, Dinccag N, Alptekin S. Salivary peroxidase activity in whole saliva of patients with insulin-dependent (type-1) diabetes mellitus. J Clin Periodontol 1996;23(9):879–81.
18. D'Aiuto F, Ready D, Tonetti MS. Periodontal disease and C-reactive protein-associated cardiovascular risk. J Periodontal Res 2004;39(4):236–41.
19. Tonetti MS, D'Aiuto F, Nibali L, et al. Treatment of periodontitis and endothelial function. N Engl J Med 2007;356(9):911–20.
20. Christodoulides N, Mohanty S, Miller CS, et al. Application of microchip assay system for the measurement of C-reactive protein in human saliva. Lab Chip 2005;5(3):261–9.
21. Loos BG, Tjoa S. Host-derived diagnostic markers for periodontitis: do they exist in gingival crevice fluid? Periodontology 2000 2005;39:53–72.
22. Kinney JS, Ramseier CA, Giannobile WV. Oral fluid-based biomarkers of alveolar bone loss in periodontitis. Ann N Y Acad Sci 2007;1098:230–51.
23. Airila-Mansson S, Soder B, Kari K, Meurman JH. Influence of combinations of bacteria on the levels of prostaglandin E2, interleukin-1beta, and granulocyte elastase in gingival crevicular fluid and on the severity of periodontal disease. J Periodontol 2006;77(6):1025–31.
24. Miller CS, King CP, Jr, Langub MC, Kryscio RJ, Thomas MV. Salivary biomarkers of existing periodontal disease: a cross-sectional study. J Am Dent Assoc 2006;137(3):322–9.
25. Birkedal-Hansen H. Role of matrix metalloproteinases in human periodontal diseases. J Periodontol 1993;64(5 Suppl):474–84.
26. Herr AE, Hatch AV, Throckmorton DJ, et al. Microfluidic immunoassays as rapid saliva-based clinical diagnostics. Proc Natl Acad Sci USA 2007;104(13):5268–73.
27. Kivela-Rajamaki M, Maisi P, Srinivas R, et al. Levels and molecular forms of MMP-7 (matrilysin-1) and MMP-8 (collagenase-2) in diseased human peri-implant sulcular fluid. J Periodontal Res 2003;38(6):583–90.
28. Teng YT, Sodek J, McCulloch CA. Gingival crevicular fluid gelatinase and its relationship to periodontal disease in human subjects. J Periodontal Res 1992;27(5):544–52.

29. Ma J, Kitti U, Teronen O, et al. Collagenases in different categories of peri-implant vertical bone loss. J Dent Res 2000;79(11):1870–73.
30. Hernandez M, Valenzuela MA, Lopez-Otin C, et al. Matrix metalloproteinase-13 is highly expressed in destructive periodontal disease activity. J Periodontol 2006;77(11):1863–70.
31. Giannobile WV. C-telopeptide pyridinoline cross-links. Sensitive indicators of periodontal tissue destruction. Ann N Y Acad Sci 1999;878:404–12.
32. Oringer RJ, Palys MD, Iranmanesh A, et al. C-telopeptide pyridinoline cross-links (ICTP) and periodontal pathogens associated with endosseous oral implants. Clin Oral Implants Res 1998;9(6):365–73.
33. Talonpoika JT, Hamalainen MM. Type I collagen carboxyterminal telopeptide in human gingival crevicular fluid in different clinical conditions and after periodontal treatment. J Clin Periodontol 1994;21(5):320–26.
34. Nakashima K, Giannopoulou C, Andersen E, et al. A longitudinal study of various crevicular fluid components as markers of periodontal disease activity. J Clin Periodontol 1996;23(9):832–8.
35. Sharma CG, Pradeep AR. Gingival crevicular fluid osteopontin levels in periodontal health and disease. J Periodontol 2006;77(10):1674–80.
36. Giannobile WV. Periodontal surveillance—implications in the promotion of public health. J Periodontol 2007;78(7):1177.
37. Yager P, Edwards T, Fu E, et al. Microfluidic diagnostic technologies for global public health. Nature 2006;442(7101):412–8.
38. Tabak LA. Point-of-care diagnostics enter the mouth. Ann N Y Acad Sci 2007;1098:7–14.

Role of saliva in detection of substance abuse

16

Uttam Garg and Lance Presley

INTRODUCTION

Substance abuse is a major social problem with its significant impact on public safety and lost productivity. Governmental, industrial, and sports agencies are increasingly involved in substance abuse control. Currently, urine and blood are the most commonly used specimen types for drugs of abuse testing. In these specimen types, commonly abused drugs and/or their metabolites can be detected from a few hours to a few days. One of the common reasons for use of these samples is their high concentration of drugs. In recent years, with the advent of sensitive methods and many other advantages, the interest in alternate samples such as hair, oral fluid, and sweat is growing. Advantages and disadvantages of these sample types are shown in Table 16.1 and approximate detection times for various sample types are shown in Figure 16.1. Of these alternate sample types, saliva is the most common alternate matrix for the detection of drug abuse. In many circumstances saliva is a preferred matrix over urine and blood as it is easy to collect on-site and provides a better indication of recent drug use. Furthermore in forensic situations, saliva can be collected under direct supervision without the need for special sample collection facility.[1] Also, the concentrations of drugs in saliva correlate better with blood concentrations as compared to urine. Although therapeutic drugs and hormones have been measured in saliva, its main application has been in drugs of abuse testing.[2,3]

A number of factors affect the concentration of drugs in saliva. Plasma pH, saliva pH, drug ionization, and protein binding are important factors in determining the drug concentration.[4] Saliva pH and volume varies under different conditions and does affect the drug concentrations. Saliva is slightly acidic, but its pH increases with increase in flow rate from a low of approximately 5.5 to a high of 7.9. Even though saliva composition changes with the flow rate, it approximately contains 90% water and 10% solutes such as electrolytes, amylase, glucose, urea, and proteins. Some of the mechanisms by which drugs incorporate into saliva include passive diffusion, ultrafiltration, and secretion. Drugs are also deposited in the oral cavity during smoking and through oral and intranasal administration.[2,3,5]

Table 16.1 Advantages and disadvantages of different specimen types for detection of substance abuse.

Specimen	Advantages	Disadvantages
Blood	• Detects recent use • Correlates better with impairment • Sample difficult to adulterate	• Needs trained person for sample collection • Lack of point-of-care devices for blood • Rapid drug clearance
Hair	• Supervised, noninvasive sample collection • Longer detection window • Sample stable for years • Sample can be obtained from mummified or exhumed bodies	• Does not detect recent use • Sample may not be available • Hair color bias issues • Expensive analysis • Environmental contamination
Oral fluid	• Detects recent use • Easy, supervised, noninvasive sample collection • Point-of-care testing available	• Shorter detection window • Contamination from passive exposure • Some individuals may not be able to provide sample
Sweat	• Provides longer and cumulative drug exposure (3–14 days) • Easy, noninvasive sample collection • Collection devices are tamper resistant	• Intersubject variation in sweat production • Expensive analysis • Requires laboratory analysis: point-of-care tests not available
Urine	• Most standardized and studied specimen • Well-established laboratory practices • Larger menu • Less expensive • Point-of-care tests available	• Sample collection needs special facility • Collection may be considered invasive • High potential for sample adulteration • Shorter detection window • Drug concentration influenced by hydration status

SAMPLE COLLECTION

Currently, the collection of saliva is not very well standardized, and there are various techniques for its collection. Prior to sample collection, supervision of donor for 10–20 min is recommended. The donor should not be allowed to put anything in his/her mouth during this period. Expectoration or spitting using nonstimulated technique produces more froth than actual liquid resulting in viscous and small sample size that can be difficult to work with in the laboratory. Also, it may get contaminated with food and other debris. Due to these reasons, stimulation of saliva by sour candy or citric acid crystals has been used. Some techniques use manual stimulation by chewing on inert material

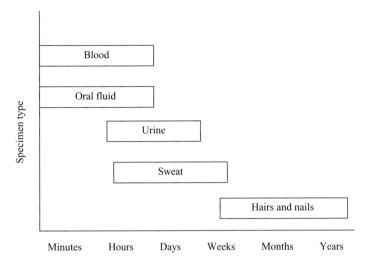

Figure 16.1   Relative detection times in various sample types.

such as Teflon. Materials such as Parafilm should not be used as it may absorb lipophilic drugs. Various commercial collectors use absorbent pad or foam for stimulation and collection of saliva. These pads may be placed in diluents before shipping the sample to the laboratory. Samples collected using collection devices generally provide cleaner, higher-volume specimens as compared to direct spitting. Collection methods for some of these commercially available devices are shown in Table 16.2.[2]

Once the saliva sample is collected, it can be screened on-site or tested in the laboratory. A number of point-of-collection devices with various collection techniques are available (Table 16.2). The point-of-care devices vary significantly for sensitivity and specificity for different drugs. Depending on the

Table 16.2   Various collection devices and their method of sampling.[2]

Name of collector	Method of sampling
DrugWipe®	Swipe only (tongue or skin)
Cozart® collector	Absorbent foam pad plus diluent
Dräger DrugTest®	Absorbent foam pad with diluent
Intercept®	Absorbent foam pad with diluent
OralScreen®	Absorbent foam pad only, drops applied to device
OralLab®	Absorbent foam pad, collector squeezed to apply oral fluid into test cartridge
OraTect®	Absorbent directly connected to device
Quantisal®	Absorbent foam pad plus diluent
SalivaScreen®	Absorbent foam pad, drops applied to device
Salivette®	Cotton wool swab which is then filtered and centrifuged
Toxiquick®	Absorbent bud, oral fluid squeezed into syringe and applied to device

Table 16.3 SAMHSA proposed initial cutoff concentrations for oral fluid samples.[10]

Analyte	Concentration (ng/mL)
THC parent drug and metabolite	4
Cocaine metabolites	20
Opiate Metabolites[a]	40
Phencyclidine	10
Amphetamines[b]	50
MDMA	50

[a] Laboratories are permitted to initially test all specimens for 6-acetylmorphine using a 4-ng/mL cutoff.
[b] Methamphetamine is the target analyte.

specific use, a particular point-of-collection device should be evaluated. Since the performance of these point-of-care devices is inconsistent, screening and confirmation of drugs using laboratory methods is preferred.

When sending samples to a laboratory, proper sample handling is important. Chain-of custody issues are similar to that of other legal samples such as blood and urine. Specimen stability is another issue. Several studies have shown that most of the drugs are stable for several days at 4°C or room temperature.[6,7] When using a particular device, recovery and stability of drugs of interest should be carried out under the conditions in which the device will be used.[8]

In the laboratory setting, screening is generally done by immunoassay, typically enzyme-linked immunosorbent assays (ELISA). While ELISA is a reliable technique for the initial testing of saliva specimens, it is more costly and time consuming than liquid immunoassays. Reagent manufactures have developed liquid immunoassay reagents traditionally used for urine testing for saliva testing (Moore C., personal communication, Immunalysis Corporation, Pomona, CA).[9] Automation of the assays will make saliva testing more cost-effective and easier to adapt on existing platforms. When used forensically, the immunoassay screen should be followed by confirmation using a chromatographic mass spectrometric technique such as gas chromatography-mass spectrometry (GC-MS) and liquid chromatography-mass spectrometry (LC-MS). Currently, GC-MS is the most widely used technique for the confirmation of drugs of abuse. Substance Abuse Mental Health Services Administration (SAMHSA) provides guidelines for initial and confirmatory cutoffs for various drugs of abuse in saliva (Tables 16.3 and 16.4).[10] Confirmation procedures must be analytically validated for performance. SAMSHA recommends the measurement of human IgG to rule out the possible sample adulteration.[10]

To compare their accuracies, laboratories participate in proficiency testing programs. In the United States, the National Laboratory Certification Program has provided saliva samples of known drug content to participating laboratories. The study has grown to 16 participant laboratories since its inception in 2000. Data from 2006 show low inter-laboratory variance.[11]

Table 16.4 SAMHSA proposed confirmatory cutoff concentrations for oral fluid samples.[10]

Analyte	Concentration (ng/mL)
THC parent drug	2
Cocaine[a]	8
Opiates	
Morphine	40
Codeine	40
6-Acetylmorphine	4
Phencyclidine	10
Amphetamines	
Amphetamine	50
Methamphetamine[b]	50
MDMA	50
MDA	50
MDEA	50

[a] Cocaine or benzoylecgonine.
[b] Specimen must also contain amphetamine at a concentration greater than or equal to the limit of detection.

Questions have been raised about the adulterants during saliva sample collection. A number of products are available on the internet that guarantee to beat oral fluid drug testing. There is no evidence that these products really work. Wong et al.[12] investigated the effects of various adulterants and foodstuffs on Oratect device and found that these products do not interfere in the testing. In addition, two commercial adulterant products "Clear Choice Fizzy Flush" and "Kleen Mouthwash" were also tested. These products had no effect in destroying the drug compounds or changing the pH of the oral fluid. The effect of these adulterants was through washing of oral cavity and was not different from a common mouthwash. In another study, a series of potential adulterants of oral fluid were evaluated on Cozart microplate EIA for opiates, and no effect of these adulterants was found.[13]

CORRELATION OF SALIVA WITH URINE AND BLOOD

For most drugs urine has the highest concentration of metabolites, whereas blood and saliva have higher concentrations of the parent drugs. For example, there is only a small amount of carboxy metabolite of δ-9-tetrahydrocannabinol (THC) in saliva. However, due to rapid metabolism of cocaine, benzoylecgonine and ecgonine methyl ester are detectable in saliva. Therefore, the drug testing in saliva should target the parent drugs. The correlation of drugs between blood and saliva depends on several factors including pH of saliva, protein binding of the drug, and its pK. For acidic drugs, the concentration is

Table 16.5 Average oral fluid to blood concentration of some drugs.[2]

Drug (type)	Average oral fluid to blood concentration ratio
Alcohol (ethanol)	1.07
Barbiturates	0.3
Buprenorphine	1
Codeine (basic)	4
Methamphetamine (basic)	2
MDMA (basic)	7
Cocaine (basic)	3
Diazepam (acidic)	0.01–0.02
Methadone (basic)	1.6
Morphine (basic)	0.8
δ-9-Tetrahydrocannabinol (neutral)	1.2

lower in saliva, whereas for basic drugs the concentration is higher in saliva. During recent use and in the absorptive phase, the drug concentrations are higher in saliva as compared to blood.[2,4] Average oral fluid to blood concentration of some drugs is shown in Table 16.5.[2]

Studies have compared the positivity rate of drugs in saliva and blood. In one large study using 77,218 specimens, rate of positivity for amphetamines, cannabinoids, cocaine, opiates, and phencyclidine (PCP) in nonregulated workplace drug testing programs was investigated.[14] The saliva samples were collected using Intercept Oral Collection device (OraSure Technologies, Bethlehem, PA). The device consists of absorbent cotton fiber pad, which is placed between the lower gum and cheek for 2–5 min for sample collection. The collected sample is placed in the preservative solution for transportation to the laboratory. In this study the samples were screened by enzyme immunoassay for THC (parent drug and metabolite), cocaine metabolites, opiate metabolites, PCP, and amphetamines at cutoffs of 3, 15, 30, 3, and 120 ng/mL, respectively. The screen positive samples were confirmed using GC-MS-MS at cutoff values of 1.5, 6, 30, 30, 3, 1.5, 120, and 120 ng/mL for THC (parent drug), benzoylecgonine, morphine, codeine, 6-acetylmorphine, PCP, amphetamine, and methamphetamine, respectively. Confirmed positive rate in this study was 5.1% (3,908 out of 77,218). Of these five drug categories, marijuana and cocaine accounted for 85.75% of the positives. The order of rate of positivity was THC > cocaine > amphetamines > opiates > PCP. Overall positive rate in this study was comparable to the urine (N > 5,200,000, urine positive rate of 4.46%). Oral fluid positivity rate, for amphetamine and cocaine, was 60% higher than urine suggesting that these drugs accumulate more efficiently in saliva as compared to urine. Another remarkable finding in this study was the presence of 6-acetylmorphine in 67% morphine-positive samples indicating the wide use of heroin. However, in another report on 114 adult arrestees, the sensitivity for THC detection in saliva was only 5% as compared to urine. Use of different cutoffs and analytical methods may be the reason for these differences.

Cocaine and heroin had sensitivity of 100 and 88% and specificity of 99 and 100%, respectively.[15]

DETECTION OF SPECIFIC DRUGS IN ORAL FLUID: AMPHETAMINE, METHAMPHETAMINE, AND RELATED SYMPATHOMIMETIC AMINES

Amphetamines and methamphetamine are central nervous system stimulants with limited legitimate use. They are used in the treatment of narcolepsy, obesity, and attention-deficit disorders. However, due to initial euphoric affects, these drugs have high potential of abuse and addiction. Other sympathomimetic drugs with very high abuse potential include designer drugs such as methylenedioxyamphetamine (MDA), methylenedioxymethamphetamine (MDMA), and methylenedioxyethamphetamine (MDEA). Although urine is the most common matrix for the detection of sympathomimetic drugs, these drugs have been detected in saliva. The analytical methods for detection of amphetamine include immunoassays, GC-MS, and LC-MS.

The concentration of sympathomimetic amines in saliva is generally much higher as compared to plasma. In a study on human volunteers, who received four doses of 10 and/or 20 mg S-(+)-methamphetamine within 7 days, oral fluid methamphetamine concentrations were higher than plasma; average 24-h area under the curve was 3.8 times higher than plasma. Although there was significant intra- and interindividual variability, there was a correlation between the dose and the drug concentration in saliva.[16] In another study, the subjects were administered four low (10 mg) and high (20 mg) daily oral doses of methamphetamine in two separate sessions. Blood, urine, and saliva samples were collected for 4 days. Although the oral fluid concentrations were higher, methamphetamine and metabolite concentrations in oral fluid and plasma followed the same pattern, and the concentration was dose dependent. Urine drug concentrations were substantially higher than those in oral fluid, and the detection times were longer.[17] Like urine, SAMHSA has proposed cutoffs for amphetamine, methamphetamine, MDMA, MDA, and MDEA for screening and confirmation (Tables 16.3 and 16.4). Also, the guidelines require the presence of amphetamine on methamphetamine-positive samples.[10]

CANNABINOIDS/MARIJUANA

Cannabinoids are a group of compounds that are found in the plant species *Cannabis sativa* and have psychoactive properties. The major psychoactive compound is δ-9-tetrahydrocannabinol. It is generally consumed by smoking and has euphoric effect. The effect occurs within minutes of smoking and persists for several hours. It is associated with loss of short-term memory and intellectual impairment. Although, marijuana is considered an illegal drug, it has some legitimate medical use. Synthetic THC, Dronabinol (Marinol), is used to treat anorexia and nausea in cancer and AIDS patients. Although marijuana trafficking is illegal under the federal law, several states in the United States have legalized the use of marijuana for medical use.

Urine is the most commonly used matrix for the detection of marijuana abuse. The target compound in urine is THC metabolite 11-nor-δ-9-tetrahydrocannabinol-9-carboxylic acid (THC-COOH). In saliva although both parent compound, THC and the metabolite THC-COOH, have been detected, the metabolite is present in much lower concentration than the parent drug. Detection of THC-COOH is preferred as it minimizes the argument for passive exposure to marijuana in drug-testing cases even though passive exposure was shown not to be the cause of positive results.[18] The presence of THC in oral fluid is mostly from smoking and ingestion as there is very little transport from blood to oral fluid. Detection of cannabinoids in oral fluid is a better indicator of recent use than detection of the metabolite in urine.

A number of methods including immunoassays and GC-MS for detection of cannabinoids in oral fluid have been described. Although currently not in wide use, several LC-MS-MS methods have been developed. Advantages of LC-MS-MS over GC-MS include less time for sample preparation and greater sensitivity. Besides laboratory analysis, several point-of-collection devices for the detection of THC are available. There are significant differences in the performance of these devices.

COCAINE

Cocaine is an alkaloid with potent central nervous system (CNS) stimulatory properties and high potential for abuse. Its effects are through inhibition of epinephrine, norepinephrine, and dopamine reuptake at nerve synapses. For recreational use cocaine is administered by snorting or intravenously. The freebase form of cocaine, commonly referred as "crack," is more volatile and easy to smoke. Cocaine and its metabolites including anhydroecgonine, benzoylecgonine, and ecgonine methyl ester are present in the saliva after inhalation, and intravenous or intranasal administration of the drug. Oral fluid being acidic and cocaine being basic, the concentration of cocaine in oral fluid is generally higher than plasma and is detectable for longer time.[2] SAMHSA proposed cutoffs are 20 ng/mL for screening (cocaine metabolites) and 8 ng/mL for confirmation (cocaine or benzoylecgonine).[10] The methods of analyses of cocaine and its metabolites include immunoassays, GC-MS, and LC-MS.

OPIOIDS/OPIATES

Opioid is a term used for all substances with morphine-like properties, whereas the term "opiates" is used to describe natural occurring alkaloids of opium. A number of studies have shown presence of opiates in oral fluid. The major opiates that have been studied in saliva include morphine, codeine, hydrocodone, hydromorphone, 6-acetylmorphine, and oxycodone. Several methods including immunoassays, GC-MS, and LC-MS have been described for the assay of opiates. When performing opiate assay, keto opiates such as hydrocodone, hydromorphone, and oxycodone may form multiple derivatives that may interfere in analysis of other opiates. To eliminate interference from keto opiates, oximization with hydroxylamine or methoxyamine has been used.[3] SAMHSA proposed initial and confirmatory cutoffs are shown in Tables 16.3 and 16.4.[10]

PHENCYCLIDINE

PCP is a potent veterinary analgesic and anesthetic, and is a common drug of abuse. The drug is structurally related to ketamine and was developed as intravenous anesthetic for human use. Overdose of PCP results in lethargy, disorientation, and hallucinations. The drug has been detected in oral fluid, and there is a good correlation between oral fluid and plasma concentrations. In a study, paired serum and saliva samples collected from 100 emergency department patients suspected of PCP intoxication were analyzed using radioimmunoassay. In this study, 74 of the oral fluid samples and 75 of the serum samples were positive for PCP. The study found no correlation between PCP concentrations and severity of intoxication.[19] There is a good correlation between oral fluid and plasma PCP concentrations, though intra- and interindividual variability are high and the ratio of oral fluid to plasma concentration varies with pH.[4] The frequently used methods for analysis of PCP in oral fluid include immunoassays, GC-MS, and LC-MS.

BARBITURATES AND BENZODIAZEPINES

Barbiturates are a class of CNS depressants that can be prescribed for ailments ranging from migraine headaches to epileptic seizures. They may be detected in saliva samples with detection times varying with the specific barbiturate.

Benzodiazepines are used as sedative hypnotics and anxiolytics. They are very similar in structure and can easily be found in saliva. A database review reported 892 benzodiazepine-positive specimens from a pool of 635,000 saliva specimens. Nordiazepam was found most often but alprazolam was not included in the study.[20]

OTHER SUBSTANCES

In addition to the drugs of abuse mentioned earlier, a number of other substances including γ-hydroxybutyrate, nicotine, and methadone are easily detected in saliva. Methadone, a synthetic opiate agonist, is extensively used in maintenance therapy of heroin addicts. A database review found 998 methadone-positive specimens from a pool of 635,000 saliva specimens. While methadone was present in all specimens, the methadone metabolite 2-ethylidene-1,5-dimethyl-3,3-diphenylpyrrolidine (EDDP) was found in only 30% of the methadone-positive specimens.[20]

In conclusion, saliva provides a good alternate matrix for substance abuse testing. However, two states, Hawaii and Maine, currently do not allow the use of saliva for employee drug testing. Despite analytical challenges, due to easy and under direct supervision sample collection, drugs of abuse testing in saliva provide additional opportunities in substance abuse detection and deterrence programs.

REFERENCES

1. Cone EJ. Oral fluid testing: new technology enables drug testing without embarrassment. J Calif Dent Assoc 2006;34:311–15.
2. Drummer OH. Drug testing in oral fluid. Clin Biochem Rev 2006;27:147–59.
3. Garg U. Hair, oral fluid, sweat and meconium testing for drugs of abuse: advantages and Pitfalls. In: Dasgupta A, ed., *Handbook of Drug Monitoring Methods: Therapeutics and Drugs of Abuse*. Totowa, NJ: Humana Press, 2008:337–64.
4. Aps JK, Martens LC. Review: the physiology of saliva and transfer of drugs into saliva. Forensic Sci Int 2005;150:119–31.
5. Cone EJ, Huestis MA. Interpretation of oral fluid tests for drugs of abuse. Ann N Y Acad Sci 2007;1098:51–103.
6. Cone EJ, Menchen SL. Stability of cocaine in saliva. Clin Chem 1988;34:1508.
7. Ventura M, Pichini S, Ventura R, Zuccaro P, Pacifici R, de la Torre R. Stability studies of principal illicit drugs in oral fluid: preparation of reference materials for external quality assessment schemes. Ther Drug Monit 2007;29:662–5.
8. Kadehjian L. Legal issues in oral fluid testing. Forensic Sci Int 2005;150:151–60.
9. Zhao Y, Ananias D, Rashid S, et al. *Automated Immunoassay for the Detection of Cocaine in Oral Fluid on Roche Instrument Platforms*. Durham, NC: Society of Forensic Toxicologists Annual Meeting; 2007.
10. Department of Health and Human Services Administration. Substance Abuse and Mental Services Administration. *Proposed Revisions to Mandatory Guidelines for Federal Workplace Drug Testing Programs*. Federal Register; 2004:19673–731.
11. Stout PR, Ropero-Miller J, Eicheldinger CR, et al. *Results of a Pilot Oral Fluids Performance Testing Program in the United States*. Durham, NC: Society of Forensic Toxicologists Annual Meeting; 2007.
12. Wong RC, Tran M, Tung JK. Oral fluid drug tests: effects of adulterants and foodstuffs. Forensic Sci Int 2005;150:175–80.
13. Cooper G, Wilson L, Reid C, Baldwin D, Hand C, Spiehler V. Validation of the Cozart microplate EIA for analysis of opiates in oral fluid. Forensic Sci Int 2005;154:240–46.
14. Cone EJ, Presley L, Lehrer M, et al. Oral fluid testing for drugs of abuse: positive prevalence rates by Intercept immunoassay screening and GC-MS-MS confirmation and suggested cutoff concentrations. J Anal Toxicol 2002;26:541–6.
15. Yacoubian GS, Jr, Wish ED, Perez DM. A comparison of saliva testing to urinalysis in an arrestee population. J Psychoactive Drugs 2001;33:289–94.

16. Schepers RJ, Oyler JM, Joseph RE, Jr, Cone EJ, Moolchan ET, Huestis MA. Methamphetamine and amphetamine pharmacokinetics in oral fluid and plasma after controlled oral methamphetamine administration to human volunteers. Clin Chem 2003;49:121–32.

17. Huestis MA, Cone EJ. Methamphetamine disposition in oral fluid, plasma, and urine. Ann N Y Acad Sci 2007;1098:104–21.

18. Niedbala RS, Kardos KW, Fritch DF, et al. Passive cannabis smoke exposure and oral fluid testing. II. Two studies of extreme cannabis smoke exposure in a motor vehicle. J Anal Toxicol 2005;29:607–15.

19. McCarron MM, Walberg CB, Soares JR, Gross SJ, Baselt RC. Detection of phencyclidine usage by radioimmunoassay of saliva. J Anal Toxicol 1984;8:197–201.

20. Cone EJ, Clarke J, Tsanaclis L. Prevalence and disposition of drugs of abuse and opioid treatment drugs in oral fluid. J Anal Toxicol 2007;31:424–33.

Head and neck cancer

Joseph A. Califano and Suhail K. Mithani

INTRODUCTION

Head and neck squamous cell cancer (HNSCC) is the sixth most common cancer in the United States. HNSCC includes all lesions of the mucosal surfaces from the internal nose and nasopharynx to the thoracic inlet level of the trachea and esophagus[1] (Table 17.1). The oral cavity is the most prevalent site of primary malignancy within the head and neck.

Fifty percent of patients present with advanced-stage disease due to the asymptomatic nature of early lesions. Half of patients with newly diagnosed oral cancer are alive 5 years from the time of diagnosis. The need for early diagnosis of HNSCC is illustrated by the 90% cure rate for stage I laryngeal cancer, compared to the <50% rate of control of stage IV laryngeal cancer.

DEMOGRAPHICS AND ETIOLOGY

HNSCC usually develops in the sixth and seventh decades of life after prolonged exposure to carcinogens, usually tobacco and alcohol. Statistical analysis of age-specific incidence data for patients with HNSCC suggests that these cancers arise after six to ten independent genetic events. Inherited genetic syndromes such as Fanconi anemia and dyskeratosis congenita have been associated with development of head and neck cancers at a younger age as have infection with Epstein-Barr virus (EBV), HIV, and human papilloma virus (HPV).[2]

TREATMENT

The mainstay of therapy for HNSCC has been surgery or primary radiotherapy with use of adjuvant chemotherapy. Often, all three modalities are employed for advanced disease.

Table 17.1 Sites and anatomic structures from which HNSCC arises.

Sites	Structures
Lip	Vermilion border, mucosal surfaces
Tongue	Tongue, lingual tonsil, Waldeyer's ring
Tonsil	Palatine tonsil, tonsillar fossa, tonsillar pillars
Oropharynx	Floor of mouth, retromolar trigone, hard and soft palate, buccal mucosa, vestibule, oropharynx, pharynx, pharyngoepiglottic folds, glossoepiglottic folds, vallecula, lingual surface of the epiglottis
Nose	Nasal cavity, nasopharynx
Hypopharynx	Pyriform sinus, postcricoid, lateral/posterior pharyngeal walls
Larynx	Laryngeal cartilage, supraglottis, glottis, subglottis, trachea above bifurcation
Cervical esophagus	Cervical esophagus, upper 1/3 of esophagus

SALIVA AS A DIAGNOSTIC TOOL FOR ORAL CANCER

HNSCC has an advantageous profile for molecular early detection and screening strategies, as it is a tumor that (1) often remains occult until later stages; (2) occurs in a specific population with a defined age-specific incidence and a defined carcinogen exposure; (3) has a long latency period; (4) has a high likelihood of successful treatment if diagnosed at an early or premalignant stage; (5) has a defined genetic progression and a premalignant precursor that can be defined as high risk by molecular markers.[3,4] The constant association of malignant and premalignant oral lesions with saliva coupled with the known propensity of this type of cancer to shed cells and genetic material makes saliva almost the ideal medium for sampling as a means for detection.

Approaches and applications of salivary diagnostics

Three applications for salivary diagnostics in HNSCC are risk prediction, screening/detection, and prognosis/surveillance.

As a population-based screening tool, a salivary diagnostic test can be utilized for early detection of disease or increased risk of disease development in an at-risk population with strictly defined risk factors. However, ability to identify a single marker for diagnostic purposes suffers because of the difficulty in producing tests with adequate sensitivity so that they are useful in detection as well as adequate specificity to not generate large amounts of false positives in the setting of low incidence.

Another potential application of salivary diagnostics lies in identification of primary recurrence after surgical resection. Again, achievement of appropriate sensitivity and specificity is problematic due to the mucosal field effect of molecular changes, in which HNSCC develops making it difficult to identify markers, which are only present in tumor but not detectable in surrounding epithelium.

Preclinical exploratory	**Phase 1**	Promising direction identified
Clinical assay and validation	**Phase 2**	Clinical assay detects established disease
Retrospective longitudinal	**Phase 3**	Biomarker detects disease early before it becomes clinical and a "screen-positive" rule is defined
Prospective screening	**Phase 4**	Extent and characteristics of disease detected by the test and the false referral rate are identified
Cancer control	**Phase 5**	Impact of screening on reducing the burden of disease on the population is quantified

Figure 17.1 Phases of biomarker development (from reference 38).

Several markers and approaches have been assessed in a limited fashion as salivary diagnostic tools, with several showing early promise. However, no clinical trials of salivary diagnostic methods have been undertaken to date to demonstrate feasibility and clinical applicability of these techniques (Fig. 17.1).

DNA-BASED TECHNIQUES

Microsatellite instability

Microsatellite instability (MSI) refers to alterations copy number of small repeats of a short nucleotide motif, which occur in tens of thousands of locations in the human genome. In MSI, these areas are aberrantly replicated or deleted leading to expansion or contraction of the specific area. MSI is thought to be related to deficits in DNA mismatch repair and replication, and multiple types of microsatellites have demonstrated alterations in a variety of human cancers. Head and neck cancers have been found to have microsatellite instability at a variety of loci in the genome,[5] and due to their propensity to shed genetic materials, DNA from salivary rinses.

MSI profiles from brushed oral mucosal samples from 44 HNSCC patients at the time of tumor resection and 43 matched controls were compared. This study demonstrated microsatellite instability of at least one marker in 11/13 primary tumors in the oral cavity with identical alterations found in the saliva samples in all cases (100% of those with markers; 85% overall). No microsatellite alterations were detected in any of the samples from the healthy control subjects.[6] Two other smaller studies demonstrated similar findings.[7,8]

p53 mutation

p53 is a powerful tumor-suppressor gene altered in many cancers. It is a transcription factor that is activated in normal cells in response to DNA damage, inducing cell cycle arrest, and either DNA repair activation or activation of apoptosis, depending on the context of the DNA injury.

Missense mutations in p53 DNA (changing the amino acid sequence of the transcribed protein) are present in around 50% of head and neck cancers. Detecting these mutations in body fluids in HNSCC patients has been the subject of a variety of studies. Early efforts used polymerase chain reaction (PCR)-based techniques to identify the same p53 mutations in DNA extracted from the salivary rinses from patients with corresponding p53 mutation in primary HNSCC in a small cohort of patients.[9]

Other approaches involve the observation that patients with cancer often generate p53 antibodies. Investigators have found that 13% (3/23) of patients with oral squamous cell carcinoma had antibodies against p53 in the saliva, by ELISA.[10]

Mitochondrial mutation

Mitochondria are the source of aerobic energy to meet a cell's demands for adenosine triphosphate (ATP) and are involved in the pathway and regulation of apoptosis and generation of free radicals. Approximately 50% of HNSCC bears mitochondrial mutation of some type.[11] Mitochondrial DNA also has the benefit of having a much higher copy number, making it easier for detection studies. As a screening tool, tumor-specific mitochondrial mutations were detectable by PCR in 67% (6 of 9) saliva samples from head and neck cancer patients that corresponded to mutations found in tumors.[12]

The overall content of cellular mitochondrial DNA increases as a proposed compensation for general mitochondrial dysfunction with increasing degrees of dysplasia and transition carcinoma.[13] This change was detected in the saliva when multivariate analysis of the saliva of patients with head and neck cancer versus screening patients showed a significant and independent association of diagnosis, age, and smoking with increasing mtDNA/nuclear DNA for Cox I and Cox II.[14]

With the advent of high-throughput resequencing arrays such as the MitoChip (Affymetrix), not only the entire mitochondrial genome can be sequenced rapidly, but also minor populations of mutated mitochondrial DNA can be detected.[15]

Methylation

Methylation takes place in the regulatory units of the genome (promoters) in CpG (cytosine-guanine dinucleotides)-rich areas that can be modified by the addition of a methyl group. Inactivation of tumor-suppressor genes in this manner has been increasingly shown to play a role in tumorigenesis. Tumors have been shown to preferentially shed DNA, and one large advantage of methylation is its ready use for screening, as DNA is stable in saliva and small levels of methylation can be detected by bisulfite sequencing, quantitative, or standard methylation-specific PCR (MSP).

Recent studies have shown correlation in the detectable presence of methylation of p16 between tumors, saliva, and serum via MSP compared to normal controls.[16] Methylation has been demonstrated in the oral rinses of patients with premalignant lesions at a rate that corresponded to oral rinse samples from cancer patients. p16 and O_6-methylguanine-DNA methyltransferase (MGMT) were observed to be methylated by MSP in 44 and 56% of the oral samples, respectively.[17] This lends potential application of this technique to early detection of lesions by saliva. A single study has assessed the application of assessment of promoter hypermethylation by MSP in saliva for surveillance after resection of cancer. In a small cohort, assessment of salivary methylation in a panel of genes predicted clinical recurrence prior to conventional diagnostic studies with a high degree of sensitivity and specificity.[18]

Human papillomavirus detection

HPV encodes for viral oncogenes that have been implicated in carcinogenesis of tumors of the oropharynx and particularly of Waldeyer's tonsillar ring.[19] New studies show promising molecular screening approaches that have increased sensitivity for detection. Real-time PCR of HPV-associated DNA is now the standard for detection at low thresholds. A cohort of patients with oral cancer demonstrated a 45.6% incidence of tumor HPV positivity. However, only 57% of these patients had detectable HPV-16 DNA in salivary rinses, a sensitivity of 32.6%. Specificity of 98.7% can be achieved with this technique.[20] Follow-up studies have demonstrated a lack of both sensitivity and specificity. In a case control study, 19% of head and neck cancer-positive patients (201 total) and 10% of control subjects (333 total) demonstrated detectable HPV16 DNA in saliva.[21]

Technologies such as competitive PCR coupled with mass spectrometry have promise to yield more specificity with positive results of one one-copy number of DNA over real-time PCR, but the issue of false-positive nonpathologic detection of HPV remains.[22] While the utility in population-based screening is still being evaluated, HPV positivity may eventually play a role in disease monitoring and surveillance.

GENOMIC EXPRESSION PROFILING

Expression microarrays utilize a small silicon chip embedded with gene-specific oligonucleotides to study mRNA expression of many genes in a sample. In oral cancer, this approach has been employed to search for early detection markers in the saliva.

Efforts to examine the mRNA expression differences in the saliva have been promising. A previous study determined 1,679 genes had differing expression levels in saliva of HNSCC and controls ($p < 0.05$). These potential salivary RNA biomarkers were IL8, IL1B, DUSP1, HA3, OAZ1, S100P, and SAT, and in combinations yielded sensitivity (91%) and specificity (91%) in distinguishing squamous cell carcinoma.[23] However, a recent study has raised issues about the validity of this technique. This study demonstrated that microarray signal derived from saliva may be a reflection of DNA contamination rather than RNA expression, and concluded that salivary extracts do not support mRNA expression studies.[24] However, subsequent studies have responded to this criticism[25,26] and conclude that RNA is present in the saliva and amenable to further study for identification of markers. Development of standards surrounding appropriate collection and management of salivary samples for RNA analysis[27] is under active investigation.

PROTEIN IDENTIFICATION AND PROTEOMIC PROFILING

Proteins found in saliva may have diagnostic value for detection of oral cancer. Several proteins have been identified with altered salivary levels in patients with oral cancer by conventional protein detection means. Salivary carcinoembryonic antigen (CEA) was found to be increased while gastrointestinal cancer antigen (GICA) was found to be decreased in patients with oral cavity lesions as compared to patients with benign oral lesions.[28] Human alpha defensin-1 (HNP-1) was found to be decreased in the saliva of head and neck cancer patients after resection and not present in the saliva of normal saliva.[29] Various chemokines and cellular molecules, TNF-α,[30,31] IL-1,[30,31] IL-8,[23] and CD44,[32] have been found to have altered protein levels in the saliva of patients of oral cancer as compared to disease-free controls.

New proteomic techniques that can quantitate protein expression in complex mixtures promise the possibility identifying novel markers for detection in saliva, which could be amenable to development of clinical assay by conventional methods.[33–35]

Initial studies have used these techniques in analysis of serum in various cancers, and their power for detection of biomarkers of disease lends credence to their application as discovery tools in saliva diagnostics. Salivary proteomic studies using surface-enhanced laser desorption ionization-time of flight (SELDI-TOF) mass spectrometry have identified biomarkers whose expression is significantly altered in the saliva of patients with oral lichen planus, a premalignant oral lesion.[36] A small pilot study has compared proteome profiles of saliva between head and neck squamous cell carcinomas and normal patients using a variety of mass spectrometry techniques and identified several proteins with expression differences.[37]

CONCLUSIONS AND FUTURE DIRECTIONS

Salivary diagnostics of oral cancer remains in a preclinical stages. At present there are many diagnostic markers and diagnostic techniques that show promise. Developing technologies, such as expression arrays, proteomic approaches (protein microarrays, SELDI/MALDI-TOF), RT-PCR, quantitative DNA PCR, and MSP, all offer hope in detecting molecular changes in saliva.

Changes studied include the detection of loss of heterozygosity, mutations, expression levels, protein levels, and presence of methylation or viral DNA.

Further studies of promising markers will be designed in a prospective fashion and subjected to rigorous analysis prior to clinical application. In order to reach significance, often times multiple markers are needed and studies addressing these combinations will be undertaken. However, there is considerable reason for optimism that in the near future novel molecular markers will exist that diagnose patients and predict clinical course and response to therapy.

REFERENCES

1. Davies L, Welch HG. Epidemiology of head and neck cancer in the United States. Otolaryngol Head Neck Surg 2006;135:451–7.
2. Gillison ML. Human papillomavirus-associated head and neck cancer is a distinct epidemiologic, clinical, and molecular entity. Semin Oncol 2004;31:744–54.
3. Califano J, van der Riet P, Westra W, et al. Genetic progression model for head and neck cancer: implications for field cancerization. Cancer Res 1996;56:2488–92.
4. Ha PK, Benoit NE, Yochem R, et al. A transcriptional progression model for head and neck cancer. Clin Cancer Res 2003;9:3058–64.
5. El-Naggar AK, Hurr K, Huff V, Clayman GL, Luna MA, Batsakis JG. Microsatellite instability in preinvasive and invasive head and neck squamous carcinoma. Am J Pathol 1996;148:2067–72.
6. Spafford MF, Koch WM, Reed AL, et al. Detection of head and neck squamous cell carcinoma among exfoliated oral mucosal cells by microsatellite analysis. Clin Cancer Res 2001;7:607–12.
7. Nunes DN, Kowalski LP, Simpson AJ. Detection of oral and oropharyngeal cancer by microsatellite analysis in mouth washes and lesion brushings. Oral Oncol 2000;36:525–8.
8. Okami K, Imate Y, Hashimoto Y, Kamada T, Takahashi M. Molecular detection of cancer cells in saliva from oral and pharyngeal cancer patients. Tokai J Exp Clin Med 2002;27:85–9.
9. Boyle JO, Mao L, Brennan JA, et al. Gene mutations in saliva as molecular markers for head and neck squamous cell carcinomas. Am J Surg 1994;168:429–32.
10. Warnakulasuriya S, Soussi T, Maher R, Johnson N, Tavassoli M. Expression of p53 in oral squamous cell carcinoma is associated with the presence of IgG and IgA p53 autoantibodies in sera and saliva of the patients. J Pathol 2000;192:52–7.
11. Zhou S, Kachhap S, Sun W, et al. Frequency and phenotypic implications of mitochondrial DNA mutations in human squamous cell cancers of the head and neck. Proc Natl Acad Sci U S A 2007;104:7540–45.
12. Fliss MS, Usadel H, Caballero OL, et al. Facile detection of mitochondrial DNA mutations in tumors and bodily fluids. Science 2000;287:2017–19.

13. Kim MM, Clinger JD, Masayesva BG, et al. Mitochondrial DNA quantity increases with histopathologic grade in premalignant and malignant head and neck lesions. Clin Cancer Res 2004;10:8512–15.

14. Jiang WW, Masayesva B, Zahurak M, et al. Increased mitochondrial DNA content in saliva associated with head and neck cancer. Clin Cancer Res 2005;11:2486–91.

15. Sui G, Zhou S, Wang J, et al. Mitochondrial DNA mutations in preneoplastic lesions of the gastrointestinal tract: a biomarker for the early detection of cancer. Mol Cancer 2006;5:73.

16. Nakahara Y, Shintani S, Mihara M, Hino S, Hamakawa H. Detection of p16 promoter methylation in the serum of oral cancer patients. Int J Oral Maxillofac Surg 2006;35:362–5.

17. Sanchez-Cespedes M, Esteller M, Wu L, et al. Gene promoter hypermethylation in tumors and serum of head and neck cancer patients. Cancer Res 2000;60:892–5.

18. Righini CA, de Fraipont F, Timsit JF, et al. Tumor-specific methylation in saliva: a promising biomarker for early detection of head and neck cancer recurrence. Clin Cancer Res 2007;13:1179–85.

19. Nair S, Pillai MR. Human papillomavirus and disease mechanisms: relevance to oral and cervical cancers. Oral Dis 2005;11:350–59.

20. Zhao M, Rosenbaum E, Carvalho AL, et al. Feasibility of quantitative PCR-based saliva rinse screening of HPV for head and neck cancer. Int J Cancer 2005;117:605–10.

21. Smith EM, Ritchie JM, Summersgill KF, et al. Human papillomavirus in oral exfoliated cells and risk of head and neck cancer. J Natl Cancer Inst 2004;96:449–55.

22. Yang H, Yang K, Khafagi A, et al. Sensitive detection of human papillomavirus in cervical, head/neck, and schistosomiasis-associated bladder malignancies. Proc Natl Acad Sci U S A 2005;102:7683–8.

23. Li Y, St John MA, Zhou X, et al. Salivary transcriptome diagnostics for oral cancer detection. Clin Cancer Res 2004;10:8442–50.

24. Kumar SV, Hurteau GJ, Spivack SD. Validity of messenger RNA expression analyses of human saliva. Clin Cancer Res 2006;12:5033–9.

25. Park NJ, Zhou X, Yu T, et al. Characterization of salivary RNA by cDNA library analysis. Arch Oral Biol 2007;52:30–35.

26. Park NJ, Li Y, Yu T, Brinkman BM, Wong DT. Characterization of RNA in saliva. Clin Chem 2006;52:988–94.

27. Park NJ, Yu T, Nabili V, et al. RNAprotect saliva: an optimal room-temperature stabilization reagent for the salivary transcriptome. Clin Chem 2006;52:2303–304.

28. Negri L, Pacchioni D, Calabrese F, Giacomasso S, Mastromatteo V, Fazio M. Serum and salivary CEA and GICA levels in oral cavity tumours. Int J Biol Markers 1988;3:107–12.

29. Mizukawa N, Sugiyama K, Fukunaga J, et al. Defensin-1, a peptide detected in the saliva of oral squamous cell carcinoma patients. Anticancer Res 1998;18:4645–9.

30. Rhodus NL, Cheng B, Myers S, Miller L, Ho V, Ondrey F. The feasibility of monitoring NF-kappaB associated cytokines: TNF-alpha, IL-1alpha, IL-6,

and IL-8 in whole saliva for the malignant transformation of oral lichen planus. Mol Carcinog 2005;44:77–82.

31. Rhodus NL, Ho V, Miller CS, Myers S, Ondrey F. NF-kappaB dependent cytokine levels in saliva of patients with oral preneoplastic lesions and oral squamous cell carcinoma. Cancer Detect Prev 2005;29:42–5.

32. Franzmann EJ, Reategui EP, Carraway KL, Hamilton KL, Weed DT, Goodwin WJ. Salivary soluble CD44: a potential molecular marker for head and neck cancer. Cancer Epidemiol Biomarkers Prev 2005;14:735–9.

33. Oppenheim FG, Salih E, Siqueira WL, Zhang W, Helmerhorst EJ. Salivary proteome and its genetic polymorphisms. Ann N Y Acad Sci 2007;1098:22–50.

34. Hu S, Li Y, Wang J, et al. Human saliva proteome and transcriptome. J Dent Res 2006;85:1129–33.

35. Drake RR, Cazare LH, Semmes OJ, Wadsworth JT. Serum, salivary and tissue proteomics for discovery of biomarkers for head and neck cancers. Expert Rev Mol Diagn 2005;5:93–100.

36. Yang MH, Chiang WC, Chou TY, et al. Increased NBS1 expression is a marker of aggressive head and neck cancer and overexpression of NBS1 contributes to transformation. Clin Cancer Res 2006;12:507–15.

37. Ohshiro K, Rosenthal DI, Koomen JM, et al. Pre-analytic saliva processing affect proteomic results and biomarker screening of head and neck squamous carcinoma. Int J Oncol 2007;30:743–9.

38. Pepe MS, Etzioni R, Feng Z, et al. Phases of biomarker development for early detection of cancer. J Natl Cancer Inst 2001;93:1054–61.

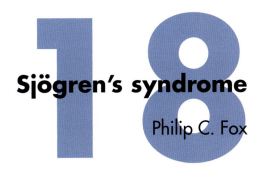

Sjögren's syndrome

Philip C. Fox

INTRODUCTION

Sjögren's syndrome is an autoimmune exocrinopathy, which affects between 2 and 4 million persons in the United States, 90% of whom are women.[1] The typical presentation includes complaints of oral and ocular dryness, a result of salivary and lacrimal dysfunction. Although Sjögren's syndrome is most often recognized by the symptoms of mouth and eye dryness, it is a systemic disorder and dryness may affect other mucosal areas (nose, throat, trachea, vagina), the skin, and involve many organ systems (e.g., thyroid, lung, and kidney).

There are primary and secondary forms of the syndrome.[1] Secondary Sjögren's syndrome occurs in conjunction with another autoimmune connective tissue disease, such as rheumatoid arthritis, systemic lupus erythematosus, systemic sclerosis, or primary biliary cirrhosis, while primary Sjögren's syndrome patients have no other autoimmune disorder. Both primary and secondary Sjögren's syndrome patients commonly have prominent serologic signs of autoimmunity, including hypergammaglobulinemia, autoantibodies, an elevated sedimentation rate, monoclonal gammopathies, and hypocomplementemia.

Among the most serious consequences of Sjögren's syndrome is an increased risk of developing malignant lymphoma, most typically B cell maltomas involving the salivary glands. It has been reported that primary Sjögren's syndrome patients have a 20–40-fold increased risk of lymphoma.[2,3] Recently, factors have been identified to help identify those patients at greatest risk. These include the presence at the time of initial diagnosis of palpable purpura, a low C4 level, mixed cryoglobulinemia, or salivary gland enlargement.[3–5]

EXOCRINE INVOLVEMENT IN SJÖGREN'S SYNDROME

The most common oral symptom in Sjögren's syndrome is xerostomia (dry mouth), a consequence of salivary dysfunction. In addition to oral dryness complaints, salivary gland dysfunction may induce complaints of dysphagia, adherence of food to the buccal or palatal surfaces, problems with dentures, a feeling of burning when eating spicy foods, an inability to eat dry foods, difficulty speaking for extended periods, and taste changes.[6] With diminished saliva production, chapped lips and dry, flaky perioral skin are common findings. Cracking and fissuring of the corners of the mouth, known as angular cheilitis, are also noted in these patients. Intraorally, the oral mucosa may be erythematous, dry, or atrophic. The tongue may appear furrowed, atrophic, and devoid of papillae. There is a marked increase in dental caries.

Opportunistic oral fungal infections are common and occur in up to 70% of patients with Sjögren's syndrome.[7] Chronic erythematous candidiasis is the most frequent type of fungal infection and may be responsible for the burning sensation and intolerance to spicy food.

Persistent or intermittent major salivary gland enlargement has been reported in up to 50% of Sjögren's syndrome patients.[6] Biopsy of the parotid gland frequently displays what are termed benign lymphoepithelial lesions, which can resemble lymphoid structures.[8] Biopsy of the minor salivary glands, which is a common diagnostic procedure for Sjögren's syndrome, reveals a focal mononuclear cell infiltration surrounding ducts, a loss of acinar structures, and the relative preservation of ductal cells. As a consequence to these histological changes and other immune-mediated changes, there is diminished salivary flow and alteration of the composition of the saliva.

Lacrimal gland involvement manifests as keratoconjunctivitis sicca, a term describing the ocular surface changes found in Sjögren's syndrome. These are a result of the reduction in tear output and altered composition of the secretion. Patients with dry eyes often complain of a gritty, scratchy sensation.[9] Other ocular symptoms include irritation, blurred vision, photophobia, and discharge at the inner canthus of the eye, especially on awakening. Corneal ulceration is a serious complication of severe dry eyes, which may develop in a small number of Sjögren's syndrome patients.

NONEXOCRINE (EXTRAGLANDULAR) INVOLVEMENT IN SJÖGREN'S SYNDROME

Dryness of the skin (xerosis) and pruritis are common cutaneous aspects of Sjögren's syndrome. Xerosis tends to be worse in the winter months, when humidity is lower. Other cutaneous manifestations include alopecia, photosensitivity lesions, erythema nodosum, lichen planus, vitiligo, cutaneous amyloidosis, cutaneous B cell lymphoma, granuloma annulare, and granulomatous panniculitis. A reaction to cold temperatures known as Raynaud's phenomenon has been reported in 13–20% of Sjögren's syndrome patients.[10] Patients may also suffer from inflammatory vascular disease. Vasculitis most commonly presents as palpable and nonpalpable purpura of the lower extremities, which can mimic Waldenström's hyperglobulinemic purpura.

A dry and persistent cough is a common symptom in patients with Sjögren's syndrome. This is due to decreased mucosal secretions from the exocrine glands and subsequent dryness in the upper airway. This condition is termed xerotrachea and is regarded as the tracheobronchial equivalent of xerostomia.

More than half of patients with primary Sjögren's syndrome complain of arthralgia, with or without evidence of arthritis. Unlike rheumatoid arthritis, the arthropathy is typically nonerosive and does not result in any deformation. Myalgia is also common in both primary and secondary Sjögren's syndrome.

Peripheral neuropathy is an extensively documented complication in primary Sjögren's syndrome.[11] Cranial nerve neuropathies are also found in patients with Sjögren's syndrome, especially in those with a preexisting peripheral neuropathy. The prevalence of central nervous system (CNS) involvement in Sjögren's syndrome is controversial. Some studies have suggested that involvement of the CNS occurs in as many as 25% of patients with primary Sjögren's syndrome.[12] Severe CNS manifestations are very uncommon in Sjögren's syndrome.

Involvement of other organ systems is not uncommon, with frequent reports of liver disease, renal involvement, and thyroid disease. Neonatal lupus and heart block in infants of mothers with Sjögren's syndrome have also been reported and are attributed to the presence of anti-SS-A (Ro) autoantibodies in the maternal circulation.[13] Adult-onset heart block can also occur in Sjögren's syndrome patients with active disease and may be associated with the production of antibodies against cardiac muscle and muscarinic receptors.

Depression and personality disorders have been found to be more common in patients with Sjögren's syndrome and many patients suffer from significant fatigue.[14] This is a debilitating condition that interferes with daily chores and social activities, thus reducing the quality of life of many patients. The fatigue is not felt to be related to depression.

LYMPHOMA AND PSEUDOLYMPHOMA IN SJÖGREN'S SYNDROME

The lymphocytic proliferation observed in the salivary glands in Sjögren's syndrome may progress from a polyclonal infiltration to a monoclonal gammopathy to a frank lymphoma. An increased frequency of circulating monoclonal immunoglobulins, increased mixed monoclonal cryoglobulins, and non-Hodgkin's lymphomas (typically MALT (mucosa-associated lymphoid tissue) lymphomas) all have been reported to be associated with Sjögren's syndrome. A recent meta-analysis concluded that there is a significantly higher risk of developing non-Hodgkin's lymphomas in patients with primary Sjögren's syndrome compared to other autoimmune diseases and healthy controls.[4] The lifetime risk is approximately 4–10%.[3]

MANAGEMENT OF SJÖGREN'S SYNDROME

Management of Sjögren's syndrome is still primarily palliative, although current research is targeting the underlying systemic autoimmunity. Palliative measures are aimed at diminishing symptoms, primarily by increasing mucosal hydration. Patients are encouraged to sip water frequently, use available rinses, gels, sprays, and mouthwashes, avoid or minimize alcohol, caffeine, and intense flavorings, and increase humidity in the environment, particularly during sleep.

Preventive measures will help to minimize the effects of salivary hypofunction and include supplemental fluoride applications, use of remineralizing solutions and xylitol-containing products, meticulous oral hygiene, and adoption of a noncariogenic diet.

Salivary secretions can be stimulated by masticatory and gustatory activity. Systemic secretogogues are used widely for salivary stimulation. These agents are FDA approved for relief of oral dryness symptoms in Sjögren's syndrome and also provide significant transient increases in salivary output for a period of 3–4 h.

Recent clinical research has focused on biological agents that are directed against the underlying autoimmune inflammatory process. Ongoing clinical studies examining the efficacy of the anti-B cell agents rituximab (anti-CD20) and epratuzumab (anti-CD22) show promise and may prove to be viable therapeutics to address this condition.[15,16]

DIAGNOSIS OF SJÖGREN'S SYNDROME

The cause of Sjögren's syndrome is not known. Diagnosis is based on evaluation of signs and symptoms. Identification of valid diagnostic biomarkers has been hampered by imprecise case definitions and nonhomogeneous study populations. Further, laboratory markers identified to date have proved to lack both sensitivity and specificity.

Classification criteria for Sjögren's syndrome were developed and validated between 1989 and 1996 by the European Study Group on Classification for Sjögren's Syndrome. These criteria were reviewed by an American-European Consensus Group, who suggested modifications, defined clearer classification rules for primary versus secondary disease, and provided more precise exclusion criteria.[17] The widespread acceptance of these classification criteria in the research community has greatly aided standardization of diagnosis and definition of patients.

At present, a large NIH-funded study is acquiring patients and has a goal of establishing definitive diagnostic criteria for Sjögren's syndrome. Initial results are expected by 2009.

SALIVARY DIAGNOSTICS IN SJÖGREN'S SYNDROME

Most diagnostic work has been done in blood and/or serum. None of the factors identified has proved to be sufficiently specific for diagnostic purposes or has shown strong correlation with disease activity measures.

Salivary measures that have been used diagnostically include measurement of saliva output (sialometry) and analyses of saliva composition (sialochemistry). Many of the same factors studied in blood have been examined in saliva, including cytokines (IL-6, TNF-α), lactoferrin, lysozyme, $\beta2$ microglobulin, and various B cell markers.[18–22] While numerous alterations have been identified in Sjögren's syndrome patients, these generally have lacked specificity, being a reflection of the altered salivary gland function rather than the autoimmune process itself. The alterations found in saliva in Sjögren's syndrome are similar to the changes that may be seen in any condition with reduced salivary output (such as following radiotherapy) or exocrine inflammatory involvement (such as parotitis). Further, there is a tremendous amount of variability in the results, as Sjögren's syndrome is progressive and patients are heterogeneous in regard to secretory dysfunction.

PROTEOMIC STUDIES OF SALIVA IN SJÖGREN'S SYNDROME

There are now four published studies that apply modern proteomic approaches to saliva in Sjögren's. The first study by Ryu et al. using surface-enhanced laser desorption ionization-time-of-flight-mass spectrometry (SELDI-TOF-MS) of parotid saliva looked at 41 primary Sjögren's syndrome patients, a smaller number of subjects with nonspecific complaints of oral dryness and five healthy controls.[23] The investigators identified a number of potential biomarkers for the condition. Both increased and decreased protein constituents were identified using two-dimensional gel electrophoresis. Proteins increased were β_2-microglobulin, lactoferrin, IgK light chain, polymeric Ig receptor, lysozyme C, and cystatin C. Decreased proteins were amylase, carbonic anhydrase VI, and two previously unidentified presumed proline-rich proteins. These findings mirror earlier results using conventional clinical chemical and immunohistochemical techniques. There were no striking differences in protein expression between patients with high or low focus scores (a measure of the extent of salivary gland infiltration). The results were interpreted as indicative of acinar cell damage, with an increase in inflammatory and immune proteins and a decrease in salivary protein products. An important consideration is that as all subjects had established disease, it cannot be determined if changes identified are a cause or an effect of the disorder.

A second study by Giusti et al. examined whole (mixed) saliva of 12 primary Sjögren's syndrome patients compared to 12 healthy controls.[24] These investigators used matrix-assisted laser desorption ionization-time of flight (MALDI-TOF) combined with quantitative two-dimensional gel electrophoresis and identified both qualitative and quantitative differences. They too found a decrease in salivary proteins and an increase in inflammatory and immune markers in Sjögren's syndrome patients. The four proteins reported to be decreased were α-amylase precursor, cystatin SN precursor, keratin 6L, and prolactin-inducible protein precursor. Increased proteins were fatty acid-binding protein, ACTB protein, an α-actin fragment, leukocyte elastase inhibitor, glutathione-S-transferase, and five unidentified proteins. They also identified a number of proteins present only in the Sjögren's syndrome samples (cal-granulin B, cyclophilin A, lipocalin-1 precursor, phosphatidyl ethanolamine-binding protein, IGKC protein, and zinc-2 glycoprotein precursor). There were four proteins found only in the control samples (carbonic anhydrase VI, and 3 cystatins: cystatins S, C precursor, and D). Although there was general agreement with the study of Ryu et al.,[23] the results for cystatins were different. These discrepancies are likely the result of the different samples (parotid vs whole saliva) utilized.

Peluso et al. examined proteins in whole saliva of nine primary and nine secondary Sjögren's syndrome patients compared to ten healthy controls using high-performance liquid chromatography (HPLC) coupled with MS electrospray ionization.[25] They also looked at the effect of treatment with pilocarpine on the salivary protein profile in a subgroup of six primary Sjögren's syndrome patients. Sixty-two salivary proteins were analyzed, with 58% found to be either decreased or absent in the primary Sjögren's syndrome samples compared to controls. Eight proteins were found at significantly lower levels than in the controls. For secondary Sjögren's syndrome patients, 18 of the 62 proteins were found in a significantly lower percentage of patients than in controls. A number of salivary cystatins (C, S, S2, SA, SN) and histatins[2–4,7,9,11,12] were identified less frequently in patients versus controls. Interestingly, this study using whole saliva found decreased cystatin expression, in agreement with the results of the work of Giusti et al.,[24] also using whole saliva. Peluso et al.[25] also found that pilocarpine stimulation partially restored the salivary protein profile to that of the healthy controls, with the best response from parotid proteins.

Most recently, Hu and coworkers examined whole saliva from ten women with primary Sjögren's syndrome to identify potential protein and mRNA biomarkers.[26] Using MALDI-TOF-mass spectrometry with validation by real-time quantitative polymerase chain reaction, they found 16 downregulated and 25 upregulated proteins compared to healthy controls. Cystatins were down-regulated, while salivary amylase, β_2-microglobulin, actin, and carbonic anhydrase I and II, were upregulated. Further, using expression microarray profiling, they found 27 mRNAs significantly upregulated, the majority of which were interferon inducible or related to lymphocyte filtration and antigen presentation. In general, the results reflected the damage to glandular cells and the activated immune response characteristic of Sjögren's syndrome. They also compared the results from whole saliva with samples of individual gland secretions and found that the whole saliva samples contained a greater array of proteins, peptides, and mRNA. Thus, whole saliva appears to be a more informative sample for future genomic and proteomic studies.

Table 18.1 summarizes the results of these four studies.

SUMMARY

The current literature of proteomics of saliva in Sjögren's syndrome must be seen as preliminary, as the number of patients studied is small, the populations are heterogeneous, studies are few, and samples vary between investigations.

Table 18.1 Summary of proteomic studies of saliva in Sjögren's syndrome.

Study	Saliva type	Techniques	Subjects	Controls	Proteins increased in patients	Proteins decreased in patients	Proteins only in patients	Proteins only in controls
Ryu et al.[23]	Parotid	SELDI-TOF-MS; 2D-DIGE	Primary Sjögren's syndrome	Xerostomia patients and healthy controls	6	4	NR	NR
Giusti et al.[24]	Whole (mixed)	MALDI-TOF; 2D-E	Primary Sjögren's syndrome	Healthy controls	10	4	6	4
Peluso et al.[25]	Whole (mixed)	HPLC; MS-electrospray ionization	Primary (1°) and secondary (2°) Sjögren's syndrome	Healthy controls	1°:2 / 2°:3	1°:8 / 2°:2	1	NR
Hu et al.[26]	Whole (mixed)	MALDI-TOF; RT-QPCR	Primary Sjögren's syndrome	Healthy controls	25	16	3	1

NR, not reported.

Also, controls should include not just healthy controls, but also other autoimmune inflammatory disorders and salivary conditions. However, the general agreement in overall results to date is encouraging and further studies are definitely in order. Care must be taken in future studies to assure adequate sample sizes, well-defined populations, and appropriate controls. It seems likely that the techniques available now (and those being developed) in proteomics will allow definition of a pattern of protein expression in saliva in Sjögren's syndrome that will provide sufficient sensitivity and specificity to be of diagnostic utility.

REFERENCES

1. Kassan SS, Moutsopoulos HM. Clinical manifestations and early diagnosis of Sjögren's syndrome. Arch Intern Med 2004;164:1275–84.
2. Kassan SS, Thomas TL, Moutsopoulos HM, et al. Increased risk of lymphoma in sicca syndrome. Ann Intern Med 1978;89:888–92.
3. Theander E, Henriksson G, Ljungberg O, Mandl T, Manthorpe R, Jacobsson LT. Lymphoma and other malignancies in primary Sjögren's syndrome: a cohort study on cancer incidence and lymphoma predictors. Ann Rheum Dis 2006;65:796–803.
4. Zintzaras E, Voulgarelis M, Moutsopoulos HM. The risk of lymphoma development in autoimmune diseases: a meta-analysis. Arch Intern Med 2005;165:2337–44.
5. Ioannidis JP, Vassiliou VA, Moutsopoulos HM. Long-term risk of mortality and lymphoproliferative disease and predictive classification of primary Sjögren's syndrome. Arthritis Rheum 2002;46:741–7.
6. Daniels TE, Fox PC. Salivary and oral components of Sjögren's syndrome. Rheum Dis Clin North Am 1992;18:571–89.
7. Soto-Rojas AE, Villa AR, Sifuentes-Osornio J, Alarcon-Segovia D, Kraus A. Oral manifestations in patients with Sjögren's syndrome. J Rheumatol 1998;25:906–10.
8. Daniels TE. Labial salivary gland biopsy in Sjögren's syndrome: assessment as a diagnostic tool criterion in 362 suspected cases. Arthritis Rheum 1984;27:147–56.
9. Friedlaender MH. Ocular manifestations of Sjögren's syndrome: keratoconjunctivitis sicca. Rheum Dis Clin North Am 1992;18:591–608.
10. Provost TT, Watson R. Cutaneous manifestations of Sjögren's syndrome. Rheum Dis Clin North Am 1992;18:609–16.
11. Hietaharju A, Yli-Kerttula U, Hakkinen V, Frey H. Nervous system manifestation in Sjögren's syndrome. Acta Neurol Scand 1990;81:144–52.
12. Alexander E. Central nervous system disease in Sjögren's syndrome. Rheum Dis Clin North Am 1992;18:637–72.
13. Borda E, Sterin-Borda L. Autoantibodies against neonatal heart M1 muscarinic acetylcholine receptor in children with congenital heart block. J Autoimmun 2001;16:143–50.
14. Barendregt PJ, Visser MRM, Smets EMA, et al. Fatigue in primary Sjögren's syndrome. Ann Rheum Dis 1998;57:291–5.

15. Pijpe J, van Imhoff GW, Spijkervet FK, et al. Rituximab treatment in patients with primary Sjögren's syndrome: an open-label phase II study. Arthritis Rheum 2005;52:2740–50.
16. Steinfeld SD, Youinou P. Epratuzumab (humanised anti-CD22 antibody) in autoimmune diseases. Expert Opin Biol Ther 2006;6:943–9.
17. Vitali C, Bombardieri S, Jonsson R, the European Study Group on classification criteria for Sjögren's syndrome. Classification Criteria for Sjögren's syndrome: a revised version of the American-European Consensus Group. Ann Rheum Dis 2002;61:554–8.
18. Grisius MM, Bermudez DK, Fox PC. Salivary and serum interleukin 6 in primary Sjögren's syndrome. J Rheumatol 1997;24:1089–91.
19. Gottenberg JE, Busson M, Cohen-Solal J, et al. Correlation of serum B lymphocyte stimulator and beta2 microglobulin with autoantibody secretion and systemic involvement in primary Sjögren's syndrome. Ann Rheum Dis 2005;64:1050–55.
20. Turkcapar N, Sak SD, Saatci M, Duman M, Olmez U. Vasculitis and expression of vascular cell adhesion molecule-1, intercellular adhesion molecule-1, and E-selectin in salivary glands of patients with Sjögren's syndrome. J Rheumatol 2005;32:1063–70.
21. Zigon P, Bozic B, Cucnik S, Rozman B, Tomsic M, Kveder T. Are autoantibodies against a 25-mer synthetic peptide of M3 muscarinic acetylcholine receptor a new diagnostic marker for Sjögren's syndrome? Ann Rheum Dis 2005;64:1247.
22. Miyazaki K, Takeda N, Ishimaru N, Omotehara F, Arakaki R, Hayashi Y. Analysis of in vivo role of alpha-fodrin autoantigen in primary Sjögren's syndrome. Am J Pathol 2005;167:1051–9.
23. Ryu OH, Atkinson JC, Hoehn GT, Illei GG, Hart TC. Identification of parotid salivary biomarkers in Sjögren's syndrome by surface-enhanced laser desorption/ionization time-of-flight mass spectrometry and two-dimensional difference gel electrophoresis. Rheumatology (Oxford) 2006;45:1077–86.
24. Giusti L, Baldini C, Bazzichi L, et al. Proteome analysis of whole saliva: a new tool for rheumatic diseases–the example of Sjögren's syndrome. Proteomics 2007;7:1634–43.
25. Peluso G, De Santis M, Inzitari R, et al. Proteomic study of salivary peptides and proteins in patients with Sjögren's syndrome before and after pilocarpine treatment. Arthritis Rheum 2007;56:2216–22.
26. Hu S, Wang J, Meijer J, et al. Salivary proteomic and genomic biomarkers for primary Sjogren's syndrome. Arthritis Rheum 2007;56:3588–600.

19

Salivary gland dysfunction associated with systemic disease

Nelson L. Rhodus

INTRODUCTION

Saliva in normal quantity and composition is likely the most important aspect of the host immune system in the protection of the oral cavity from disease and deterioration. However, when saliva is reduced in volume and/or changes in its chemical composition, the mouth becomes very susceptible to painful inflammation, lesions, infections, and tremendous increase in dental caries and periodontal disease.[1]

Xerostomia is the symptomatic lack of saliva (dry mouth), whereas hyposalivation is the reduction in salivary flow irrespective of symptoms and may be the result of many causes or the combination of several etiological factors, including many systemic diseases.[2,3]

Common causes of hyposalivation include side effects of over 1,100 medications, radiation or chemotherapy for head and neck cancer, and several systemic diseases. Systemic diseases associated with salivary hypofunction include autoimmune diseases (Sjögren's syndrome, systemic lupus erythematosus, systemic sclerosis, rheumatoid arthritis, fibromyalgia, and others), metabolic diseases (diabetes, renal, or liver disease), infectious diseases (HIV and others), organ or bone marrow transplants, and others.[4,5]

This chapter reviews the systemic diseases (except for Sjögren's syndrome that has been presented in detail in Chapter 18) associated with salivary gland dysfunction and hyposalivation.

DIAGNOSIS OF SALIVARY GLAND DYSFUNCTION

Sialometry

Sialometry (measuring salivary flow) is useful both as an initial screening tool for hyposalivation, regardless of etiology, and to assess xerostomia and its treatment. To be diagnostically valuable, salivary flow collection must be performed precisely, according to the type of gland, and over a period of at least 5 min (often up to 15 min).

Pathology

The precise diagnosis for the related conditions should be made to determine whether a chronic inflammatory condition, such as Sjögren's syndrome (SS) is present. The diagnosis of many of these conditions remains controversial.

The antinuclear antibodies (ANA) are the SS-A(Ro) and SS-B(La). The former is present in approximately 70% of patients with primary SS (pSS) and 15–90% with secondary SS (sSS). The latter is present in approximately 50% of patients with pSS and 5–30% with sSS. Both of these ANA may also be found in other autoimmune disorders.

Labial or other salivary gland biopsies or other tests may help arrive at a specific diagnosis. Labial salivary gland histopathology has almost universally been accepted as the prima facie indicator of SS, as well as practically every other type of salivary gland disorder. In the case of SS, the lymphocyte infiltrates are numerous, arranged periductally, and may ultimately invade the acinar cells. Of course, in benign or malignant neoplastic disease, it is critical to obtain a representative histological specimen. For suspected infectious disease causing the salivary gland disorder, cultures from saliva may be of some limited use, but most commonly a biopsy is indicated.

These diagnostic tests are critical for identifying salivary gland dysfunction associated with systemic disease, not only to rule out SS or another autoimmune inflammatory disease, but also to determine the true nature of the underlying disease.

Imaging

Radiographic findings may appear in advanced stages of fibrosis of the salivary glands. Sialograms are performed by injecting a radiocontrast dye into the salivary ductal system prior to conventional radiography. Sialograms may reveal punctate radio-opaque calcifications or, in more advanced cases, larger, lobular calcifications. MRI sialography is much more accurate in demonstrating the level of salivary gland destruction in some conditions.

SYSTEMIC DISEASES AFFECTING SALIVARY GLAND FUNCTION

Epidemiology, pathophysiology, and essential clinical and diagnostic features of several systemic disease categories will be discussed. Those entities which contribute to salivary gland hypofunction due to neoplasia will not be discussed here.

Chronic inflammatory rheumatic disorders

More than 100 arthritic (or rheumatic) diseases affect different parts of the body. Some of the more common types include rheumatoid arthritis,[5–26] osteoarthritis, systemic lupus erythematosus,[4,6,16,21] juvenile arthritis,[9,13,14] scleroderma,[13,14,20,27] Sjögren's syndrome (see Chapter 18), gout ankylosing spondylitis, Lyme disease, fibromyalgia,[15,28] vasculitis,[8,22,29] polymyositis,[6,19] synovitis,[30] primary biliary cirrhosis,[31–34] and psoriatic arthritis.[35] According to the Arthritis Foundation, more than 40 million Americans suffer from the various forms of arthritis, and more than 8 million of these are disabled. For most of these conditions, the estimates of prevalence range from 1 to 2% of the general population.[35]

Many of these chronic autoimmune inflammatory disorders have salivary gland involvement ranging from 10 to 60% depending on the particular disease. The leading example of such a condition is Sjögren's syndrome in which 100% of affected patients will have salivary gland dysfunction.

Several other conditions resemble SS in lymphocytic infiltration into the parenchyma of the salivary glands. In fact, it is a diagnostic challenge to determine whether indeed the condition is SS (particularly secondary SS) versus another primary autoimmune inflammatory disorder (rheumatoid arthritis, systemic lupus erythematosus, systemic sclerosis, scleroderma, fibromyalgia, vasculitis, polymyositis, or primary biliary cirrhosis).

Consequently, many other inflammatory autoimmune disorders that affect salivary glands may be actually undiagnosed SS, particularly secondary SS. However, some of these diseases appear to have some capacity to affect salivary glands on their own.[6]

Autoimmune-mediated musculoskeletal disorders are characterized by circulating pathogenic autoantibodies and autoreactive T cells. These antibodies may be used for prognosis, to monitor response to treatment, or to predict relapse of disease. Certain autoantibody assays are considered clinically most relevant. These include rheumatoid factor (RF), anti-cyclic citrullinated antibody (anti-CCP), antinuclear autoantibodies (ANA), anti-doublestranded DNA antibodies, antibodies to extractable nuclear antigens (ENA), and antineutrophil cytoplasmic autoantibodies (ANCA). Consequently, the accurate diagnosis of such conditions as rheumatoid arthritis, systemic lupus erythematosus, Sjögren's syndrome, systemic sclerosis/CREST (calcinosis, Raynaud's, esophagitis, scleroderma, telangectasia (syndrome)), polymyositis/dermatomyositis, and vasculitis is imperative in determining the nature of the presenting salivary gland dysfunction.[6]

Some studies have utilized such testing and found that the diagnosed condition does indeed involve a salivary gland component. For example, a significant percentage (17%) of a large cohort of well-characterized patients ($n = 587$) with rheumatoid arthritis (not secondary SS) demonstrated salivary gland histopathology and dysfunction.[7] Even in patients diagnosed with secondary SS with different disorders such as rheumatoid arthritis, systemic lupus erythematosus, systemic sclerosis/CREST, and polymyositis/dermatomyositis, the presence and level of salivary gland histopathology and dysfunction varies. Further, some studies, such as that reported by Helenius and colleagues, demonstrated that those separate conditions alone independent of secondary SS can involve salivary gland histopathology and dysfunction.[11]

In another study by Wangkaew et al.,[14] salivary gland histopathology and dysfunction was found more commonly in systemic lupus erythematosus (22% vs 0%, $p < 0.01$) and scleroderma (16% vs 4%, $p < 0.05$) than in the controls, but there was no statistical difference in patients with rheumatoid arthritis. Again, these finding were independent of SS.

Primary biliary cirrhosis (PBC) has been associated with salivary gland histopathology and dysfunction independent of SS as well. In one such study,[33] 75% of the subjects had salivary changes associated with PBC. In another study, 60% of the PBC subjects demonstrated salivary gland dysfunction, but that study did not control for SS.[33] Indeed the overlap of PBC and these other autoimmune inflammatory conditions with SS is well-documented. Other studies have shown that autoimmune inflammatory conditions such as fibromyalgia, rheumatoid arthritis, vasculitis, and polymyositis may demonstrate salivary gland histopathology and dysfunction independent of SS.

Other autoimmune inflammatory disorders

Some other autoimmune inflammatory disorders that present similar to SS in lymphocytic infiltration into the parenchyma of the salivary glands include autoimmune thyroiditis,[36–41] autoimmune hepatitis,[42–44] chronic pancreatitis,[45,46] and Lyme disease.[17] As mentioned previously, it is a diagnostic challenge to determine whether indeed the condition is SS (particularly secondary SS) versus another primary autoimmune inflammatory disorder.

Thyroiditis is common in SS (30–60%) and, therefore, testing for autoantibodies is important.[38] However, thyroid dysfunction on its own may have associated salivary gland histopathology and dysfunction.[40] The study by Soy et al.[41] reported an incidence of 30% of xerostomia symptoms in patients with autoimmune thyroiditis. Autoimmune hepatitis has been shown to be associated with salivary gland histopathology and dysfunction independent of SS.[40,41]

Sarcoidosis

Sarcoidosis is a granulomatous disease of unknown cause, which can essentially affect any organ system. Evidently, the pathophysiology involves inadequate degradation of antigenic material that accumulates in tissues and causes progressive noncaseating granulomatous inflammation. Sarcoidosis has an ethnic predilection for African Americans, who are 17 times more susceptible than Caucasians.

Although any organ system can be affected, the most common are the lungs, lymph nodes, eyes, skin, and salivary glands. Salivary gland dysfunction is common but may occur insidiously without major clinical manifestations. Often the saliva displays mucous extravasation. Diagnosis is made by histopathology. Many cases spontaneously resolve within 2 years.[19,47–50]

Diabetes mellitus

The literature is replete with references to diabetes mellitus and salivary histopathology and dysfunction.[2,51–78]

GENETIC AND DEVELOPMENTAL DISEASES AFFECTING SALIVARY GLAND DYSFUNCTION

Many genetic and developmental diseases have been related to salivary gland dysfunction. These include ectodermal dysplasia,[79–81] cleft palate,[82] Allgrove syndrome,[83] Down's syndrome,[84] CREST syndrome,[6] cystic fibrosis,[85] Cowden's syndrome,[86] Levi–Hollister syndrome,[87] systemic amyloidosis,[88–91] familial amyloidotic polyneuropathy,[92] myotonic dystrophy,[5] sphingolipid storage disease, Gaucher disease,[5] Pader–Willi syndrome,[93] Papillion–Lefevre syndrome,[94] and Waldenstrom's macoglobulenemia.[95]

Ectodermal dysplasia is an inherited disorder in which certain tissues fail to mature completely during development. The tissues most likely to experience agenesis include the salivary gland, the teeth, and the lacrimal glands. Of course, these patients will manifest salivary gland dysfunction.[79–81] Among the other conditions, cystic fibrosis, cleft palate, and Down's syndrome have also been reported to occasionally manifest a genesis of the salivary glands and therefore salivary gland dysfunction.[82]

METABOLIC AND OTHER CONDITIONS RESULTING IN HYPOSALIVATION

These include celiac disease,[96] other gastrointestinal disorders[97] dehydration,[23] anorexia/bulimia,[5] ESRD[98–102] pulmonary diseases,[32,103–106] chronic lymphocytic leukemia,[107] lymphoma,[108–110] thalassemia,[111] nutritional deficiencies,[23,112–114] neurological disease,[110,115–118] allergies,[51,119] depression,[23,116,120,121] bone marrow transplants,[122] solid organ transplants,[123–126] and breast implants.[127]

Obviously, one of the earliest and most conspicuous manifestations of dehydration is the loss of water and salivary gland hypofunction. This condition may result from many pharmacological agents and other therapies (i.e., cancer chemotherapy, hemodialysis, etc.), and several systemic diseases: gastrointestinal (malabsorption, vomiting), renal, hematologic, neurologic, allergies. Transplantation may result in some level of dehydration and/or hypovolemia, the loss of water (absolute or failure of reabsorption) and, therefore, salivary gland hypofunction.[116–127] Studies have reported salivary gland hypofunction in end-stage renal disease,[98–102] hematological conditions (thalassemia),[111] or leukemia.[107]

Several reports have also associated allergies and pulmonary problems (asthma, pneumonia, etc.) with salivary gland hypofunction.[32,51,103–106,119] It is difficult to know the precise relationship because in most cases there was no control for medications, associated autoimmune diseases, or other potential contributory factors to the salivary gland hypofunction. The conditions may also be associated with other inflammatory or infiltrative pathologies that may further contribute to and complicate the salivary gland dysfunction. These examples further illustrate the likelihood of several diseases overlapping and contributing to salivary gland dysfunction. Therefore, accurate diagnosis of all contributing conditions is imperative.

INFECTIOUS DISEASES AFFECTING SALIVARY GLAND DYSFUNCTION

Infectious diseases that affect salivary gland dysfunction include HIV,[9,108,128–134] hepatitis C,[44,51,135–150] hepatitis G,[151] cytomegalovirus,[129,152] Epstein-Barr virus,[153–155] retroviruses,[156,157] paramyxovirus,[5] bacterial infection (parotitis),[158,159] *Helicobacter pylori*,[160] tuberculosis,[161] parvovirus.[162,163]

Human immunodeficiency virus

Patients with human immunodeficiency virus (HIV) may have a salivary gland involvement with enlargement of one or more of the major salivary glands. This involvement may be due to the HIV itself or another HIV-associated disease, such as cytomegalovirus or lymphoepithelial cyst. It has been shown[133] that these patients may have a significant change in several salivary components— decreased protein, increased IgA, lysozyme, albumin, and salivary gland inflammatory infiltrate. The observed changes are similar to those of SS, but less pronounced.

HIV-positive patients with salivary gland enlargement had lower-stimulated parotid salivary flow than HIV patients without salivary gland enlargement.[93] Several studies found that salivary flow rates were affected in HIV patients. There has been some ambiguity as to how much of this is induced by medication. In two recent studies, HIV was identified as a significant risk factor for xerostomia and salivary gland hypofunction measured as unstimulated whole saliva ≤ 0.1 mL/min.[92,93]

Several studies have reported salivary gland enlargement in children and adults with HIV infection.[90,92,93] The salivary gland enlargement may involve all the major salivary glands. These patients may have xerostomia. The HIV-associated salivary gland disease (HIV-sgd) is similar histologically to Sjögren's syndrome, but without autoantibodies that are found in Sjögren's. Of the patients seen at the Oral AIDS Center at the University of California, San Francisco, 6% had HIV-sgd. No evidence has been found of direct invasion of the salivary glands by HIV-1. Non-Hodgkin's lymphoma, Kaposi's sarcoma, benign lymphoepithelial cysts, and benign lymphoepithelial lesions have been reported in the major salivary glands of HIV-infected individuals.[93]

There is really no treatment other than to palliate the xerostomia symptoms or to stimulate salivary flow via secretogogues.

Hepatitis C

It has been suggested that up to 50% of patients with hepatitis C virus (HCV) infection have reduced salivary flow.[164] A possible etiologic role of HCV in primary SS has been suggested.[165] In a study on 45 chronic HCV patients,[166]

53% had a certain or probable diagnosis of Sjögren's syndrome according to the European criteria.[167] In this study, 47% had a focal lymphocytic infiltration score of a grade III or IV on a minor salivary gland biopsy. A conflicting study showed no association between whole salivary flow in 74 chronic HCV infection patients compared to healthy controls.[168] In that study, patients with confounding signs of underlying diseases, which could produce xerostomia, such as Sjögren's syndrome and other autoimmune diseases, as well as diabetes mellitus, were excluded.

In summary, many systemic diseases may cause or be associated with salivary gland dysfunction. It is imperative to perform comprehensive diagnostic testing in order to determine the nature of the problem, whether primary or secondary and only then may the appropriate therapeutic strategy be planned.

REFERENCES

1. Mandel ID. Sialochemistry in diseases and clinical situations affecting salivary glands. Crit Rev Clin Lab Sci 1980;12(4):321–66.
2. Sreebny LM, Yu A, Green A, Valdini A. Xerostomia in diabetes mellitus. Diabetes Care 1992;15(7):900–904.
3. Rhodus NL. Xerostomia and the geriatric patient. Dentistry 1988;8(2):12–17.
4. Rhodus NL. Sjogren's syndrome. Quintessence Int 1999;30(10):689–99.
5. von Bultzingslowen I, Sollecito TP, Fox PC, et al. Salivary dysfunction associated with systemic diseases: systematic review and clinical management recommendations. Oral Surg Oral Med Oral Pathol Oral Radiol Endod 2007;103(Suppl S57):e1–15.
6. van Paassen P, Damoiseaux J, Tervaert JW. Laboratory assessment in musculoskeletal disorders. Best Pract Res Clin Rheumatol 2003;17(3):475–94.
7. Cimmino MA, Salvarani C, Macchioni P, et al. Extra-articular manifestations in 587 Italian patients with rheumatoid arthritis. Rheumatol Int 2000;19(6):213–17.
8. Doyle MK. Vasculitis associated with connective tissue disorders. Curr Rheumatol Rep 2006;8(4):312–16.
9. Flaitz CM. Parotitis as the initial sign of juvenile Sjögren's syndrome. Pediatr Dent 2001;23(2):140–42.
10. Scofield RH, Bruner GR, Harley JB, Namjou B. Autoimmune thyroid disease is associated with a diagnosis of secondary Sjogren's syndrome in familial systemic lupus. Ann Rheum Dis 2007;66(3):410–13.
11. Helenius LM, Meurman JH, Helenius I, et al. Oral and salivary parameters in patients with rheumatic diseases. Acta Odontol Scand 2005;63(5):284–93.
12. Shimoyama K, Ogawa N. Salivary gland examinations in patients with rheumatoid arthritis. Nippon Rinsho 2005;63(Suppl 1):386–9.
13. Walton AG, Welbury RR, Thomason JM, Foster HE. Oral health and juvenile idiopathic arthritis: a review. Rheumatology (Oxford) 2000;39(5):550–55.

14. Wangkaew S, Kasitanon N, Sivasomboon C, Wichainun R, Sukitawut W, Louthrenoo W. Sicca symptoms in Thai patients with rheumatoid arthritis, systemic lupus erythematosus and scleroderma: a comparison with age-matched controls and correlation with disease variables. Asian Pac J Allergy Immunol 2006;24(4):213–21.
15. Ostuni P, Botsios C, Sfriso P, et al. Fibromyalgia in Italian patients with primary Sjogren's syndrome. Joint Bone Spine 2002;69(1):51–7.
16. Rhodus NL, Johnson DK. The prevalence of oral manifestations of systemic lupus erythematosus. Quintessence Int 1990;21(6):461–5.
17. Rhodus NL, Falace DA. Oral concerns in Lyme disease. Northwest Dent 2002;81(2):17–18.
18. Rhodus N. Xerostomia and glossodynia in patients with autoimmune disorders. Ear Nose Throat J 1989;68(10):791–4.
19. Koarada S, Uchida M, Tada Y, et al. A case of Sjogren's syndrome complicated by polymyositis and sarcoidosis with HLA-B7 and DR 8: common causes of susceptibility for these diseases. Nihon Rinsho Meneki Gakkai Kaishi 2000;23(2):141–7.
20. Maeda M, Ichiki Y, Aoyama Y, Kitajima Y. Surfactant protein D (SP-D) and systemic scleroderma (SSc). J Dermatol 2001;28(9):467–74.
21. Magnusson V, Nakken B, Bolstad AI, Alarcon-Riquelme ME. Cytokine polymorphisms in systemic lupus erythematosus and Sjogren's syndrome. Scand J Immunol 2001;54(1–2):55–61.
22. Makino H, Wada J. History of nephrology in the past 100 years: collagen disease and vasculitis. Nippon Naika Gakkai Zasshi 2002;91(5): 1492–7.
23. Astor FC, Hanft KL, Ciocon JO. Xerostomia: a prevalent condition in the elderly. Ear Nose Throat J 1999;78(7):476–9.
24. Benitha R, Tikly M. Functional disability and health-related quality of life in South Africans with rheumatoid arthritis and systemic lupus erythematosus. Clin Rheumatol 2007;26(1):24–9.
25. Carmona L, Gonzalez-Alvaro I, Balsa A, Angel Belmonte M, Tena X, Sanmarti R. Rheumatoid arthritis in Spain: occurrence of extra-articular manifestations and estimates of disease severity. Ann Rheum Dis 2003;62(9):897–900.
26. Moen K, Bertelsen LT, Hellem S, Jonsson R, Brun JG. Salivary gland and temporomandibular joint involvement in rheumatoid arthritis: relation to disease activity. Oral Dis 2005;11(1):27–34.
27. Watanabe Y, Mizukami T, Egawa T, et al. A case of progressive systemic sclerosis complicated by idiopathic portal hypertension with severe anemia. Ryumachi 1999;39(3):586–90.
28. Rhodus NL, Fricton J, Carlson P, Messner R. Oral symptoms associated with fibromyalgia syndrome. J Rheumatol 2003;30(8):1841–5.
29. Magro CM, Crowson AN. A clinical and histologic study of 37 cases of immunoglobulin A-associated vasculitis. Am J Dermatopathol 1999;21(3):234–40.
30. Brennan MT, Pillemer SR, Goldbach-Mansky R, El-Gabalawy H, Schumacher HR, Jr, Fox PC. Focal sialadenitis in patients with early synovitis. Clin Exp Rheumatol 2001;19(4):444–6.

31. Burnevich EZ, Lopatkina TN. System manifestations of primary biliary cirrhosis. Klin Med (Mosk) 2006;84(12):42–6.

32. Hiraoka A, Kojima N, Yamauchi Y, et al. An autopsy case of primary biliary cirrhosis with severe interstitial pneumonia. Intern Med 2001;40(11):1104–108.

33. Ikuno N, Mackay IR, Jois J, Omagari K, Rowley MJ. Antimitochondrial autoantibodies in saliva and sera from patients with primary biliary cirrhosis. J Gastroenterol Hepatol 2001;16(12):1390–94.

34. Valera MJ, Smok SG, Poniachik TJ, et al. Primary biliary cirrhosis: a thirteen years experience. Rev Med Chil 2006;134(4):469–74.

35. Arthritis Foundation. *Primer on the Rheumatic Diseases.* Atlanta, GA: Arthritis Foundation; 2005.

36. Belgodere X, Viraben R, Gorguet B, Allaouchiche B, Lieutaud O, Maestracci D. Guess what! Cutaneous sarcoidosis, Sjogren's syndrome and autoimmune thyroiditis associated with hepatitis C virus infection. Eur J Dermatol 1999;9(3):235–6.

37. Biro E, Szekanecz Z, Czirjak L, et al. Association of systemic and thyroid autoimmune diseases. Clin Rheumatol 2006;25(2):240–45.

38. D'Arbonneau F, Ansart S, Le Berre R, Dueymes M, Youinou P, Pennec YL. Thyroid dysfunction in primary Sjogren's syndrome: a long-term followup study. Arthritis Rheum 2003;49(6):804–809.

39. Kerimovic-Morina D. Autoimmune thyroid disease and associated rheumatic disorders. Srp Arh Celok Lek 2005;133(Suppl 1):55–60.

40. Mason DK, Harden RM, Alexander WD. The salivary and thyroid glands. A comparative study in man. Br Dent J 1967;122(11):485–9.

41. Soy M, Guldiken S, Arikan E, Altun BU, Tugrul A. Frequency of rheumatic diseases in patients with autoimmune thyroid disease. Rheumatol Int 2007;27(6):575–7.

42. Biasi D, Caramasch P, Carletto A, et al. Sjogren's syndrome associated with autoimmune hepatitis. A case report. Clin Rheumatol 1997;16(4):409–12.

43. Ishikawa Y, Cho G, Yuan Z, Inoue N, Nakae Y. Aquaporin-5 water channel in lipid rafts of rat parotid glands. Biochim Biophys Acta 2006;1758(8):1053–60.

44. Sorrentino D, Ferraccioli GF, DeVita S, Labombarda A, Boiocchi M, Bartoli E. Hepatitis C virus infection and gastric lymphoproliferation in patients with Sjogren's syndrome. Blood 1997;90(5):2116–17.

45. Itazu T, Takai S, Tono Y, Yasuda K, Hashimoto H, Hirose S. Case of subclinical sicca with acute pancreatitis and insulin dependent diabetes mellitus. Nippon Naika Gakkai Zasshi 1994;83(10):1831–3.

46. Yule AJ. Fibrocystic disease of the pancreas (mucoviscidosis). Case report. Aust Dent J 1970;15(6):519–20.

47. Kelly DR, Spiegel JC, Maves M. Benign lymphoepithelial lesions of the salivary glands. Arch Otolaryngol 1975;101(1):71–5.

48. Kelly IM, Lees WR, Watts RW. Case report: grey scale and colour Doppler ultrasound appearance of acute sarcoidosis of the parotid gland. Clin Radiol 1994;49(6):425–6.

49. Vasil'ev VI, Logvinenko OA, Simonova MV, et al. Sicca syndrome in sarcoidosis and involvement of the salivary and lacrymal glands. Ter Arkh 2005;77(1):62–7.
50. Neville BWDD, Allen CM, Bouquot JE. *Oral and Maxillofacial Pathology*. Philadelphia, PA: W.B. Saunders; 1995.
51. Frieri M. Identification of masqueraders of autoimmune disease in the office. Allergy Asthma Proc 2003;24(6):421–9.
52. Alavi AA, Amirhakimi E, Karami B. The prevalence of dental caries in 5–18-year-old insulin-dependent diabetics of Fars Province, southern Iran. Arch Iran Med 2006;9(3):254–60.
53. Belazi M, Velegraki A, Fleva A, et al. Candidal overgrowth in diabetic patients: potential predisposing factors. Mycoses 2005;48(3):192–6.
54. Ben-Aryeh H, Serouya R, Kanter Y, Szargel R, Laufer D. Oral health and salivary composition in diabetic patients. J Diabetes Complications 1993;7(1):57–62.
55. Benucci MDS, Saviola G, Manfredi M. Modifications of markers of bone resorption in patients affected by glucocorticoid induced osteoporosis (GIOP) treated with neridronate. Recenti Prog Med 2006;97(1):24–7.
56. Benucci M, Li Gobbi F, Del Gobbo A, Gambacorta G, Mannoni A. Association between serum amyloid A (SAA) in salivary glands and high levels of circulating beta 2-microglobulin in patients with Sjögren syndrome. Reumatismo 2003;55(2):98–101.
57. Bernardi MJ, Reis A, Loguercio AD, Kehrig R, Leite MF, Nicolau J. Study of the buffering capacity, pH and salivary flow rate in type 2 well-controlled and poorly controlled diabetic patients. Oral Health Prev Dent 2007;5(1):73–8.
58. Carda C, Mosquera-Lloreda N, Salom L, Gomez de Ferraris ME, Peydro A. Structural and functional salivary disorders in type 2 diabetic patients. Med Oral Patol Oral Cir Bucal 2006;11(4):E309–14.
59. Chavez EM, Taylor GW, Borrell LN, Ship JA. Salivary function and glycemic control in older persons with diabetes. Oral Surg Oral Med Oral Pathol Oral Radiol Endod 2000;89(3):305–11.
60. Cherry-Peppers G, Sorkin J, Andres R, Baum BJ, Ship JA. Salivary gland function and glucose metabolic status. J Gerontol 1992;47(4):M130–34.
61. Finney LS, Finney MO, Gonzalez-Campoy JM. What the mouth has to say about diabetes. Careful examinations can avert serious complications. Postgrad Med 1997;102(6):117–26.
62. Golla K, Epstein JB, Rada RE, Sanai R, Messieha Z, Cabay RJ. Diabetes mellitus: an updated overview of medical management and dental implications. Gen Dent 2004;52(6):529–35; quiz 36, 27–28.
63. Guggenheimer J, Moore PA. Xerostomia: etiology, recognition and treatment. J Am Dent Assoc 2003;134(1):61–9; quiz 118–9.
64. Guggenheimer J, Moore PA, Rossie K, et al. Insulin-dependent diabetes mellitus and oral soft tissue pathologies. I. Prevalence and characteristics of non-candidal lesions. Oral Surg Oral Med Oral Pathol Oral Radiol Endod 2000;89(5):563–9.

65. Kimura I, Sasamoto H, Sasamura T, Sugihara Y, Ohgaku S, Kobayashi M. Reduction of incretin-like salivatin in saliva from patients with type 2 diabetes and in parotid glands of streptozotocin-diabetic BALB/c mice. Diabetes Obes Metab 2001;3(4):254–8.
66. Lamey PJ, Darwazeh AM, Frier BM. Oral disorders associated with diabetes mellitus. Diabet Med 1992;9(5):410–16.
67. Meurman JH, Collin HL, Niskanen L, et al. Saliva in non-insulin-dependent diabetic patients and control subjects: the role of the autonomic nervous system. Oral Surg Oral Med Oral Pathol Oral Radiol Endod 1998;86(1):69–76.
68. Moore PA. The diabetes-oral health connection. Compend Contin Educ Dent 2002;23(Suppl 12):14–20.
69. Moore PA, Guggenheimer J, Etzel KR, Weyant RJ, Orchard T. Type 1 diabetes mellitus, xerostomia, and salivary flow rates. Oral Surg Oral Med Oral Pathol Oral Radiol Endod 2001;92(3):281–91.
70. Muzyka BC. Diabetes mellitus: a clinical update of terminology, prevalence, and economics. Pract Proced Aesthet Dent 2004;16(7):522.
71. Narhi TO, Meurman JH, Odont D, Ainamo A, Tilvis R. Oral health in the elderly with non-insulin-dependent diabetes mellitus. Spec Care Dentist 1996;16(3):116–22.
72. Rhodus NL. Detection and management of the diabetic patient. Compendium 1987;8(1):73–9.
73. Rhodus NL, Vibeto BM, Hamamoto DT. Glycemic control in patients with diabetes mellitus upon admission to a dental clinic: considerations for dental management. Quintessence Int 2005;36(6):474–82.
74. Stegeman CA. Oral manifestations of diabetes. Home Healthc Nurse 2005;23(4):233–40; quiz 41–2.
75. Vernillo AT. Diabetes mellitus: relevance to dental treatment. Oral Surg Oral Med Oral Pathol Oral Radiol Endod 2001;91(3):263–70.
76. Wollner D. Oral implications of diabetes mellitus. Pac Health Dialog 2003;10(1):98–101.
77. Zachariasen RD. Xerostomia and the diabetic patient. J Gt Houst Dent Soc 1996;67(7):10–13.
78. Zielinski MB, Fedele D, Forman LJ, Pomerantz SC. Oral health in the elderly with non-insulin-dependent diabetes mellitus. Spec Care Dentist 2002;22(3):94–8.
79. McDonald FG, Mantas J, McEwen CG, Ferguson MM. Salivary gland aplasia: an ectodermal disorder? J Oral Pathol 1986;15(2):115–17.
80. Prager TM, Finke C, Miethke RR. Dental findings in patients with ectodermal dysplasia. J Orofac Orthop 2006;67(5):347–55.
81. Singh P, Warnakulasuriya S. Aplasia of submandibular salivary glands associated with ectodermal dysplasia. J Oral Pathol Med 2004;33(10):634–6.
82. Matsuda C, Matsui Y, Ohno K, Michi K. Salivary gland aplasia with cleft lip and palate: a case report and review of the literature. Oral Surg Oral Med Oral Pathol Oral Radiol Endod 1999;87(5):594–9.
83. Vucicevic-Boras V, Juras D, Gruden-Pokupec JS, Vidovic A. Oral manifestations of triple A syndrome. Eur J Med Res 2003;8(7):318–20.

84. Ferguson MM, Ponnambalam Y. Aplasia of the parotid gland in Down syndrome. Br J Oral Maxillofac Surg 2005;43(2):113–17.
85. Slomiany BL, Murty VL, Slomiany A. Salivary lipids in health and disease. Prog Lipid Res 1985;24(4):311–24.
86. Chaudhry SI, Shirlaw PJ, Morgan PR, Challacombe SJ. Cowden's syndrome (multiple hamartoma and neoplasia syndrome): diagnostic dilemmas in three cases. Oral Dis 2000;6(4):248–52.
87. Fierek O, Laskawi R, Bonnemann C, Hanefeld F. The Levy-Hollister syndrome: a syndrome of dysplasias with ENT-manifestations. HNO 2003;51(8):654–7.
88. Basak PY, Ergin S, Sezer MT, Sari A. Amyloidosis of the tongue with kappa light chain disease. Australas J Dermatol 2001;42(1):55–7.
89. Jardinet D, Westhovens R, Peeters J. Sicca syndrome as an initial symptom of amyloidosis. Clin Rheumatol 1998;17(6):546–8.
90. Koloktronis A, Chatzigiannis I, Paloukidou N. Oral involvement in a case of AA amyloidosis. Oral Dis 2003;9(5):269–72.
91. Odell EW, Lombardi T, Shirlaw PJ, White CA. Minor salivary gland hyalinisation and amyloidosis in low-grade lymphoma of MALT. J Oral Pathol Med 1998;27(5):229–32.
92. Jaskoll T, Zhou YM, Chai Y, et al. Embryonic submandibular gland morphogenesis: stage-specific protein localization of FGFs, BMPs, Pax6 and Pax9 in normal mice and abnormal SMG phenotypes in FgfR2-IIIc(+/Delta), BMP7(−/−) and Pax6(−/−) mice. Cells Tissues Organs 2002;170(2–3):83–98.
93. Young W, Khan F, Brandt R, Savage N, Razek AA, Huang Q. Syndromes with salivary dysfunction predispose to tooth wear: case reports of congenital dysfunction of major salivary glands, Prader-Willi, congenital rubella, and Sjogren's syndromes. Oral Surg Oral Med Oral Pathol Oral Radiol Endod 2001;92(1):38–48.
94. Eronat N, Ucar F, Kilinc G. Papillon Lefevre syndrome: treatment of two cases with a clinical microbiological and histopathological investigation. J Clin Pediatr Dent 1993;17(2):99–104.
95. Malaviya AN, Kaushik P, Budhiraja S, et al. Hypergammaglobulinemic purpura of Waldenstrom: report of 3 cases with a short review. Clin Exp Rheumatol 2000;18(4):518–22.
96. Collin P, Reunala T, Pukkala E, Laippala P, Keyrilainen O, Pasternack A. Coeliac disease—associated disorders and survival. Gut 1994;35(9):1215–18.
97. Boyce HW, Bakheet MR. Sialorrhea: a review of a vexing, often unrecognized sign of oropharyngeal and esophageal disease. J Clin Gastroenterol 2005;39(2):89–97.
98. Chaby G, Viseux V, Poulain JF, De Cagny B, Denoeux JP, Lok C. Topical silver sulfadiazine-induced acute renal failure. Ann Dermatol Venereol 2005;132(11 Pt 1):891–3.
99. Adam FU, Torun D, Bolat F, Zumrutdal A, Sezer S, Ozdemir FN. Acute renal failure due to mesangial proliferative glomerulonephritis in a pregnant woman with primary Sjogren's syndrome. Clin Rheumatol 2006;25(1):75–9.

100. Bayraktar G, Kazancioglu R, Bozfakioglu S, Ecder T, Yildiz A, Ark E. Stimulated salivary flow rate in chronic hemodialysis patients. Nephron 2002;91(2):210–14.

101. Postorino M, Catalano C, Martorano C, et al. Salivary and lacrimal secretion is reduced in patients with ESRD. Am J Kidney Dis 2003;42(4): 722–8.

102. Schiodt FV, Clemmesen JO, Hansen BA, Larsen FS. Cerebral edema due to hemodialysis in paracetamol-induced fulminant hepatic failure. Scand J Gastroenterol 1995;30(9):927–8.

103. Aiello M, Chetta A, Marangio E, Zompatori M, Olivieri D. Pleural involvement in systemic disorders. Curr Drug Targets Inflamm Allergy 2004;3(4):441–7.

104. Lambert M, Hebbar M, Viget N, Hatron PY, Hachulla E, Devulder B. Bronchiolitis obliterans with organized pneumonia: a rare complication of primary Gougerot-Sjogren syndrome. Rev Med Interne 2000;21(1):74–7.

105. McGrath-Morrow S, Laube B, Tzou SC, et al. IL-12 overexpression in mice as a model for Sjogren lung disease. Am J Physiol Lung Cell Mol Physiol 2006;291(4):L837–46.

106. Todea D, Ariesanu N. Diagnostic problems in pleural involvement in systemic diseases. Pneumologia 2006;55(3):119–22.

107. Airoldi M, Crespi D, Puricelli S, Pelucco L. Chronic lymphatic leukemia and large granular lymphocytes. Recenti Prog Med 1998;89(2):74–8.

108. Marsot-Dupuch K, Quillard J, Meyohas MC. Head and neck lesions in the immunocompromised host. Eur Radiol 2004;14(Suppl 3):E155–67.

109. Singh B, Poluri A, Shaha AR, Michuart P, Har-El G, Lucente FE. Head and neck manifestations of non-Hodgkin's lymphoma in human immunodeficiency virus-infected patients. Am J Otolaryngol 2000;21(1):10–13.

110. Sugai S. Sjogren's syndrome associated with liver and neurological disorders, and malignant lymphoma. Intern Med 2000;39(3):193–4.

111. Borgna-Pignatti C, Cammareri V, De Stefano P, Magrini U. The sicca syndrome in thalassaemia major. Br Med J (Clin Res Ed) 1984;288(6418):668–9.

112. Enwonwu CO. Ascorbate status and xerostomia. Med Hypotheses 1992;39(1):53–7.

113. Rhodus NL, Brown J. The association of xerostomia and inadequate intake in older adults. J Am Diet Assoc 1990;90(12):1688–92.

114. Rhodus NL. Qualitative nutritional intake analysis of older adults with Sjogren's syndrome. Gerodontology 1988;7(2):61–9.

115. Frezzini C, Pabari S, Chaudhry S, Hodgson T, Porter S. Trigeminal neuropathy and autonomic neuropathy—a rare combination: OC7. Oral Dis 2006;12(s1):11.

116. Graham CH, Meechan JG. Dental management of patients taking methadone. Dent Update 2005;32(8):477–8, 81–2, 85.

117. Saini T, Edwards PC, Kimmes NS, Carroll LR, Shaner JW, Dowd FJ. Etiology of xerostomia and dental caries among methamphetamine abusers. Oral Health Prev Dent 2005;3(3):189–95.

118. Sandberg GE, Wikblad KF. Oral dryness and peripheral neuropathy in subjects with type 2 diabetes. J Diabetes Complications 2003;17(4):192–8.

119. Rothstein. Allergic reaction to thioridazine. N Engl J Med 1974;63:6.

120. Akhondzadeh S, Fallah-Pour H, Afkham K, Jamshidi AH, Khalighi-Cigaroudi F. Comparison of *Crocus sativus* L. and imipramine in the treatment of mild to moderate depression: a pilot double-blind randomized trial [ISRCTN45683816]. BMC Complement Altern Med 2004;4:12.

121. Valtysdottir ST, Gudbjornsson B, Lindqvist U, Hallgren R, Hetta J. Anxiety and depression in patients with primary Sjogren's syndrome. J Rheumatol 2000;27(1):165–9.

122. Rhodus NL, Little JW. Dental management of the bone marrow transplant patient. Compendium 1992;13(11):1040, 2–50.

123. Diaz-Ortiz ML, Mico-Llorens JM, Gargallo-Albiol J, Baliellas-Comellas C, Berini-Aytes L, Gay-Escoda C. Dental health in liver transplant patients. Med Oral Patol Oral Cir Bucal 2005;10(1):72–6; 66–72.

124. Guggenheimer J, Eghtesad B, Close JM, Shay C, Fung JJ. Dental health status of liver transplant candidates. Liver Transpl 2007;13(2):280–86.

125. Rhodus NL, Little JW. Dental management of the renal transplant patient. Compendium 1993;14(4):518–24, 26, 28 passim; quiz 32.

126. Schiodt FV, Atillasoy E, Shakil AO, et al. Etiology and outcome for 295 patients with acute liver failure in the United States. Liver Transpl Surg 1999;5(1):29–34.

127. Brinton LA, Buckley LM, Dvorkina O, et al. Risk of connective tissue disorders among breast implant patients. Am J Epidemiol 2004;160(7):619–27.

128. Okoje VN, Obiechina AE, Aken'Ova YA. Orofacial lesions in 126 newly diagnosed HIV/AIDS patients seen at the University College Hospital, Ibadan. Afr J Med Med Sci 2006;35(1):97–101.

129. Fleck M, Kern ER, Zhou T, Lang B, Mountz JD. Murine cytomegalovirus induces a Sjogren's syndrome-like disease in C57Bl/6-lpr/lpr mice. Arthritis Rheum 1998;41(12):2175–84.

130. Ceballos-Salobrena A, Gaitan-Cepeda LA, Ceballos-Garcia L, Lezama-Del Valle D. Oral lesions in HIV/AIDS patients undergoing highly active antiretroviral treatment including protease inhibitors: a new face of oral AIDS? AIDS Patient Care STDS 2000;14(12):627–35.

131. LIttle J, Rhodus N. HIV and AIDs: update for dentistry. Gen Dent 2007;55(3):184–96.

132. Schiodt M. HIV-associated salivary gland disease: a review. Oral Surg Oral Med Oral Pathol 1992;73(2):164–7.

133. Schiodt M, Atkinson JC, Greenspan D, et al. Sialochemistry in human immunodeficiency virus associated salivary gland disease. J Rheumatol 1992;19(1):26–9.

134. Zeitlen S, Shaha A. Parotid manifestations of HIV infection. J Surg Oncol 1991;47(4):230–32.

135. Abraham S, Begum S, Isenberg D. Hepatic manifestations of autoimmune rheumatic diseases. Ann Rheum Dis 2004;63(2):123–9.

136. Boscagli A, Hatron PY, Canva-Delcambre V, et al. Sicca syndrome and hepatitis C virus infection: a Gougerot-Sjogren pseudo-syndrome? Rev Med Interne 1996;17(5):375–80.

137. Cacoub P. Treatment of extrahepatic manifestations associated with hepatitis C virus infection. Gastroenterol Clin Biol 2002;26(Spec No 2):B210–19.

138. Cacoub P. Extrahepatic manifestations associated with hepatitis C virus. Nephrologie 2001;22(6):295–6.
139. Carrozzo M, Gandolfo S. Oral diseases possibly associated with hepatitis C virus. Crit Rev Oral Biol Med 2003;14(2):115–27.
140. Casals MR, Garcia-Carrasco M, Cervera R, Font J. Sjogren syndrome and hepatitis C virus infection. Med Clin (Barc) 1999;112(18):718–9.
141. Coates EA, Brennan D, Logan RM, et al. Hepatitis C infection and associated oral health problems. Aust Dent J 2000;45(2):108–14.
142. De Vita S, De Re V, Sansonno D, et al. Gastric mucosa as an additional extrahepatic localization of hepatitis C virus: viral detection in gastric low-grade lymphoma associated with autoimmune disease and in chronic gastritis. Hepatology 2000;31(1):182–9.
143. Drucker Y. Hepatitis C virus infection in patients with Sjogren's syndrome and non-Hodgkin's lymphoma: comment on the article by Voulgarelis et al. Arthritis Rheum 2000;43(5):1187.
144. Garcia-Carrasco M, Escarcega RO. Extrahepatic autoimmune manifestations of chronic hepatitis C virus infection. Ann Hepatol 2006;5(3):161–3.
145. Garcia-Carrasco M, Ramos M, Cervera R, et al. Hepatitis C virus infection in "primary" Sjogren's syndrome: prevalence and clinical significance in a series of 90 patients. Ann Rheum Dis 1997;56(3):173–5.
146. Gordon SC. Extrahepatic manifestations of hepatitis C. Dig Dis 1996;14(3):157–68.
147. Gumber SC, Chopra S. Hepatitis C: a multifaceted disease. Review of extrahepatic manifestations. Ann Intern Med 1995;123(8):615–20.
148. Jorgensen C, Legouffe MC, Perney P, et al. Sicca syndrome associated with hepatitis C virus infection. Arthritis Rheum 1996;39(7):1166–71.
149. Nagao Y, Sata M. HCV and extrahepatic manifestations. Nippon Rinsho 2004;62(Suppl 7)(Pt 1):561–8.
150. Ramos-Casals M, Cervera Segura R. Sjogren syndrome and hepatitis C virus: casual or etiopathogenic relationship. Rev Clin Esp 2001;201(9):515–7.
151. Font J, Tassies D, Garcia-Carrasco M, et al. Hepatitis G virus infection in primary Sjogren's syndrome: analysis in a series of 100 patients. Ann Rheum Dis 1998;57(1):42–4.
152. Greenberg MS, Glick M, Nghiem L, Stewart JC, Hodinka R, Dubin G. Relationship of cytomegalovirus to salivary gland dysfunction in HIV-infected patients. Oral Surg Oral Med Oral Pathol Oral Radiol Endod 1997;83(3):334–9.
153. Dawson TM, Starkebaum G, Wood BL, Willkens RF, Gown AM. Epstein-Barr virus, methotrexate, and lymphoma in patients with rheumatoid arthritis and primary Sjogren's syndrome: case series. J Rheumatol 2001;28(1):47–53.
154. Fox RI. Clinical features, pathogenesis, and treatment of Sjogren's syndrome. Curr Opin Rheumatol 1996;8(5):438–45.
155. Nagata Y, Inoue H, Yamada K, et al. Activation of Epstein-Barr virus by saliva from Sjogren's syndrome patients. Immunology 2004;111(2):223–9.
156. Christensen T, Moller-Larsen A. Human endogenous retroviruses and disease? Ugeskr Laeger 2003;165(6):556–61.

157. Mason AL, Xu L, Guo L, Garry RF. Retroviruses in autoimmune liver disease: genetic or environmental agents? Arch Immunol Ther Exp (Warsz) 1999;47(5):289–97.
158. Ericson S ZB, Ohman J. Recurrent parotitis and sialactesis in childhood. Ann Otol, Rhino, Laryngol 1991;100(2):25–56.
159. Raad SM, II, Caranasos GF. Acute bacterial sialadenitis. Rev Inf Dis 1990;12(12):591–5.
160. Sato R, Fujioka T, Murakami K, Kodama M. *Helicobacter pylori* eradication therapy for extragastrodudenal diseases. Nippon Shokakibyo Gakkai Zasshi 2003;100(11):1295–301.
161. Correa PA, Gomez LM, Cadena J, Anaya JM. Autoimmunity and tuberculosis. Opposite association with TNF polymorphism. J Rheumatol 2005;32(2):219–24.
162. Battino M, Ferreiro MS, Gallardo I, Newman HN, Bullon P. The antioxidant capacity of saliva. J Clin Periodontol 2002;29(3):189–94.
163. De Stefano R, Manganelli S, Frati E, et al. No association between human parvovirus B19 infection and Sjogren's syndrome. Ann Rheum Dis 2003;62(1):86–7.
164. Coates E, Brennan D, Logan R, et al. Hepatitis C infection and associated oral health problems. Aust Dent J 2000;45(2):108–14.
165. Haddad J, Deny P. Lymphocytic sialoadenitis of Sjogren's syndrome associated with chronic hepatitis C virus liver. Lancet 1992;339(8789):321.
166. Loustaud-Ratti V, Riche A, Liozon E, et al. Prevalence and characteristics of Sjogren's syndrome or Sicca syndrome in chronic hepatitis C virus infection: a prospective study. J Rheumatol 2001;28(10):2245–51.
167. Vitali C, Bombardieri S, Moutsopoulos HM, et al. Assessment of the European classification criteria for Sjogren's syndrome in a series of clinically defined cases: results of a prospective multicentre study. The European Study Group on Diagnostic Criteria for Sjogren's Syndrome. Ann Rheum Dis 1996;55(2):116–21.
168. Ferreiro MC, Prieto MH, Rodriguez SB, Vazquez RL, Iglesias AC, Dios PD. Whole stimulated salivary flow in patients with chronic hepatitis C virus infection. J Oral Pathol Med 2002;31(2):117–20.

20

Progression and treatment evaluation in diseases affecting salivary glands

Jiska M. Meijer, Cees G.M. Kallenberg, and Arjan Vissink

INTRODUCTION

Many diseases and conditions can affect salivary glands resulting in a reduced or increased salivary flow. Treatment for these and other disorders can affect salivary secretion as well. Frequent causes of long-lasting reduced salivary flow are drugs, systemic conditions like Sjögren's syndrome, and radiation injury to salivary gland tissue.

The sensation of a dry mouth (xerostomia) is not always accompanied by a reduced salivary secretion (hyposalivation). In about one-third of the patients with xerostomia, there is no good correlation between actual mouth dryness and level of salivary secretion. The discrepancy between salivary secretion status and level of complaints is even more striking in drooling. Usually, salivary secretion is normal or even reduced, but swallowing of saliva is impaired. Well-known causes of the inability to empty the mouth of saliva are an infantile swallowing pattern, a disturbed sensibility of the oral tissues, and anatomic limitations due to trauma and ablative surgery. Thus, many factors have to be considered when selecting a salivary evaluation tool for the subset of patients or healthy subjects.

Notwithstanding the above, salivary research provides powerful tools to diagnose diseases affecting salivary glands, to assess disease progression, and to evaluate treatment. In progressive diseases like Sjögren's syndrome (SS), salivary secretion generally diminishes with time (Fig. 20.1). This progression is not so obvious when monitoring whole saliva, but becomes much clearer when measuring gland-specific saliva.[1] While sialometry is a robust tool for evaluating disease progression, analysis of salivary composition (sialochemistry) differentiates between salivary gland diseases, and measures the disease activity (Table 20.1)[2] and the effect of intervention treatment.[3] Additional tools are sialography (imaging of the extent of destruction of the ductal system), salivary scintigraphy (imaging of the glandular secretory activity), salivary gland biopsy (glandular pathology underlying the observed changes), and the imaging of the anatomical structures with CT, MRI, or ultrasound.

The six above-mentioned variables (sialometry, sialochemistry, sialography, salivary scintigraphy, biopsy, and imaging) are gland-specific and can measure disease progression and/or activity. Other essential information might come

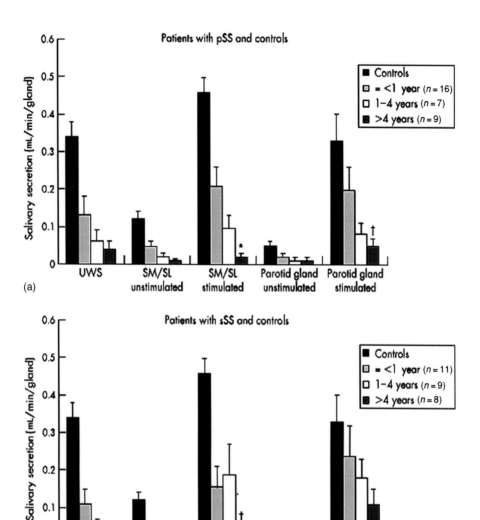

Figure 20.1 Relationship between disease duration (time from first complaints induced by or related to oral dryness until referral) and standard error of mean (SEM) salivary flow rates in patients with (a) primary Sjögren's syndrome (pSS) and in those with (b) secondary Sjögren's syndrome (sSS). Normal values are derived from historic controls ($n = 36$). SM/SL, submandibular/sublingual glands; UWS, unstimulated whole saliva. *Significant difference versus patients with early Sjögren's syndrome (<1 year oral complaints; $p < 0.005$) by the Mann–Whitney U test. †Significant difference versus patients with early Sjögren's syndrome ($p < 0.05$) by the Mann–Whitney U test. (Modified after Pijpe et al.[1])

Table 20.1 Salivary gland parameters and clinical data of some disorders affecting the salivary glands (van den Berg et al., 2007).[2]

	SS (pSS/sSS)	Sialosis	Sodium retention syndrome	Medication-induced xerostomia
Sialometry	UWS ≤1.5 mL in 15 min	Normal, increased, or decreased	Normal or decreased	UWS decreased; SWS (sub)normal
Sialochemistry	Na and Cl increased	K increased	Na decreased	Normal
Sialography	Sialectasia	Thin duct system, enlarged gland	Usually normal, but a thin duct system and enlarged gland may be present	Normal
Complaints	Mouth dryness in rest and during eating or speaking Need for drinks to swallow (dry) food Eye dryness. Swelling of the salivary glands	Persistent, bilateral swelling of the parotid glands	Often mouth dryness Recurrent, short lasting (usually at most some hours), mostly unilateral swellings of the parotid gland	Mouth dryness in rest
Schirmer's test	≤5 mm/5 min	Unknown, but reduction is not uncommon	Unknown, but reduction is not uncommon	Unknown, but reduction is not uncommon
Associated diseases	sSS: associated with another connective tissue/autoimmune disease	Endocrine disorder Metabolic disorder Dysfunction ANS	Cardiovascular disease Disorder of the fluid or electrolyte balance	Use of xerogenic medication

Sjögren's syndrome is an autoimmune disorder affecting the exocrine glands including the salivary glands. Sialosis is a salivary condition characterized by persistent swelling of the parotid glands related to a metabolic disorder as diabetes, alcohol abuse, anorexia, and bulimia. Sodium retention syndrome is characterized by mostly unilateral, incidental, short-lasting (hours) swelling of the parotid gland often related to cardiovascular disorders (hypotension, hypertension). SS, Sjögren's syndrome; pSS, primary Sjögren's syndrome; sSS, secondary Sjögren's syndrome; UWS: unstimulated whole saliva; SWS, stimulated whole saliva; SM/SL, saliva from sublingual/mandibular gland; ANS, autonomic nervous system.

from the pattern of complaints, medical history, the clinical picture, serology, and questionnaires. Serological parameters and subjective questionnaire responses can add important information on the disease progression and treatment outcome.

This chapter discusses the main tools for evaluation of disease progression and treatment including applications to clinical research and practice.

TOOLS TO MEASURE SALIVARY GLAND FUNCTION AND DISEASE ACTIVITY

Sialometry

Saliva collection provides sound clinical information. Accurate measures of salivary flow rate and composition are essential for many diagnostic, therapeutic, and research protocols. Saliva collection is a noninvasive tool of assessing a variety of disease characteristics and levels of certain drugs and hormones. Whole saliva is a mixture of not only salivary secretions, but also fluids, debris, and cells not originating in the salivary glands. Therefore, the analysis of individual gland saliva is usually a more reliable procedure for diagnosing diseases of the salivary glands than analysis of whole saliva. However, for certain diagnostic procedures whole saliva might be more useful, for example, when assessing specific roles of saliva in the oral cavity or when whole saliva is used as a diagnostic fluid for conditions relying on leakage of serum products or gingival crevicular fluid into saliva. For the various methods that can be applied to collect saliva, see Chapter 4.

In healthy subjects and patients in whom both glands are affected simultaneously (e.g., Sjögren's syndrome), flow rates of the left and right parotid glands are similar. Therefore, sorting out discrepancies between the observed flow of the left and right parotid glands assures the reliability of the samples collected. This is a very powerful internal control of the reliability of the saliva sample collected and outweighs the effect of repeated sampling of a parotid gland to get a reliable baseline sample. Increasing the number of collections has been shown to have a negligible effect on the reliability of baseline parotid flow rates for clinical trials. Consequently, one reliable baseline sample is sufficient for clinical studies evaluating the progression of disease or the effect of a therapy.[4] Moreover, salivary flow rates are not constant and exhibit a considerable amount of variability. Therefore, salivary collections should be performed under well-defined conditions and, for repeated collections, at the same time of the day to minimize intrapatient variability. Nevertheless, even if the circadian rhythm is ruled out and the samples are indeed collected under well-defined conditions, the measured increase or decrease of salivary flow has to exceed about one-quarter to one-third of the parotid flow rate at baseline before an observed effect related to a given therapy can be assessed as a "real" effect in an individual patient. This information is in addition to subjective assessments of such an effect.[4]

Sialochemistry

Saliva is an attractive diagnostic fluid because salivary testing provides several key advantages including low cost, noninvasiveness, and easy sample collection and processing. Human saliva collection is less invasive than phlebotomy and is clinically relevant because many, if not all, blood components are reflected in saliva. Among others, sodium, potassium, chloride, calcium, phosphate, urea, total protein, and a number of enzymes (e.g., amylase, lysozyme, and lactoferrin) can be detected in saliva and have diagnostic potential (Table 20.1). In addition, a large range of more or less disease-related changes in protein composition of saliva have been reported. A new method to assess the protein composition in health and disease is salivary proteomics—the identification of the entire spectrum of proteins in human saliva. Saliva also harbors diagnostic RNA biomarkers (detection of RNA biomarkers); see Chapters 11 and 12 (salivary proteomics and genomics).

Sialography

Through retrograde infusion of oil- or water-based iodine contrast, the architecture of the salivary duct system is visualized radiographically. It is a low morbidity, well-accepted technique. Sialography should not, however, be performed in patients with a history of iodine allergy. The sialographic procedure can be performed in 10–15 min.

Inflammation appears on sialograms as diffuse collections of contrast fluid at the terminal acini of the ductal tree. This condition, known as sialectasia, can be classified into punctate (<1 mm), globular (uniform and 1–2 mm), cavitary (coalescent and >2 mm), and destructive (normal ductal structures are no longer visible). Sialectasia is thought to result from progressive acinar atrophy and dilatation, which, in turn, is caused by increasing intraluminal pressure resulting from the presence of periductal lymphocytic infiltrates with secondary duct narrowing. So, these four grades of sialectasia are thought to represent increasing glandular damage, caused by chronic salivary gland inflammation.

Salivary scintigraphy

Salivary scintigraphy is based on the ability of parotid and submandibular glands to trap the radionuclide isotope technetium-sodium (Tc99m) pertechnetate. This ability is due to the fact that Tc99m substitutes for chloride in the active sodium/potassium/chloride cotransport in the striated ducts. After intravenous injection of Tc99m, scintigraphy may reveal functional abnormality of the salivary glands through photographically recording with a gamma scintillation camera, the radiation from salivary isotope accumulation and excretion.

Improvements of salivary scintigraphy include salivary single-photon emission computed tomography (SPECT) and human immunoglobulin G (HIG) scintigraphy. Salivary SPECT creates a three-dimensional image with a rotating gamma camera without marking an ROI (region of interest) as it uses a single pixel as the ultimate ROI. Scintigraphy is a valuable tool to measure activity of the glands, and it can be performed in the same gland at different time periods to assess progression. Unfortunately, the diagnostic accuracy is low.

Computer tomography and magnetic resonance imaging

Magnetic resonance imaging (MRI) depicts lesions more accurately because soft tissue contrast resolution is better in MRI than computer tomography

(CT). Detailed knowledge of the anatomy of the parotid gland and surrounding structures is necessary for evaluating and diagnosing lesions. Bilateral imaging and comparison between right and left glands is essential. CT and MRI are of less value as diagnostic tools for such salivary gland disorders as Sjögren's syndrome, sialadenosis, and bacterial or viral sialadenitis.

Ultrasound

Ultrasound has no known contraindications and is a quick and well-accepted, noninvasive procedure. With color Doppler sonography, the complex vascular anatomy can be accurately recorded.[5] Its potential in routine salivary diagnostics is restricted as tissue penetration depth is limited and proper interpretation of salivary sonograms requires a great deal of experience.

Histopathology

The labial and parotid glands are accessible for histopathological evaluation, and biopsies from these glands are often performed routinely. In Sjögren's syndrome, a disease affecting the salivary glands in which biopsies most often are taken as a routine procedure, the parotid and labial gland biopsies are diagnostically comparable. However, a parotid biopsy is preferred, due to lower morbidity than labial biopsies in which sensory loss may occur, easier access to larger tissue samples, and earlier detection of lymphomas.[6] In addition, repeated biopsies can be taken from the same parotid gland, making parotid biopsies an important tool in treatment evaluation (the outcomes can even be compared with saliva samples obtained from the same gland).

Cytology

A cytological puncture (ultrasound guided) can distinguish salivary gland disorders from lymph nodes disorders, and inflammation from malignancy.

Subjective evaluation

VAS

A visual analog scale (VAS) is a line of, for example, 10 mm on which the patient can mark the severity of the complaint. For Sjögren's syndrome, VAS scores are available for oral dryness, oral dryness during the day, oral dryness at night, difficulty swallowing *dry* food without any additional liquids, difficulty swallowing *any* food without any additional liquids, difficulty speaking without drinking liquids, and dry eyes (sensation of sand or gravel in the eyes).

MFI

The multidimensional fatigue index (MFI) is a 20-item self-report instrument designed to objectively measure fatigue, including the dimensions of general fatigue, physical fatigue, mental fatigue, reduced motivation, and reduced activity. This validated questionnaire detects expected differences in fatigue between groups, within groups, and between conditions.[7] A higher score (range 4–20) indicates a higher level of fatigue. Fatigue is a complaint not uncommon to patients suffering from salivary gland disorders, particularly patients with salivary gland disorders related to an autoimmune disease or as a result of cancer treatment.

SF-36

The 36-item short form (SF-36) is constructed to survey health status and was designed for use in clinical practice and research, health policy evaluations, and general population surveys. The SF-36 includes one multi-item scale that assesses eight health concepts. The questionnaire has been developed for self-administration by persons 14 years of age and older or for administration by a trained interviewer. A higher score indicates a higher level of well-being.[8] Health status can severely be impaired in patients suffering from salivary gland disorders particularly in patients with salivary gland disorders related to an autoimmune disease or as a result of cancer treatment.

Dry mouth questionnaires

Objective salivary gland function is not always consistent with the subjective perception. Whether the patient reports sipping liquids to aid in swallowing dry foods, dry mouth when eating a meal, or difficulties swallowing any foods is highly predictive of salivary gland function and, therefore, clinically useful in patients who report oral dryness.[9]

Serological parameters

In systemic diseases affecting the salivary glands, serological parameters can be useful in evaluating activity and progression of the disease and in evaluating treatment. For example, C-reactive protein (CRP) and erythrocyte sedimentation rate (ESR) are general parameters in peripheral blood for inflammation and are elevated in most autoimmune diseases. IgM-Rf (rheumatoid factor) and IgA correlate with B-cell activity and are elevated in SS. IgM-Rf is also elevated in patients with rheumatoid arthritis and some other conditions. Antinuclear antibodies (ANA), anti-Ro/SSA and anti-La/SSB, can be detected in SS (anti-SSB is the most specific antibody).

APPLICATION OF THESE TOOLS IN CLINICAL RESEARCH AND CLINICAL PRACTICE

The clinical application of the above-mentioned variables in treatment evaluation will be illustrated for patients with a reduced salivary flow due to head and neck radiotherapy and Sjögren's syndrome.

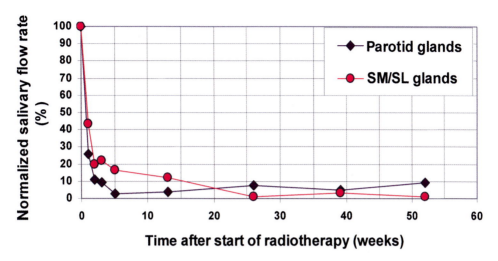

Figure 20.2 Flow rate of parotid and submandibular/sublingual saliva (SM/SL) as a function of time after start of radiotherapy (conventional fractionation schedule, 2 Gy per day, 5 days per week, total dose 60–70 Gy). The parotid, submandibular, and sublingual glands are located in the treatment portal. Initial flow rates were set to 100%. (Adapted from Burlage et al.[12])

Radiotherapy

Xerostomia is a common and disturbing side effect of head and neck radio-therapy, leading to considerable morbidity, including severe oral discomfort, problems with speaking, dysphagia, and an increased incidence of caries and mucosal infections. Although new radiation techniques enabled significant sparing of the parotid glands, the amount of normal salivary gland tissue irra-diated may still be substantial resulting in clinically relevant radiation-induced xerostomia.[10,11]

Although salivary gland tissue is a well-differentiated tissue and, theoret-ically, should be relatively radioresistant, studies have shown a rapid decline in parotid and submandibular/sublingual salivary flow, even after low doses of radiotherapy (Fig. 20.2). In humans, it has been reported that the TD_{50} (i.e., the dose to the whole organ leading to a complication probability of 50%) for parotid glands varies from 28.4 to 31 Gy at 6 weeks increasing to 39 Gy at 1 year after completion of radiotherapy.

Sjögren's syndrome

Sjögren's syndrome (SS) is a chronic lymphoproliferative autoimmune disease with disturbances of T-lymphocytes, B-lymphocytes, and exocrine glandular cells. SS can be primary (pSS) or secondary (sSS), the latter being associated with another autoimmune disease (e.g., rheumatoid arthritis and systemic lu-pus erythematosus). The main symptoms of SS are xerostomia, dry eyes (ker-atoconjunctivitis sicca), increased caries activity, fatigue, and arthralgia (sys-temic features). The disease can have a great impact on the quality of life of

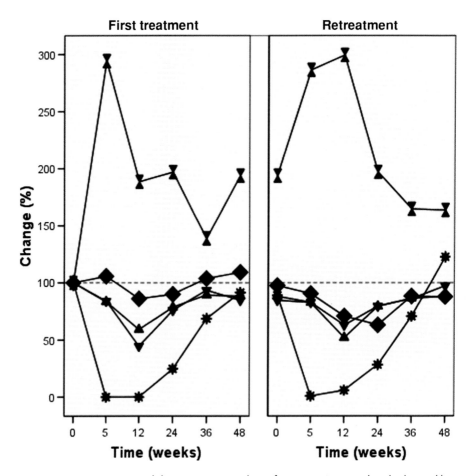

Figure 20.3   Increase and decrease (mean values of 5 patients) in stimulated submandibular/sublingual flow rate, IgM-RF, B cells, VAS score for dry mouth during the night and multidimensional fatigue inventory (MFI) score for fatigue following rituximab (re)treatment (baseline is 100%). Baseline values (week 0, first treatment) were stimulated submandibular/sublingual flow rate 0.09 mL/min (SD 0.07), IgM-RF 339 (SD 329), B cells 0.19 10^9/L (SD 0.09), VAS score for dry mouth during the night 85 (SD 12), MFI score for fatigue 16 (SD 3). (Modified after Meijer et al.[13]). ●, stimulated submandibular/sublingual salivary flow rate; ♦, IgM-RF; ∗, B cells; ▲, VAS score for dry mouth during the night; ▼, score for fatigue.

the patients. There are no causal treatment options, and treatment used today is mainly symptomatic. Dry eyes are treated with eyedrops or gel, and sometimes anti-inflammatory or immunosuppressive medication is indicated. Dry mouth is treated with saliva-stimulating medication (pilocarpine) or with saliva substitutes. Currently, drug trials are evaluating biological agents with promising early results (Fig. 20.3).

Sialometry and sialochemistry

Salivary flow rates have diagnostic and prognostic value in SS. Since the amount and composition of saliva reflects the autoimmune process in the salivary glands, analysis of saliva may also be valuable in diagnosis, prognosis, and evaluation of treatment. SS is characterized by high sodium and high chloride concentration and a low phosphate concentration in parotid saliva.

Sialometry and sialochemistry, easily performed and tolerated, are valuable in measuring disease progression (Fig. 20.1) and treatment outcome. For example, rituximab significantly increased salivary secretion (Fig. 20.3) and nearly normalized salivary sodium concentration.

A pilot study of ten SS patients and ten age- and sex-matched controls demonstrated that pSS patients' saliva contains proteomic and genomic diagnostic biomarker candidates (see Fig. 4 in reference 14).

Proteomics of saliva may also be useful in diagnosis, disease progression, and treatment evaluation, but further research is necessary to precisely assess its value.

Histopathology

In SS, widely accepted criteria for histologic confirmation is focal lymphocytic sialoadenitis in labial salivary glands and lymphoepithelial lesions in parotid salivary glands.

Moreover, repeated salivary gland biopsies might offer an objective method for evaluating treatment, in addition to serological and functional parameters. The parotid gland is the primary site to study changes after systemic therapy since SS lymphoproliferation occurs especially in these glands. Repeated parotid biopsies in SS patients treated with rituximab show redifferentiation of lymphoepithelial lesions into regular ducts, which is in line with the sialochemical changes in parotid saliva.

Subjective evaluation

Fatigue is one of the most disabling complaints in SS, and it leads to a substantial decrease in health-related quality of life. By using the MFI, patients with pSS reported more fatigue than healthy controls on all the dimensions of the MFI and, when controlling for depression, significant differences remain on the dimensions of general fatigue, physical fatigue, and reduced activity. VAS scores have been used to assess subjective sicca complaints and have been validated for patients with xerostomia. After rituximab treatment, in patients with early pSS, assessment of mouth dryness, arthralgia, physical functioning, vitality, and most domains of the MFI significantly improved.[3]

Serological parameters

Polyclonal expansion and secretory hyperactivity of B cells is an early event in pSS. This is demonstrated in the blood by increased amounts of different autoantibodies and by increased amounts of total Ig (primarily IgG). The more serious systemic complications occur mainly in patients with increased IgM-Rf levels, and levels of circulating IgM-Rf correlate positively with the number of extraglandular disease manifestations. Other researchers also reported an association between a high B-cell autoreactivity (production of ANA, anti-Ro/SSA, and anti-La/SSB) and the development of complications or more severe manifestations like neuropathy, kidney, and pulmonary involvement. Rituximab treatment resulted in pSS patients in a rapid decrease in peripheral B cells, accompanied by a decrease in IgM-Rf levels (Fig. 20.3).

CONCLUSION

Salivary research provides powerful tools to diagnose diseases affecting the salivary glands, to assess disease progression, and to evaluate treatment. Important gland-specific parameters are sialometry, sialochemistry, and histopathology. More general tools are subjective questionnaires (e.g., VAS, MFI, SF-36) and serological parameters.

REFERENCES

1. Pijpe J, Kalk WWI, Bootsma H, Spijkervet FKL, Kallenberg CGM, Vissink A. Progression of salivary gland dysfunction in patients with Sjögren's syndrome. Ann Rheum Dis 2007;66(1):107–12.
2. van den Berg I, Pijpe J, Vissink A. Salivary gland parameters and clinical data related to the underlying disorder in patients with persisting xerostomia. Eur J Oral Sci 2007;115(2):97–102.
3. Pijpe J, van Imhoff GW, Spijkervet FKL, et al. Rituximab treatment in patients with primary Sjögren's syndrome: an open-label phase II study. Arthritis Rheum 2005;52(9):2740–50.
4. Burlage FR, Pijpe J, Coppes RP, et al. Accuracy of collecting stimulated human parotid saliva. Eur J of Oral Sci 2005;113(5):386–90.
5. Martinoli C, Derchi LE, Solbiati L, Rizzatto G, Silvestri E, Giannoni M. Color Doppler sonography of salivary glands. Am J Roentgenol 1994;163(4):933–41.
6. Pijpe J, Kalk WWI, van der Wal JE, et al. Parotid gland biopsy compared with labial biopsy in the diagnosis of patients with primary Sjögren's syndrome. Rheumatology (Oxford) 2007;46(2):335–41.
7. Smets EM, Garssen B, Bonke B, De Haes JC. The Multidimensional Fatigue Inventory (MFI) psychometric qualities of an instrument to assess fatigue. J Psychosom Res 1995;39(3):315–25.
8. Ware JE, Jr, Sherbourne CD. The MOS 36-item short-form health survey (SF-36). I. Conceptual framework and item selection. Med Care 1992; 30(6):473–83.
9. Fox PC, Busch KA, Baum BJ. Subjective reports of xerostomia and objective measures of salivary gland performance. J Am Dent Assoc 1987;115(4): 581–4.
10. Terhaard CH, Lubsen H, Rasch CR, et al. The role of radiotherapy in the treatment of malignant salivary gland tumors. Int J Radiat Oncol Biol Phys 2005;61(1):103–11.
11. Vissink A, Burlage FR, Spijkervet FK, Jansma J, Coppes RP. Prevention and treatment of the consequences of head and neck radiotherapy. Crit Rev Oral Biol Med 2003;14(3):213–25.

12. Burlage FR, Coppes RP, Meertens H, Stokman MA, Vissink A. Parotid and submandibular/sublingual salivary flow during high dose radiotherapy. Radiother Oncol 2001;61(3):271–4.

13. Meijer JM, Pijpe J, Vissink A, Kallenberg CGM, Bootsma H. Treatment of primary Sjögren's syndrome with rituximab: extended follow-up, safety and efficacy of retreatment. Ann Rheum Dis, in press.

14. Hu S, Wang J, Meijer J, et al. Salivary proteomic and genomic biomarkers for primary Sjogren's syndrome. Arthritis Rheum 2007;56(11):3588–600.

21

The uses of saliva in forensic genetics

Jack Ballantyne and Jane Juusola

WHY SALIVA IS FOUND IN FORENSIC CASEWORK

Transfer of body fluids

Forensic science can be defined as the application of science to the solution of certain problems that arise in connection with the administration of justice. It is science exercised in the service of the law. The subdiscipline of forensic genetics concerns itself with the identification and analysis of biological material that provides probative information to law enforcement investigators, the defense, and to the triers of fact (i.e., the judiciary). The commission of a violent crime often results in a number of different types of biological material being transferred in a unidirectional or bidirectional manner between the victim, the perpetrator, the crime scene, or the weapon.[1] A genetic analysis of such biological material by the forensic biologist may associate or exclude a particular individual with the crime in question. Such analysis may also aid in the reconstruction of the sequence of events that occurred before, during, or after the commission of the crime. The types of biological material encountered at crime scenes include body fluids such as blood, semen, saliva, and vaginal secretions as well as a variety of other tissues such as hair, teeth, bone, brain, muscle, and adipose.[1] More recently invisible dermal tissue secretions colloquially referred to as "touch DNA" have become excellent sources of probative genetic information.[1]

Persistence and location of saliva on evidence

Saliva, the subject of this chapter, is found in a variety of guises at crime scenes. Some of the most common sources included discarded cigarette butts and drink containers. Saliva is also found commonly in sexual assault cases that involve oral intercourse and is often admixed with other body fluids such as vaginal secretions or semen.[2] Saliva stains in the dried state are reasonably stable and, if the environmental conditions are not too extreme, can be detected months or years after deposition.[3] However, a simple wash cycle with biological detergents will remove all traces of the dried saliva stain.[3]

Importance of saliva

DNA profiling

Due to the presence of significant numbers of nucleated buccal epithelial cells in saliva, it is an excellent source of DNA from which a genetic profile of the donor is relatively easily obtained.[4] This is accomplished using standard DNA isolation methods followed by routine short tandem repeats (STR) DNA analysis of the resulting extracts.[5] Approximately 0.5–1.0 ng of DNA is required for such analysis, which represents approximately 80–160 cells.[5]

The identification of saliva

The ability to positively identify the presence of saliva stains at the crime scene is important in two ways. First, in order to obtain a DNA profile, one must first actually locate the deposited stain itself. While this may be a facile exercise with a single cigarette butt, it poses a more challenging exercise when one has to sift through dozens or even hundreds of items seized from the crime scene. Thus, methods to screen evidence for the presence of saliva stains are required in order to obtain the relevant stains for subsequent DNA analysis. Such screening methods need to be sensitive (to ensure no false-negative results) but not necessarily highly specific, since a small false-positive error rate is often an acceptable byproduct of a rapid and cheap high-throughput screening method. As detailed below, detection of the α-amylase enzyme is commonly used to screen evidence for the presence of saliva stains. Second, the positive identification of the stain as being saliva may be important evidence in itself. For example, a DNA profile matching a cohabiting male suspect on the nightdress of a child living in an extended family home may have differing degrees of probity depending on whether the source of the DNA was saliva versus semen. The remainder of the chapter describes in some detail the molecular genetics methods that are likely to be used in the near future for the identification of saliva in the forensic context.

SALIVA DIAGNOSTICS IN FORENSICS

Classical methods

Saliva is a secretion that acts as a digestive aid and that contains secretions from the salivary gland. There is currently no definitive test for the positive identification of saliva, although there are a number of substances present in higher concentration in saliva than elsewhere. These include the enzymes alkaline phosphatase and α-amylase and the inorganic anions thiocyanate and nitrite.[6] The presence of significant levels of α-amylase is strongly indicative of the presence of saliva, and the detection of α-amylase is the most commonly used test for it.[6]

Molecular genetic methods

In recent years, the development of new assays that are compatible with current polymerase chain reaction (PCR)-based DNA analysis techniques has become desirable. Particularly, the development of mRNA-based assays for the identification of body fluid stains has gained momentum, with new research emerging at a steady pace each year. In addition to being compatible with current DNA analysis procedures, an mRNA-based approach offers other advantages over conventional methods of body fluid identification, which use labor-intensive, technologically diverse techniques that are costly in terms of time and sample, and can be difficult to automate.[1] Additionally, there is no definitive test for saliva, since conventional methods rely on the detection of α-amylase, which is also expressed in a variety of other tissues.[6] The potential benefits of using an RNA-based approach for body fluid stain or tissue identification include greater specificity, improved timeliness, decreased sample consumption, simultaneous and semi-automated analysis through a common assay format, and compatibility with current DNA analysis procedures[7,8] (Fig. 21.1). Apart from the application in body fluid identification, the ability to detect mRNA in body fluids may have additional uses, in which novel phenotypic information about the donor of the body fluid could be obtained directly from the stain

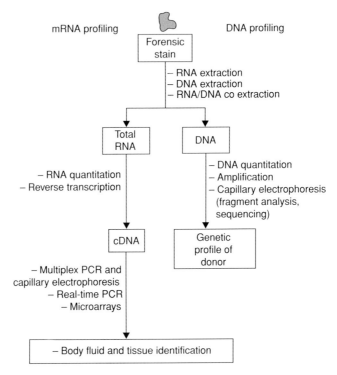

Figure 21.1 Concept of mRNA profiling for body fluid and tissue identification and its compatibility with current DNA analysis technology.

itself. Theoretically, the genetic sequences present in a stain at the DNA, RNA, or protein levels should somewhat reflect the phenotypic characteristics of the stain donor. Useful phenotypic characteristics for forensic purposes include such traits as race, age, sex, height, body stature, eye color, hair color, and facial features.

Concept of multicellular transcriptome in forensic body fluid identification

Messenger RNA is the molecular intermediate between genomic DNA and expressed protein. Terminally differentiated cells exhibit a gene expression profile, or transcriptome, that is unique to each cell type and is defined by the presence and relative abundance of specific mRNAs.[9,10] The typical body fluids encountered in forensic casework (saliva, blood, semen, vaginal secretions) consist of cells and secretions from multiple tissues. The collection of genes expressed within a body fluid or tissue has been called a "multicellular transcriptome."[11] These genes comprise ubiquitously expressed housekeeping genes and cell-type-specific genes. Theoretically, mRNA expression patterns can provide cell- and tissue-specific information that can be used to positively identify a tissue source. Until recently, no systematic studies had been carried out on the possibility of detecting and analyzing RNA sequences in biological stains of forensic significance.[11,12]

mRNA stability and recovery from dried body fluid stains including saliva

In order for an RNA-based analytical system to be successful, it must be demonstrated that it is possible to obtain RNA from biological stains. Despite its reputation for being highly unstable, RNA itself is actually a relatively stable molecule, targeted for degradation by ubiquitously present ribonucleases (RNases).[13] Several reports indicate that mRNA can be detected in postmortem tissues.[14–17] Although relatively little data exist on mRNA abundance and stability in stains of forensic importance, published results indicate that mRNA of sufficient quality and quantity can be recovered from physiological stains for analysis.[11,12,18] Dried stains may provide microenvironments that, in the dehydrated state, serve to protect the RNA from further degradation by RNases, and careful rehydration of the stain in the presence of strong RNase inhibitors seems to protect the RNA from degradation during the analytical process.

Saliva-specific gene transcripts

Forensic applications require robust and validated assays. The specificity and sensitivity of saliva identification assays are dependent on its constituent markers. Microarray data on gene expression in saliva stains are more readily available today with the wide-range use of Affymetrix Gene Chip Arrays (Affymetrix, Santa Clara, CA).[18] Candidate genes for saliva have also been identified through a combination of literature and database searches and consideration of the physiology and biochemistry of each body fluid.[11,19,20]

Molecular genetics methods used for mRNA profiling of body fluid stains

Several platforms are available for the analysis of gene expression patterns in different body fluids and tissues, including technologies that are currently used in forensic casework analysis.

Fragment analysis by capillary electrophoresis

Similarly to DNA profiling methods,[21] multiplex PCR systems that use capillary electrophoresis-laser-induced fluorescence (CE-LIF) as the method of detection can be developed for body fluid identification. Some benefits of CE over other methods is the ability to include multiple marker genes for each body fluid by using a combination of different fluorescent dyes and varied amplicon sizes, availability of amplicon size information, and ease of technology transfer due to the routine use of the ABI 310 and 3130 CE systems in crime laboratories today.

A multiplex PCR assay with eight body fluid-specific genes that uses CE-LIF as the method of amplicon detection has been described for the parallel identification of blood, saliva, semen, and vaginal secretions.[19] The octaplex system is able to reproducibly identify each of the four body fluids when present as single or mixed body fluid stains.[19] The sensitivity of the system (<200 pg to 12 ng of total RNA input) is suitable for forensic casework use, since typical sized body fluid stains (~50 μL) yield hundreds of nanograms of total RNA even in aged stains.[11] The advantage of including two markers per body fluid in one multiplex reaction is the built-in redundancy; this provides to account for possible biological variation in gene expression levels.

Quantitative PCR

Real-time quantitative PCR (qPCR) technology has wide applications in DNA quantitation and gene expression analysis. The qPCR instrument is capable of simultaneously detecting four different fluorophores, including a passive reference. As a result, multiplexes can be developed to detect up to two body fluid-specific genes and one housekeeping control gene at the same time. The ability of qPCR to quantitate target sequences is important in establishing the tissue specificity of a gene product, particularly when the relative abundance of a number of different mRNAs can demonstrate a unique or restricted pattern of expression. Several groups have developed qPCR singleplex and multiplex assays for the identification of saliva.[18,20,22] The qPCR platform offers a more quantitative approach, is more sensitive than the CE platform, and virtually eliminates the need for postamplification processing of the sample.

CONCLUSIONS

Classical protein-based markers for the forensic diagnostic indication of saliva possess limited specificity and are inefficiently compatible with DNA profiling. Studies have shown that both DNA and RNA can be isolated from biological stains, including saliva, in sufficient quantity and quality for analysis. Saliva-specific mRNA candidates have been identified by several research groups.

A select number of these candidates have been incorporated into multiplex PCR assays for body fluid identification using two different platforms (CE and qPCR) that are compatible with current methods of forensic DNA analysis. Messenger RNA-based methods show great potential for providing a reliable and sensitive approach to body fluid stain identification and, conceivably, could supplant the battery of serological and biochemical tests currently employed in the forensic serology laboratory.

REFERENCES

1. Ballantyne J. Serology: overview. In: Payne James, J, ed., *Encyclopedia of Forensic and Legal Medicine*. Oxford: Elsevier; 2005:53–63.
2. Keating SM, Higgs DF. The detection of amylase on swabs from sexual assault cases. J Forensic Sci Soc 1994;34(2):89–93.
3. Rushton C, Kipps A, Quarmby V, Whitehead PH. The distribution and significance of amylase-containing stains on clothing. J Forensic Sci Soc 1979;19(1):53–8.
4. Lee HC, Ladd C, Scherczinger CA, Bourke MT. Forensic applications of DNA typing: part 2: collection and preservation of DNA evidence. Am J Forensic Med Pathol 1998;19(1):10–18.
5. Butler JM, Buel E, Crivellente F, McCord BR. Forensic DNA typing by capillary electrophoresis using the ABI Prism 310 and 3100 genetic analyzers for STR analysis. Electrophoresis 2004;25(10–11):1397–412.
6. Gaensslen RE. *Sourcebook in Forensic Serology, Immunology, and Biochemistry*. Washington, D.C.: NIJ, US Government Printing Office; 1983.
7. Alvarez M, Juusola J, Ballantyne J. An mRNA and DNA co-isolation method for forensic casework samples. Anal Biochem 2004;335:289–98.
8. Gerhold D, Rushmore T, Caskey CT. DNA chips: promising toys have become powerful tools. Trends Biochem Sci 1999;24(5):168–73.
9. Alberts B, Bray D, Lewis J, Raff M, Roberts K, Watson JD. *Molecular Biology of the Cell*, 3rd edn. New York: Garland Publishing; 1994.
10. Caron H, van Schaik B, van der Mee M, et al. The human transcriptome map: clustering of highly expressed genes in chromosomal domains. Science 2001;291(5507):1289–92.
11. Juusola J, Ballantyne J. Messenger RNA profiling: a prototype method to supplant conventional methods for body fluid identification. Forensic Sci Int 2003;135(2):85–96.
12. Bauer M, Kraus A, Patzelt D. Detection of epithelial cells in dried blood stains by reverse transcriptase-polymerase chain reaction. J Forensic Sci 1999;44(6):1232–6.
13. Meyer S, Temme C, Wahle E. Messenger RNA turnover in eukaryotes: pathways and enzymes. Crit Rev Biochem Mol Biol 2004;39(4):197–216.
14. Finger JM, Mercer JFB, Cotton RGH, Danks DM. Stability of protein and mRNA in human postmortem liver-analysis by two-dimensional gel electrophoresis. Clin Chim Acta 1987;170:209–18.
15. Johnson SA, Morgan DG, Finch CE. Extensive postmortem stability of RNA from rat and human brain. J Neurosci Res 1986;16(1):267–80.

16. Phang TW, Shi CY, Chia JN, Ong CN. Amplification of cDNA via RT-PCR using RNA extracted from postmortem tissues. J Forensic Sci 1994;39(5):1275–9.

17. Schramm M, Falkai P, Tepest R, et al. Stability of RNA transcripts in postmortem psychiatric brains. J Neural Transm 1999;106(3–4):329–35.

18. Zubakov D, Hanekamp E, Kokshoorn M, van Ijcken W, Kayser M. Stable RNA markers for identification of blood and saliva stains revealed from whole genome expression analysis of time-wise degraded samples. Int J Legal Med 2007; 122(2):135–42.

19. Juusola J, Ballantyne J. Multiplex mRNA profiling for the identification of body fluids. Forensic Sci Int 2005;152(1):1–12.

20. Juusola J, Ballantyne J. mRNA profiling for body fluid identification by multiplex quantitative RT-PCR. J Forensic Sci 2007;52:1252–62.

21. Butler J. *Forensic DNA Typing: Biology, Technology, and Genetics of STR Markers*, 2nd edn. Burlington, MA: Elsevier Academic Press; 2005.

22. Nussbaumer C, Gharehbaghi-Schnell E, Korschineck I. Messenger RNA profiling: a novel method for body fluid identification by real-time PCR. Forensic Sci Int 2006;157(2–3):181–6.

22

SPKB—salivary proteome knowledge base: A platform for collaborative proteomics research

Weihong Yan, Weixia Yu, Shawn Than, Renli Qiao,
D. Stott Parker, Joseph A. Loo, and David T. Wong

INTRODUCTION

This chapter describes a salivary proteome knowledge base (SPKB) that was initially constructed for the National Institute of Dental and Craniofacial Research (NIDCR)-supported Human Salivary Proteome (HSP) Project. The SPKB consists of three data management systems: the salivary clinical sample database, the management system for proteomics experimental data (MS-PED), and the central repository for the centralization and integration of data collected by the HSP Project participating groups. The SPKB has been used in the collaborative HSP Project and is a dedicated resource for salivary proteomics research (http://www.hspp.ucla.edu).

BACKGROUND

Proteome-wide study of the protein components in a biological sample, such as that of a cell, a type of tissue, or a body fluid, has become possible from the development of mass spectrometry (MS)-based proteomics technologies. To date, proteome-scale studies of human body fluids have been performed, for example, in plasma, tears, and urine.[1–3] To fully characterize the protein components of a sample, it is necessary to implement diverse approaches in every step of the experimental strategy. However, the diversity of methodologies used usually goes far beyond what any single laboratory can achieve. Therefore, collaborative efforts have been common in proteome-wide projects. For example, the plasma proteome study involved collaboration of 35 laboratories across 13 countries, and their collaborative effort created a consensus plasma proteome with 3,020 identifications.[1,4] In a collaborative effort of this scale, centralization and standardization of data across all sources are vitally important.

It has been long postulated that human salivary fluid could contain valuable information for medical diagnostics and health screening. For saliva to be of medical diagnostic value, a critical first step is to comprehensively catalog the protein components and an understanding of their functions. A number of studies have been aimed at characterizing salivary proteins,[5–7] but no consensus or complete list of the salivary proteome has been established. Recently, the NIDCR funded the HSP Project, a collaborative effort of three research groups (the Scripps Research Institute, the University of California—Los Angeles, and the University of California—San Francisco) toward producing a comprehensive salivary proteome.

Proteome-scale studies produce a tremendous amount of data. Like other proteome projects, a key issue facing the HSP Project has been the development of data management systems for salivary proteomics research, the integration of the datasets collected by the HSP research groups, and the systematic analysis of the data. The SPKB is a component of the HSP Project and has been nourished by the salivary proteomics datasets from the three NIDCR-funded research groups. The SPKB was developed and proved to be highly valuable during the HSP Project.

ARCHITECTURE OF THE SPKB

Three data management systems were constructed under the SPKB: the salivary clinical sample database, MS-PED, and the central repository for the centralization and integration of the human salivary proteomics datasets. The systems were designed to capture the data flow from three major stages involved in the characterization of the salivary protein identifications (Fig. 22.1). The first stage covers salivary sample collection procedures. The second stage refers to procedures involved in an MS-based proteomics experiment. The third stage includes the centralization, standardization, and integration of salivary

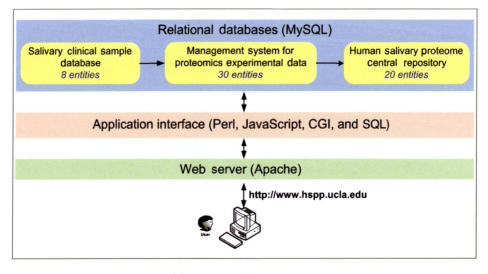

Figure 22.1   Overview of the structure of SPKB.

proteome identifications derived from multiple experiments and multiple laboratories.

The structure of SPKB is mainly composed of three layers (Fig. 22.1). The front-end layer contains web interfaces for users to submit, query, search, and download data. The back-end layer contains three relational databases, in which all data derived from these three stages reside. The intermediate layer is a number of application programs developed for communication between the user, web interface, and databases. Tools built in the intermediate layer are used to perform jobs including capturing data from the web interface, checking data integrity, writing data to the database, searching, querying and extracting data from database, and displaying data on the web interface. In addition, computational tools were developed to manage the flow of data among the three databases.

UNIQUE FEATURES OF THE SPKB FOR SALIVARY PROTEOMICS

As with all biosamples, validation and characterization of specificities existing across samples are mandatory for identification, which is required for comparison of component distinctions among sources of saliva. Human saliva is produced by three paired major exocrine glands: the parotid gland, submandibular (SM) gland, and sublingual (SL) gland. Previous studies indicated that components from these three glands can be distinct.[8] Differences can also exist among saliva donors with respect to racial, gender, and health status. Furthermore, characterization of saliva components can be influenced by the sample collection protocol and storage process. Because of the complexity intrinsic to saliva samples and sample collections, the salivary clinical sample information database was constructed to store and secure salivary sample source information. This database was designed to function as a laboratory information management system and to capture sample details (e.g., saliva donor information, donor heath status, collecting protocol, and storage information).

Like gene expression studies, proteomics experiments also produce large datasets. MS-PED is a web-based data storage and analysis package containing features for storing, annotating, and mining proteomics experimental data. It captures and stores information involved in proteomics experiments, including sample source, sample treatment, sample separation, MS experiment conditions, and MS result analysis for peptide and protein identification. Compared to existing proteomics databases, such as SWISS-2DPAGE[9] and SBEAMS (http://www.sbeams.org/Proteomics/), MS-PED takes both gel-based and liquid chromatography (LC)-based proteomics experimental data and accommodates both top-down and bottom-up proteomics. The back-end relational database design of MS-PED is in symphony with the proposed standard from proteomics initiatives,[10] and is as comprehensive as the PEDRo design.[11]

Web-based graphic interfaces and applications of MS-PED were developed that allow users to enter, edit, view, query, search, and download data. Multiple features, such as uploading of MS analysis results and templates for repeatedly used protocols, were built into the web interfaces to facilitate data entry and reduce manual data entry. An automatic tool allows users to download and disseminate proteomics experimental data from MS-PED to public proteomics database, such as PRIDE, in XML format. Security of data in MS-PED is managed and authorized through an administrative web interface. In addition, mining tools were developed for comparison of data from different experiments.

All computing tools for the construction of the three databases are open source. The system runs in a Linux environment with MySQL as the relational database server, Apache as the web server, and Perl, CGI, and Javascript as the main scripting languages. The schemas of the three databases are posted at http://www.hspp.ucla.edu.

DATA STANDARDIZATION, INTEGRATION, ANALYSIS, AND THE CENTRAL REPOSITORY OF THE HSP PROJECT

The NIDCR-HSP Project aims to comprehensively identify and characterize protein components in ductal parotid saliva and SM/SL saliva. One component of the SPKB centralizes experimental datasets collected by the three participating groups and consolidates proteomes of parotid and SM/SL saliva based on the combined datasets.

Integration of the datasets from the three groups and consolidation of the parotid and SM/SL salivary proteomes were performed in three consecutive steps:

1. Establishment of minimal information required for the exchange of the datasets, which involves designing and constructing a relational database to store the datasets and defining a data format for data exchange;
2. Standardization of the protein identifications in reference to a given version of a protein database and integration of these protein identifications;
3. Development of a web interface and tools to display, query, and disseminate the HSP datasets.

Figure 22.2 shows the structure of the HSP central repository and its web interface.

Standardized information, the format for data exchange, and the construction of a central HSP repository

Given the diversified technologies implemented by the three research groups in saliva sample collection, preparation, separation, mass spectrometry, and subsequent protein sequence search, it was critical to standardize the information necessary for data exchange and submission to the central repository. Data obtained and submitted to the central repository should be sufficiently detailed for integration and comparison, acceptable by the proteomics research community, and compatible with public proteomics databases such as PRIDE.[12] The

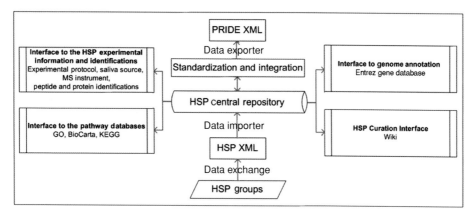

Figure 22.2 Structure of the data standardization, integration, analysis, and the central repository of the HSP Project.

SPKB data exchange standard was based on proposed guidelines for reporting mass spectrometry data (for the purpose of protein and peptide identification) and on the standard implemented in the Human Proteome Organization (HUPO) initiative project, the Human Plasma Proteome Project.[1,13] The schema of the HSP central database shows the entities with the information stored and the relationship between the entities (http://www.hspp.ucla.edu).

The extensible markup language (XML) was selected and used to submit the data to the central database. XML was chosen over other data formats because it is a simple text format and offers scalability, interoperability, and flexibility with complex data type. XML format has also been used in a wide array of biological applications, including exchange of microarray data (http://xml.coverpages.org/geml.html), biological sequence data (http://xml.coverpages.org/bsml.html), and 2D-PAGE data.[14]

Standardization, integration, and analysis of the salivary protein identifications

The purpose of integrating the salivary protein identifications identified by the three groups is to permit a consolidated catalog of the salivary proteome. A total of 2,153 distinct proteins identified from different versions of the IPI protein sequence database were submitted to the central database. Besides the variations in the saliva collection and protein/peptide separations, diversities are also seen in the MS instruments, DB search program, and sequence database. The confidence of the identifications was estimated by limiting the identification of false-positive rate (FPR) below 3%. The process of standardization and integration was performed in a similar way as described in the plasma proteome project.[1] The procedure of standardization includes standardization of the submitted protein identifications to a reference protein sequence database (IPI v3.24, December 2006 release) through inferring protein identifications from the submitted peptide identifications, clustering of the redundant (or ambiguity) protein identifications that were derived from a common set of peptide identifications, and selection of a representative protein from each cluster.

The integration process resulted in a total of 1,166 distinct protein identifications from the parotid and SM/SL saliva. Within them, 914 were identified from parotid and 917 were identified from SM/SL, with an overlap of 665 between the parotid and SM/SL proteomes. The proteins were classified based on the group(s) that identified the proteins, the annotation of the proteins, the sequence coverage, and the saliva source. The classified information was mined as a matrix and can be visualized through an array viewer software.[15] The viewer shows that the highly abundant proteins indicated by high sequence coverage can, in general, be confirmed by all three groups. In contrast, proteins identified by only one group are generally less abundant proteins.[16]

Web interface of the HSP central database, and dissemination of the HSP datasets

The data stored in the HSP central database can be accessed through a web-based interface. Tools are provided in the web interface to allow query of the database based on the saliva source, data contributor (group), protein identifier, and description. Besides experimental information that was used to derive the protein identifications, the annotation information of the HSP proteins can also be explored through the interface. The functionality of the HSP proteins was annotated with their links to a few biological pathway databases including gene ontology, Biocarta, and KEGG. Gene annotation of the HSP proteins can be explored on the web interface through their links to the Entrez gene database. The download site is provided in the web interface to allow download of salivary proteome identifications as well as their annotations. To maximize dissemination of the HSP data to the general public, a tool was developed that renders the data stored in the HSP central database exchangeable to the PRIDE database, a proteomics standards initiative-compliant public repository of protein and peptide identifications.[12] The tool was developed to convert the XML file of the HSP central database to the XML format defined by the PRIDE database. In addition, a WIKI web interface was provided with the aim of gaining feedback from experts in the salivary research field and for evaluating confidence in protein identifications.

CONCLUSION AND FUTURE DIRECTIONS

In this chapter, the SPKB was introduced as a comprehensive data management and integration system. Together with its web resources, it is an important new resource for salivary biomedical research. The SPKB system is also an example of the use of information integration technology for managing collaborative research projects in proteomics. It has been used to capture, integrate, and disseminate the data from all stages of the HSP Project.

The complexity of the salivary biological system demands extensive exploration of multidimensional data. High-throughput proteomics research is an important technology that provides insights of the protein components of saliva. Other approaches such as transcriptomics through gene expression array are also useful and have been utilized to characterize saliva beyond its protein features. The data and information derived from these –omics-based studies have not been integrated or investigated systemically. Work is underway to incorporate datasets from other saliva –omics studies into a multidimensional Salivaomics Knowledge Base (SKB). To provide systematic and integrative insights into saliva, a genome browser tool will be plugged into the SKB. All the –omics study datasets will be viewed and explored simultaneously using the genome browser. Considering the volume of data from each –omics study, incompatible data formats, and ambiguity of terminology used, it might sound too ambitious at present to mine all the datasets from the variety of –omics studies. However, the recent launch of WIKI for professionals may shed light even in this direction of our future work. Given the tremendous interest and potentials in using saliva for medical diagnostics, the SPKB and the SKB will become powerful resources for salivary research.

REFERENCES

1. Adamski M, Blackwell T, Menon R, et al. Data management and preliminary data analysis in the pilot phase of the HUPO Plasma Proteome Project. Proteomics 2005;5(13):3246–61.
2. Adachi J, Kumar C, Zhang Y, Olsen JV, Mann M. The human urinary proteome contains more than 1500 proteins, including a large proportion of membrane proteins. Genome Biol 2006;7(9):R80.
3. de Souza GA, Godoy LM, Mann M. Identification of 491 proteins in the tear fluid proteome reveals a large number of proteases and protease inhibitors. Genome Biol 2006;7(8):R72.
4. Omenn GS, Paik YK, Speicher D. The HUPO Plasma Proteome Project: a report from the Munich congress. Proteomics 2006;6(1):9–11.
5. Hu S, Xie Y, Ramachandran P, et al. Large-scale identification of proteins in human salivary proteome by liquid chromatography/mass spectrometry and two-dimensional gel electrophoresis-mass spectrometry. Proteomics 2005;5(6):1714–28.
6. Guo T, Rudnick PA, Wang W, Lee CS, Devoe DL, Balgley BM. Characterization of the human salivary proteome by capillary isoelectric focusing/nanoreversed-phase liquid chromatography coupled with ESI-tandem MS. J Proteome Res 2006;5(6):1469–78.
7. Xie H, Rhodus NL, Griffin RJ, Carlis JV, Griffin TJ. A catalogue of human saliva proteins identified by free flow electrophoresis-based peptide separation and tandem mass spectrometry. Mol Cell Proteomics 2005;4(11):1826–30.
8. Chisholm DM, Mason DK. Salivary gland disease. Br Med Bull 1975; 31(2):156–8.

9. Hoogland C, Mostaguir K, Sanchez JC, Hochstrasser DF, Appel RD. SWISS-2DPAGE, ten years later. Proteomics 2004;4(8):2352–6.

10. Orchard S, Hermjakob H, Julian RK, Jr, et al. Common interchange standards for proteomics data: public availability of tools and schema. Proteomics 2004;4(2):490–91.

11. Garwood K, McLaughlin T, Garwood C, et al. PEDRo: a database for storing, searching and disseminating experimental proteomics data. BMC Genomics 2004;5(1):68.

12. Jones P, Cote RG, Martens L. PRIDE: a public repository of protein and peptide identifications for the proteomics community. Nucleic Acids Res 2006;34(database issue):D659–63.

13. Carr S, Aebersold R, Baldwin M, Burlingame A, Clauser K, Nesvizhskii A. The need for guidelines in publication of peptide and protein identification data: working group on publication guidelines for peptide and protein identification data. Mol Cell Proteomics 2004;3(6):531–3.

14. Ravichandran V, Lubell J, Vasquez GB, Lemkin P, Sriram RD, Gilliland GL. Ongoing development of two-dimensional polyacrylamide gel electrophoresis data standards. Electrophoresis 2004;25(2):297–308.

15. Sturn A, Quackenbush J, Trajanoski Z. Genesis: cluster analysis of microarray data. Bioinformatics 2002;18(1):207–208.

16. Denny P, Hagen FK, Hardt M, et al. The proteomes of human parotid and submandibular/sublingual gland salivas collected as the ductal secretions. J Proteome Res 2008; 7(5):1994–2006.

Part III

Saliva Diagnostics—
A New Industry

23
Commercialization of oral fluid products and technologies

R. Sam Niedbala

COMMERCIAL PRODUCTS FOR ORAL DIAGNOSTICS OVERVIEW

Today, in various parts of the globe, a variety of commercial tests are being performed using a sample collected from the mouth. Just a few years ago, the vast majority of oral-based testing was relegated to the research laboratory. Today, major human clinical challenges such as HIV, substance abuse, and genetic testing are often accomplished from an oral sample at clinical laboratories and mobile roadside-testing facilities, to name two alternate settings.

The history of oral-based diagnostics is rich and contains a variety of ideas from scientists and entrepreneurs. Hundreds of years ago, kings used a simple oral test to determine guilt or innocence. The accused was asked to chew and swallow a handful of dry rice in a short period of time. The guilty could not do it and were therefore punished.[1] In some ways this reflects the history of oral diagnostics. Many diagnostic professionals desire that the testing be highly accurate and reliable, yet simple to administer, a combination of attributes not easily attained in one neat package since the royal rice test.

For example, diabetes is one of the greatest challenges of our time, as more and more humans are obese. Some have long discussed the idea of diagnosing diabetes from an oral sample. Many attempts have been made to attain this goal. Although a good idea, diabetes testing using an oral sample has failed to date because of the basic function and physiology of fluids within the mouth.

Thus, the first historical step—to determine the composition and dynamics of the oral cavity and the fluids present—still remains a challenge. The mouth is a complicated cavity affected by environmental insult and disease. It acts as a barrier to invasion of the body and, at a basic level, helps facilitate the initial intake and digestion of foods.[2] Thus, the creation of commercial products is made difficult by the complexity and transience of fluids within the mouth. For example, humans will produce between 0.5 and 1.5 L of saliva per day. Saliva production varies according to the time of day as well as hydration. The mouth also responds to stimulus such as chewing to produce more saliva. Finally, the pH of the mouth influences the way compounds cross the blood/oral cavity barrier, also making the detection of some target analytes difficult.[3]

Even with these hurdles and challenges, a number of commercial products are now firmly entrenched and commercially viable. Future products are in the pipeline and are expected to compete with blood- and urine-based tests. In the majority of cases, existing tests are mirror reflections of the blood or urine tests that are performed. However, in the case of an oral sample, the metabolites are often present in concentrations that are much lower than blood and in some cases with different ratios of metabolites.[4,5] Thus, an oral fluid sample is often described as a fuzzy mirror reflection of blood.

This is both an opportunity and challenge to commercial test developers. A competent test must be reliable and diagnostically accurate. The relationship between blood levels and oral fluid levels for the same analytes is often not well defined. Thus, commercial developers must work to understand the clinical relationship to concentration for each analyte. New analytes, however, are now being looked at solely from the perspective of the oral cavity. Recently funded projects by the National Institutes for Health are, for the first time, measuring the proteome of the mouth. These early efforts are helping to identify the normal protein signatures found solely in the oral cavity and, in the future, may be a window to the abnormal protein signatures of disease or infection. Such an approach would dramatically change the use of an oral sample from comparisons to blood to a stand-alone matrix. It would also capitalize on the ease of collection possible with an oral fluid sample.

THE BASICS OF ORAL DIAGNOSTIC PRODUCT DEVELOPMENT

The analysis of any human matrix requires sample collection techniques that ensure the analyte is properly collected and handled before analysis. Blood glucose, for example, is affected by the posture of the subject during collection. Fasting is another critical issue to many measurements, which ensures proper interpretation of clinical chemistry parameters.

Similarly, the collection and analysis of oral fluids is dependant on a number of factors to ensure reliable and meaningful results. In this section these key factors for oral-based diagnostics are discussed. Each topic identified must be addressed for the whole system to work as a reliable diagnostic for commercial applications.

PHYSIOLOGY

The first item of importance is the physiology of the oral cavity. The oral cavity is composed of a number of glands producing high-viscosity and low-viscosity fluids. In addition, the buffering capacity of these fluids varies, introducing the issue of ion concentrations that can affect analytes entering the oral cavity.[6]

To overcome this, commercial collectors have been developed and are often specified or included in diagnostic test kits. Table 23.1 provides a summary of the various collectors available. For research purposes, many clinicians will

Table 23.1 Commercial oral fluid collection devices.

Collection device	Manufacturer	Utility	Diluted sample	Collector
Intercept®	OraSure Tech.	Drug testing	Yes	Absorbent
OraSure	OraSure Tech.	HIV	Yes	Absorbent
Salivette	Sarstedt	Research	Yes	Absorbent
OralScreen/ OralConfirm	Avitar	Drug testing	Yes	Absorbent
Quantisal	Immunalysis/ Saliva Diagnostic Systems	Drug testing and HIV	Yes	Absorbent
OralStat	ABMC	Drug testing	Yes	Absorbent
Versi.Sal	Bamburgh Marsh	Drug testing	Yes	Absorbent
Salicule	AcroBiotech	Drug testing	Neat	Direct

A list of many of the available oral fluid collection devices. They are used for a variety of purposes including detection of abused substances or infectious diseases. Note that almost all devices utilize a buffer to dilute the sample following collection. Generic collectors such as a cotton swab were not included.

simply have subjects "spit" into a tube. The collected fluid is then centrifuged and the supernatant sent on for further analysis. However, "spitting" into a tube is not practical for routine laboratory or on-site testing.

Existing commercial collectors gather samples based on placement in the mouth. It is reasonable to say that there are three basic approaches to collecting an oral sample. The first is to place the collector under the tongue. This fluid will primarily be of low viscosity. The second is to place or swipe the collector in the buccal cavity between the cheek and gums. Here a combination of viscous oral fluids will be gathered onto the collector. This fluid will be diluted with a buffer prior to analysis, since the material is too viscous when first collected and cannot be pipetted. The third method involves placing a collector in the buccal cavity that has been treated with salts. As the pad wets the salts, they encourage the enhanced collection of certain target analytes. This fluid has been called oral mucosal transudate (OMT). For most commercial collectors, the term "oral fluids" is now used to describe any specimens collected from the mouth.

In summary, the oral cavity is complex and produces fluids that are not always easy to collect for analysis. Most oral-based collection is done by unsophisticated operators who are collecting and sending the specimen back to a laboratory for analysis. Therefore, whatever the collection method, it must be simple, reliable, and accurate. In addition, it should ideally collect a metered volume of fluids. At this time there are no oral fluid collection devices that can meet all these attributes. This is a potential area for improvement in the future.

POTENTIAL ANALYTES IN THE ORAL CAVITY

The question then becomes what analytes are actually in an oral sample? This question is not always easy to answer because it relates to an important challenge for oral-based diagnostics. Analytes that exist in the oral cavity are often found in low concentrations that do not allow routine detection or measurement. In the preceding section, we discussed the possible methods of collecting an oral sample. One very important point to understand is that currently there are no devices that can collect an accurate volume of sample. In order to match the accuracy of pipetting, the variation must be <5%. This inherently limits oral-based testing to qualitative measurements, which then further dictates the types of analytes that may be targeted and their uses.

Currently, there exists a broad array of analytes that are tested in specialty commercial laboratories or in general clinical laboratories using manufacturer's kits.

Specialty commercial laboratories are often focused on tests that are not easily performed if collected with commercial devices that cannot provide accurate volumes. In these cases the laboratory will often use "spitting" as the method of collection. The sample is sent back to the laboratory, and it is carefully analyzed following centrifugation. One such laboratory is Salimetrics, State College, PA, which focuses on the use of saliva to measure hormones. Some of the in-house assays developed for use with oral fluids include testosterone, progesterone, cortisol, and estriol. This laboratory through its academic roots created the scientific and clinical basis used to measure target hormones. Physicians then use the laboratory's services as part of their patient management plan. This is an excellent pathway to create oral-based diagnostics since it builds a database that can support oral testing as a viable alternative to blood-based tests.

The more traditional route for assay commercialization has been through kit manufacturers. In this case a diagnostic kit manufacturer will identify analytes of interest to an audience broad enough to support commercial development. This is an important consideration for each commercial company. In many cases potential analytes may only be used in niche markets and are therefore of little commercial interest. Alternatively, oral diseases, such as Sjögren's, are not well understood and lack specific biomarkers.

Assuming however that a new test is for human clinical use, it will require that the kit be approved by the US Food and Drug Administration (FDA) prior to sale. In Europe other certifications will be required, such as the CE Mark. So in order for a new marker to be implemented for oral-based diagnostics, it must be clinically defined and relevant, cost-effective to develop, and potentially useful to a large audience.

A recent conference on oral-based diagnostics was sponsored by the New York Academy of Sciences.[7] This meeting gathered many who are working to commercialize oral-based tests. Existing commercial tests that dominate markets today include infectious disease testing and substance abuse testing. In both cases, there are a large number of peer reviewed publications supporting the utility of a number of analytes. Today, millions of these assays are performed in laboratories around the world. In contrast, only 10 years earlier a similar meeting was sponsored by the New York Academy of Sciences. At the time

Breakdown of oral diagnostics literature

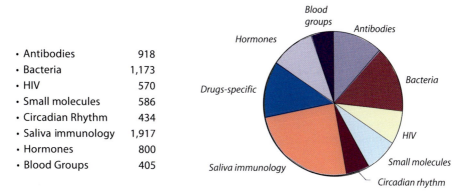

- Antibodies — 918
- Bacteria — 1,173
- HIV — 570
- Small molecules — 586
- Circadian Rhythm — 434
- Saliva immunology — 1,917
- Hormones — 800
- Blood Groups — 405

Figure 23.1 A summary of the literature related to potential oral diagnostic markers. The majority of the literature can be summarized into infectious disease, substance abuse, and hormone detection.

many ideas for testing were proposed, but few were actually in routine use. Looking through the proceedings of this earlier meeting, it is clear that many of today's routine tests were yesterday's ideas or concepts.[8]

As part of preparing this chapter, a survey of the literature pertaining to oral diagnostics or biological markers in oral fluids was conducted examining the areas studied between 1966 and 2002. A total of 20,371 articles were identified and sorted according to subject matter. Figure 23.1 shows a breakdown of the topics mentioned in the literature. There are a number of items that Figure 23.1 communicates. First is the fact that there has been and continues to be a great deal of interest in oral-based diagnostics. The most cited areas are those that identify antibodies, small molecule drugs, and hormones. If one examines available commercial products, it is evident that there is a correlation between the literature and commercial success.

Further analysis of the same literature was performed to see what methods were used to analyze oral samples. Figure 23.2 shows this breakdown. Much of the analysis of oral fluids has been conducted using chromatography, immunoassay and, in some cases, self-reports. While immunoassay is an excellent method for commercial products, it is primarily associated with research settings. This shows the underlying issues or, perhaps, the opportunities for oral-based diagnostics. Those pursuing development of products need to consider the great wealth of research already done and whether it supports pursuit of new markers in an oral sample.

HURDLES SPECIFIC TO COMMERCIALIZATION OF ORAL DIAGNOSTICS

As mentioned earlier in this chapter, oral fluids present unique physical challenges to those developing commercial test kits: viscosity of glandular fluids in the mouth, the inaccuracy of existing collection devices, and the low

Methods for studying oral fluid

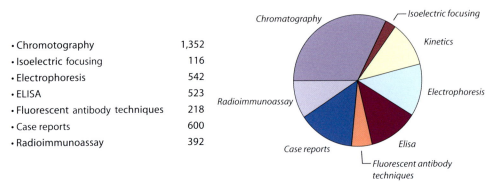

- Chromotography   1,352
- Isoelectric focusing   116
- Electrophoresis   542
- ELISA   523
- Fluorescent antibody techniques   218
- Case reports   600
- Radioimmunoassay   392

Figure 23.2   A summary of the methods commonly used to study potential analytes found in oral fluids. Many of the methods are labor-intensive and therefore appropriate for research laboratories. Thus, the challenge for diagnostic kit developers is to translate these research methods into convenient, reliable test kits.

concentration of analytes within the oral cavity. Finally, any test developed must also compare to existing tests in blood or urine.

As each oral-based test has been developed, it must also be reviewed by government bodies that permit new products to be sold. In the United States, the FDA is responsible for ensuring the safety and effectiveness of all medical devices used within the United States. Any product must be reviewed by the FDA prior to being offered for commercial sale within the United States. There are a number of pathways taken by test developers to demonstrate safety and effectiveness.[9] The two main pathways involve submission of a 510(k) application or a premarket approval application (PMA). The 510(k) path is named for the Code of Federal Regulations section that deals with this type of medical device submission. Simplified, a 510(k) application is submitted to the FDA when a new product's safety and efficacy can be compared with a product that has already been cleared for sale by the FDA. The already cleared product is called the "predicate" product. When submitting a new product to FDA as a 510(k), the new product may have different characteristics or performance, but the end result or indication must be the same. This is important since existing oral-based commercial tests were compared to blood or urine as part of FDA's review. Knowing that the metabolism and deposition of substances into the oral cavity may differ from other compartments within the human body, one should recognize that at times it may be difficult to convince the FDA that an oral-based test is viable using the 510(k) pathway to approval.

The second pathway to obtaining FDA approval to sell a medical device within the United States is called a premarket approval application or PMA. The PMA route is used when a predicate device is not available or the device is of sufficient concern to society that the FDA requires the commercial sponsor to produce a higher level of evidence for safety and efficacy. HIV tests are always

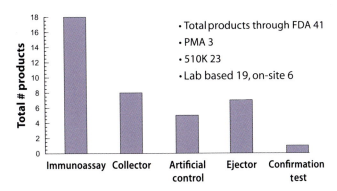

Oral-based FDA-reviwed products since 1976

- Total products through FDA 41
- PMA 3
- 510K 23
- Lab based 19, on-site 6

Figure 23.3 A summary of FDA-cleared or approved products. Most of the products approved are collectors for oral fluids and corresponding test kits. A total number of 41 approvals is an extremely small number and underscores the challenge of commercializing oral-based diagnostics.

reviewed by the FDA as PMAs. This has been true for oral collection devices and test kits that claim utility in detecting HIV.

In 1976, the FDA enacted the Medical Device Act that required all medical devices to be reviewed by the FDA prior to sale in the United States. Examination of the records at FDA since 1976 reveals 41 oral-based medical devices. Figure 23.3 shows a summary of these devices and their uses. It can be seen from Figure 23.3 that a great majority of the devices cleared or approved by the FDA for sale have been oral fluid collection devices or test kits. The additional devices are controls used in kits or other types of medical devices, which are not diagnostic in intended use.

EXISTING COMMERCIAL PRODUCTS

It would be useful at this point to examine some of the existing commercial products that involve testing of oral fluids. The products examined here are those that are offered as kits for commercial distribution and not through specialty laboratories. The most ubiquitous tests have been those to detect substance abuse and infectious diseases.

Drugs of abuse testing have primarily been an industry within the United States. It is driven by a presidential executive order created almost two decades ago.[10] This law primarily covers federal government workers, but its authority has been extrapolated to other uses such as preemployment testing in private companies or within jails or probation situations. The primary medium for testing has been urine. This is due to the fact that urine immunoassays were most readily available at the time the law was implemented. Over time the advantages and disadvantages of urine testing have been debated in courts to the point where most questions of utility and accuracy have been answered. Today, approximately 59 million drug tests are performed annually within the United States. Costing over 1 billion dollars per year, half of the monies spent are used for collecting a urine specimen in a controlled access location.

In 1997, Substance Abuse and Mental Health Services Administration (SAMHSA), the substance abuse and mental health arm of the Department of Health and Human Services, began exploring alternatives to urine testing. A number of early scientific studies had been conducted using oral fluids and suggested that it might be a viable alternative to urine. Additionally, collectors for oral fluids had already been introduced for infectious disease and could be adapted for drugs of abuse tests. The economic driver is that collection of oral fluids does not require a special location and therefore minimizes sample collection costs.

Since these initial meetings, a number of companies invested resources to develop systems for collection and testing for drugs of abuse. Today, oral-based testing for drugs of abuse are used for insurance risk assessment, nonfederally regulated preemployment testing, criminal justice, and roadside testing by law enforcement. The use of drug testing using oral fluids is growing in some markets in excess of 20% each year.

To achieve this kind of adoption, questions comparing urine results and oral sample results had to be resolved. A large number of studies have been conducted and published in peer reviewed journals.[11] In addition, population studies have shown that positivity rates between oral fluid and urine results are nearly the same.[12] The outcome of this scientific base has been the widening adoption of oral fluids and its legal defensibility for performing drug testing.[13]

Outside the United States, drugs of abuse testing with an oral sample has grown in a different arena. In Europe and Australia, lawmakers and law enforcement officials are implementing roadside tests to identify those positive for alcohol and drugs of abuse. A number of sponsored studies have been conducted examining the performance of on-site oral-based drugs of abuse tests.[14] In this situation, law enforcement officers are responsible for testing motorists suspected for drugs of abuse. Oral fluid is the preferred medium due to its ease of collection. The challenge to product developers has been the varied environments used by law enforcement. In these situations the test must be reliable and accurate in diverse weather, humidity, and light. The test format used provides a visual result for as many as nine target drugs. This has been difficult for commercial companies to develop, especially for marijuana. It is expected that issues of analytical sensitivity will be overcome as technology develops further.

The other area of clinical medicine that has been impacted by oral-based tests is infectious disease detection. Numerous infectious agents have been identified using an oral sample.[15] The primary basis for all these tests is the detection of antibodies in an oral sample. It is well established that a number of antibody subtypes will be present in the mouth with the majority being IgA. Developers and researchers have long used this to create screening tests. The advantage is always the simplicity of collecting an oral sample and the associated cost savings.

In addition to measuring pathogenic infections, measurement of immunity is also possible through detection of antibodies in the oral cavity. Measles, mumps, and rubella are good examples of how some governments are measuring immunity levels of children within their countries' populations.[16]

It is a fact that commercial entities will focus their resources on the greatest business opportunities. In the area of oral-based infectious disease testing, this has encouraged the development of HIV screening tests. It was in the early 1980s that a company called Epitope, Beaverton, OR, and Saliva Diagnostic Systems, Redmond, OR, first developed two collection devices still in use today. Table 23.1 lists the OraSure and Quantisal devices. Both were initially targeted to collect a sample of oral fluid that was shipped back to a laboratory for testing. It took many years and a great deal of funding until the OraSure collector was PMA approved for use in the detection of HIV antibodies. In addition to the collector, the company had to develop a Western blot confirmation test that could be used with OraSure samples. The company successfully introduced the products to life insurance and public health laboratories within the United States. It further spurred the development of additional assays for analytes such as hepatitis and drugs of abuse. Thus, the cost savings of collecting an oral sample along with demonstrated accuracy compared to blood created a unique use for oral-based diagnostics.

Over time the reliability of an oral-based sample was confirmed by numerous independent studies.[17,18] In parallel, the spread of HIV was still continuing around the globe. By the year 2000, close to 1 million people were infected in the United States alone with millions more in less developed countries. The US Centers for Disease Control (CDC) determined that the way to combat the spread of HIV was to find a way to take testing to locations where undiagnosed infections could be more easily identified. The problem was that no reliable rapid test had been developed for use with saliva to detect HIV antibodies.

The CDC along with FDA encouraged commercial developers to pursue developing a rapid test to fulfill the need for a rapid HIV screening test. In 2002, the OraQuick test was PMA approved by the FDA for use with blood and eventually oral fluids. The product was given approvals that allowed it to be used in remote locations allowing on-site, rapid detection of HIV-positive individuals. The product has been validated through numerous studies and found to be robust when properly used. Additional HIV tests are becoming available as other manufacturers work to meet the need. The rapid tests for HIV allow immediate intervention, so that preliminarily positive individuals can be counseled, thus stopping the spread of the virus. In this example, oral-based diagnostics were driven by societal need, technology innovation, and extensive validation evidenced through historical use. All government and private stakeholders in such efforts benefited from the commercialization outcome.

FUTURE STRATEGIES AND OPPORTUNITIES

Oral fluid-based testing using commercial products has flourished in areas such as drug testing and infectious disease testing. At this point in history, both lab-based and on-site technologies have been demonstrated. In the

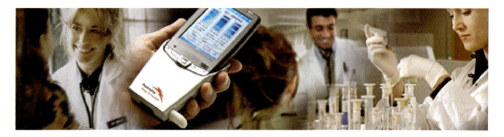

Figure 23.4 A version of the RDx reader from Alerix Inc. The instrument is small, hand-held, and inexpensive. Coupled with an oral fluid collector and rapid test, it may provide a path to future product development in oral diagnostics.

future it is expected that the focus of many commercial efforts will be to further expand on-site testing. This again brings up the issues that have limited oral diagnostics, specifically, that analytes are present in low concentrations in the mouth and that interpretation of visual rapid tests is challenging. One way this may be solved is through the use of advanced yet inexpensive instrumentation.

In the past, diagnostic companies have developed their own in-house capabilities to develop instrumentation to go along with assays. This adds financial burden to development costs and often slows commercialization. A recent solution has been the availability of inexpensive instrumentation that uses components such as simple cameras. One example is the RDx instrument from Alerix, San Jose, CA. The instrument is composed of simple electronics capable of interpreting reflectance or fluorescence. The cost of the reader is less than $100, and the company will package the electronics in whatever housing is appropriate. Commercial assay developers can access this "a la carte" approach to instrumentation. The benefit to oral-based diagnostics is that the instrument can be battery powered and disposable. Thus, remote locations do not require servicing of instruments, rather just a replacement. Figure 23.4 shows one image of the RDx reader.

In developing oral diagnostics, it was stated earlier that new tests are often demonstrated by comparing blood or urine results to oral fluids. The problem with this approach is that the marker may appear as a different metabolite in each fluid. It may also be at extremely low concentrations in an oral sample. So the question becomes, will future tests ever be developed differently?

Perhaps the answer will come from newer fields of clinical investigation. As reported in other chapters in this book, the field of oral-based proteomics and genomics is expanding. Studies are underway to define the proteome of the mouth. The results over time may generate information that specifically defines new signatures of disease using an oral sample. In addition, genomic measurements may also be performed easily by collecting cells from the mouth. In the case of proteomics and genomics, a completely new approach may be in the future for oral diagnostics.

The road to commercial success, whether based on blood, urine, or oral fluids, is long and tortuous. Assay developers face many technical hurdles as well as other issues such as regulatory approvals, patents, or finance. To successfully bring a product to market in oral-based diagnostics, the idea must work physiologically, be collected efficiently, tested at a level of appropriate analytical sensitivity, and have clear clinical utility. This is challenging when one considers the most basic functions of oral fluids to be moistening food for digestion. The hope is that as time progresses, oral-based diagnostics will move beyond comparisons to blood and urine and truly establish its own domain of tests.

REFERENCES

1. Mandel ID. The diagnostic uses of saliva. J Oral Pathol Med 1990;19(8):119–25.
2. Levine M. *Salivary Macromolecules, in Saliva as a Diagnostic Fluid*, Malamud D, ed. New York Academy of Science; 1993;694:11–16.
3. Sreebny L. Saliva flow in health and disease. Compend Contin Enduc Dent 1989;(Suppl) 13:461–9.
4. Bremen H. The Application of saliva in laboratory medicine, workshop report. J Clin Chem Clin Biochem 1989;27:221–52.
5. Kidwell D, Holland J, Athanaselis S. Testing for drug of abuse in saliva and sweat. J Chrom 1998;713:111–35.
6. Shanker A, Rastogi SK, Jain UC. A study on salivary flow rate, sodium, potassium, bicarbonate and amylase in congestive cardiac failure. Indian Heart J 1977;29(3):152–3.
7. Malamud D, Niedbala RS. *Oral-Based Diagnostics*. New York Academy of Sciences, Vol. 1098; 2007.
8. Malmud D, Tabak L. *Saliva as a Diagnostic Fluid*. New York Academy of Sciences, Vol. 694; 1993.
9. Whitmore E. *Development of FDA-Regulated Medical Products*, 2nd edn. Boca Raton Florida: ASQ Quality Press; 2004.
10. Reagan Ronald. Executive Order 12564; 1986.
11. Cone E, Huestis M. Interpretation of oral fluid tests for drug of abuse. Proc N Y Acad Sci 2007;1098:51–103.
12. Cone E, Presley L, Lehrer M, et al. Oral fluid testing for drugs of abuse: positive prevalence rates by Intercept™ immunoassay screening and GC-MS-MS confirmation and suggested cutoff concentrations. J Anal Toxicol 2002;26:541–6.
13. Kadehjian L. Legal sections in oral fluid testing. Forensic Sci Int 2005;150:151–60.
14. Verstraete AV. Detection times of drugs of abuse in blood, urine, and oral fluid. Ther Drug Monit 2004;26:200–205.
15. George JR, Fitchen JH. Future applications of oral fluid technology. Am J Med 1997;102(4A):21–5.

16. Thieme T, Piacentini S, Davidson S, Steingart K. Determination of measles, mumps, and rubella immunization status using oral fluid samples. JAMA 1994;272(3):219–21.

17. AIDS Diagnosis via Saliva. Clinica World Medical Device News. July 13; No. 308; 1988.

18. Granade TC, Phillips SK, Parekh B, et al. Detection of antibodies to human immunodeficiency virus type 1 in oral fluids: a large scale evaluation of immunoassay performance. Clin Diagn Lab Immunol 1998;5(2):171–5.

24

Coverage and reimbursement for salivary diagnostic tests

James J. Crall

INTRODUCTION

Diagnostic tests are an important element of healthcare delivery and the healthcare economy. Laboratory diagnostic tests play an integral role in good healthcare, helping clinicians to diagnose and treat patients and monitor their conditions over time.[1] Inherently, diagnostic tests are designed to inform or guide decisions regarding further testing, prevention, or treatment—decisions that ultimately influence the course of illness and cost of healthcare.[2]

A growing body of literature suggests that, in a variety of situations, salivary diagnostic testing holds considerable potential as an alternative to traditional diagnostic tests[3]; however, relatively little has been published with respect to the economics of salivary diagnostic testing. As with other types of health services, decisions concerning insurance coverage and reimbursement for salivary diagnostic tests ultimately will have a great bearing on their use in healthcare and other settings. Therefore, this chapter provides an overview of several key considerations concerning the economic aspects of salivary diagnostic tests.

THE BUSINESS OF DIAGNOSTIC TESTING

Laboratory diagnostic services accounted for an estimated $56 billion in healthcare expenditures in 2005.[2] Although $56 billion represents a relatively small portion of overall US healthcare spending, the overall impact of diagnostic tests is typified by reports that estimate that diagnostics influence 60–70% of "downstream" treatment decisions.[4,5] Medicare, the federal program providing coverage of healthcare services for the elderly and disabled, is the largest payer of clinical laboratory services, paying approximately 30% of the nation's bill for inpatient and outpatient laboratory services. Outpatient services account for approximately one-third of total Medicare laboratory expenditures.[4,6] Hospital laboratories and large independent laboratories represent about 8% of all diagnostic laboratory facilities, but account for nearly 80% of the volume of laboratory tests, with the remainder being provided in physicians' offices and other types of facilities.[1]

The field of diagnostic testing is changing rapidly because of major technological innovations. Mapping of the human genome and other scientific advances have led laboratory experts to expect major advances in clinical tests and methodologies in the near future. Particular interest is focused in the areas of genetic testing, surface markers to identify specific types of cancers, pharmacogenomics to individualize drug treatments, and molecular-level tests. These technological advances offer the prospect of substantial new opportunities for diagnostic improvements. However, changes of this nature are often associated with expensive new laboratory tests and testing methodologies that will place an increasing burden on payment systems and necessitate increasing attention to determinations of which services are to be covered and the appropriateness of payment levels.[1] Technological changes also carry the prospect of shifting the location where diagnostic testing is conducted—that is, away from central laboratory facilities to "point-of-care" locations such as outpatient treatment facilities or even home-based testing areas that may hold significant promise for applications of salivary diagnostic testing.

COVERAGE AND REIMBURSEMENT POLICIES FOR DIAGNOSTIC TESTS

Public and private healthcare benefits generally include coverage for a wide range of diagnostic tests. Healthcare insurers pay for tests performed in laboratories that meet standards certified under the Clinical Laboratory Improvement Amendments (CLIA) of 1988, according to Current Procedural Terminology (CPT) codes.[7] In cases where a CPT code does not exist, health insurers sometimes reimburse the new test by using a CPT code for an existing test, a process known as "mapping."[8–10] Once a CPT code is established, test payments are established by cross-walking or gap-filling. In cross-walking, a new test is determined to be similar to an existing test, multiple existing test codes, or a portion of an existing test code. Payment is set at an appropriate percentage of the payment for the existing test.[11] In gap-filling, insurers are left to determine an appropriate payment amount for the new code.

Dental benefits generally include coverage for diagnostic services related to diseases and conditions affecting teeth and related oral structures. However, a review of the diagnostic procedures that correspond to Current Dental Terminology (CDT) codes reveals little in the way of specific references to salivary diagnostics.

The contracts that specify the scope of services covered under various health benefits plans generally do not provide detailed descriptions of every service that will and will not be reimbursed within a category of eligible covered services; rather they usually state that the insurer will reimburse all "medically necessary" goods and services. The interpretation of the term *medically necessary* has varied over time and across health plans, but today generally rests on the application of evidence standards.[12] Such standards have two critical components: a determination about what that evidence implies about effectiveness (magnitude of benefit) and a determination about whether enough evidence is available to support conclusions about the effectiveness of the intervention in question (adequacy of evidence). Although different groups do not always reach the same conclusion about a particular technology, and the specific processes that they use to evaluate evidence vary, there has been a remarkable convergence in the acceptance of the principle that coverage determinations should be guided by the results of rigorously designed studies rather than expert opinion or the most common forms of practice.[12]

At present, coverage under both Medicare and most commercial health insurance plans for therapeutic products is based on a determination that a product has proved to be effective.[7] Laboratory tests, however, are developed under a different regulatory structure and, as a result, diagnostic tests may come to market with little information supporting their role in clinical decision making or evidence regarding their impact on patient outcomes.[2]

Medicare payment policy for outpatient laboratory services was designed in the 1980s and is now generally considered to be outdated. Payments are not consistently related to costs, and while payment rates have been modestly adjusted for inflation, neither the prevailing rates nor the basic payment methodology has evolved to take into account technology, market, and regulatory changes.[1]

COVERAGE AND REIMBURSEMENT IN THE EMERGING ERA OF DIAGNOSTIC TECHNOLOGIES

A report issued by the Institute of Medicine of the National Academy of Sciences in 2000[1] suggested that the process of establishing reimbursement levels for novel laboratory tests is out of date and not equipped to handle emerging diagnostic and genomic tests. Attention to these inadequacies has highlighted the argument that reimbursement must more accurately reflect clinical and economic value.[2] Clinical and economic value for diagnostic tests can be established through a hierarchy of evaluation criteria that includes:

1. technical feasibility and optimization (ability to produce consistent results);
2. diagnostic accuracy (based on assessments of sensitivity, specificity, and positive and negative predictive values);
3. impact on diagnostic thinking (changes in clinicians' diagnoses after testing);
4. impact on therapeutic choice (changes in planned therapy after testing);
5. impact on patient outcomes (health improvements with testing vs without testing); and
6. impact on society (cost-effectiveness).[2]

The definition of *value* for diagnostic tests is similar to that which applies to the value of other health technologies—that is, an intervention (in this case, a diagnostic test) provides an overall benefit to a patient at an acceptable cost. Recognized criteria for establishing an intervention as cost-effective include being:

- less costly and at least as effective as other interventions;
- more effective and more costly, with the added benefit worth the added cost;
- less effective and less costly, with the added benefit of the alternative intervention not worth the added cost; or
- cost saving with an outcome equal to or better than that of the alternative.[12]

Implementing a more rational basis for coverage and reimbursement decisions is a major priority for public and private third-party payers in light of the rapidly changing field of diagnostic testing. Experts note that manufacturers and laboratory service providers simply cannot expect coverage and appropriate reimbursement for every new test that comes to market, nor can payers expect to have the same level of evidence for every candidate test.[2] Development of transparent payment processes and a standard format for documenting and evaluating evidence on the diagnostic effectiveness and cost-effectiveness of testing procedures are urgently needed to help address the shortcomings of the outdated policies and decision-making processes currently in place.

REIMBURSEMENT FOR GENETIC TESTING

Literature from the field of managed care generally supports the notion that requirements for reimbursement of genetic tests should be no less stringent than those governing the reimbursement of pharmaceuticals and other diagnostics. The primary rationale for this position is that genetic tests can be expensive and misinterpreting their results can lead to unwarranted medical care, exposing the patient to unnecessary risk and the managed care organization to additional costs.[2]

As with diagnostic tests, criteria have been developed for assessing the effectiveness of genetic tests. Suggested criteria for assessing the cost-effectiveness of genetic tests include the following:

- Genotype–phenotype association (strong association between gene variants and clinically relevant outcomes);
- Genetic variant prevalence (variant allele prevalence is high enough to warrant testing and specified according to racial subgroups—since the cost-effectiveness of genetic testing is highly dependent on the prevalence of the target genetic variation);
- Clinical outcome characteristics (genetic testing results in improved clinical outcomes measured as a significant impact on quality of life, mortality, or medical care expenses);
- Intervention for the variant group (incremental use of genetic testing vs standard care provides a significant reduction in overall event rate/attributable risk); and
- Assay characteristics (rapid, reliable, and relatively inexpensive assay is available and the sensitivity, specificity, and all costs associated with the assay have been identified).[13]

The final criterion above underscores the necessity of accounting for the total costs of genetic testing, including a variety of indirect "downstream" costs to the payer, patient, and possibly the patient's family. Potential indirect costs to the payer include counseling or therapy costs subsequent to a positive result. Changes in functional, emotional, or social status may result from knowing one's genetic predisposition toward severe and debilitating diseases such as Alzheimer's disease, Huntington's disease, or breast cancer. These potential adverse effects of genetic testing on patient quality of life and payer costs will vary based on the gravity of the disease in question. However, they should be explicitly identified and incorporated into economic analyses.[13]

Disease risk and pharmacogenomic tests have enormous potential to provide a low-cost, rapid, and reliable way to screen populations for disease risk and drug response. However, these tests will also require sufficient clinical, epidemiologic, and economic data to support their use in a safe, effective, and cost-effective manner. Although some genetic tests may move rapidly from laboratory testing to clinical use, the ultimate course and longevity of a particular test will be decided by the healthcare marketplace. As genetic tests become more ubiquitous, decision makers will need to develop appropriate tools and sound criteria to create and maintain appropriate levels of reimbursement over time.

SALIVARY TESTING: AN ALTERNATIVE TO MORE EXPENSIVE, INVASIVE TESTING PROCEDURES

Recent reviews[3,14,15] suggest that certain diagnostic uses of saliva hold considerable promise in the field of healthcare. Monitoring of immune responses to viral infections, including hepatitis and HIV, may prove valuable in the identification of infected individuals, nonsymptomatic carriers, and immune individuals. Saliva also can be useful in the monitoring of therapeutic drug levels and the detection of illicit drug use. Analysis of saliva may provide valuable information regarding certain endocrine disorders. And whole saliva contains locally produced as well as serum-derived markers that have been found to be useful in the diagnosis of a variety of systemic disorders including cancer, diabetes, arthritis, and heart disease.[15]

Saliva offers an alternative to serum as a biological fluid that can be analyzed for diagnostic purposes. Whole saliva can be collected in a noninvasive manner by individuals with modest training, including patients themselves—a feature that holds considerable potential for the development and introduction of screening tests that can be performed by patients at home.[16] Many have suggested that analysis of saliva can offer a cost-effective approach for the screening of large populations and may represent an alternative for patients in whom blood drawing is difficult or when compliance is a problem.[14–16]

Owing to these advantages, salivary diagnostics provides a potentially attractive alternative to more invasive, time-consuming, complicated, and expensive diagnostic approaches. However, before salivary diagnostic tests can replace more conventional approaches, the diagnostic value of new salivary tests has to be compared with accepted diagnostic methods. The usefulness of a new test has to be determined in terms of sensitivity, specificity, correlation with established disease diagnostic criteria, and reproducibility. Health plans also have to be convinced that saliva-based tests are highly accurate as well as cost-effective—that is, that they meet the extant criteria for coverage and reimbursement outlined earlier.

BARRIERS TO THE DEVELOPMENT AND WIDESPREAD USE OF SALIVARY DIAGNOSTICS

At the 1999 National Institute of Dental and Craniofacial Research (NIDCR) workshop on development of new technologies for saliva and other oral fluid–based diagnostics, it was noted that there were three general types of barriers to wide-scale implementation of salivary diagnostics:

- The need for additional basic and applied research—for example, the need to design and develop microsensors capable of accurate measurements in small volumes and standardization of collection methods;
- The need for product development; and
- Third-party acceptance and associated legal issues.[3]

Considerable progress has been made in the intervening eight years since the NIDCR workshop toward overcoming the first barrier, primarily as a result of a considerable investment by NIDCR in salivary diagnostic technology development and salivary proteome research groups. These initiatives have led to collaboration among researchers from the fields of nanotechnology, proteomics, and genomics and those involved in the production of biosensors for real-time, ultrasensitive, and ultraspecific detection of salivary diagnostic analytes.[15] These same efforts have also led to the development of practical products such as hand-held salivary biomarker detectors that can be used in the office by dentists or other healthcare providers for point-of-care disease screening and detection. Such devices may soon be available for development and distribution through commercial channels. Thus, the barriers associated with the scientific underpinnings and commercial potential of widespread salivary diagnostic testing appear to be diminishing rapidly, leaving acceptance of these "nontraditional" approaches by clinicians and third-party payers as the final remaining challenge to widespread adoption and diffusion. Because the implications of salivary diagnostics applications for the field of medicine will likely be more considerable than for dentistry, medical insurance companies will have to be convinced that saliva-based tests are highly accurate as well as cost-effective.[3] That notwithstanding, salivary diagnostics are also likely to emerge as an important area of interest for dentists and the dental benefits industry.

SUMMARY AND COMMENTS ON THE IMPORTANCE OF REIMBURSEMENT FOR SALIVARY TESTING

Scientific and technological advances have laid the foundation for expanded clinical applications of salivary diagnostic testing, but it remains to be seen how the new developments will be applied in the healthcare marketplace. Research demonstrating that salivary assays meet the coverage and reimbursement criteria used in the private and public sectors and/or have ease-of-collection advantages compared with serum, whole blood, or other biological specimens undoubtedly will have a positive influence on the use of salivary diagnostic testing. However, it would seem that questions concerning the future of point-of-care diagnostic testing and the role of salivary diagnostics in the point-of-care and home therapy arenas are equally if not more relevant to the future of salivary diagnostics.

A recent expert review[17] noted that point-of-care diagnostics have been proposed as the latest development in clinical diagnostics several times in the past 30 years but have not yet fully developed into a business sector to match the projections. As stated earlier, recent advances have effectively removed technology as a major barrier to the development of point-of-care testing. Moreover, regulatory procedures regarding diagnostic product development and substantiation appear to have been established as a result of global healthcare economics and "consumer pressures" from patients. The final obstacles to significant transformation of the business of diagnostics relate to the conflict between two forces: the emerging ability to render a diagnosis and provide immediate treatment based on tests conducted in a wide array of nontraditional point-of-care settings on one hand and the entrenched positions of central laboratories, suppliers, and their established distribution chains and the way in which healthcare budgets are allocated on the other. In the end, the expert providing the review concluded that "the ultimate hurdle that encapsulates all of these issues is reimbursement, which is the final barrier to a significant point-of-care diagnostics market—without reimbursement there will be no market for point-of-care diagnostic testing."[17] Similarly, it appears that forthcoming decisions and policies concerning reimbursement are likely to be major determinants of the fate of salivary diagnostic testing.

REFERENCES

1. National Academy of Sciences. In: Wolman DM, Kalfoglou AL, LeRoy L, eds., *Medicare Laboratory Payment Policy: Now and in the Future—Executive Summary.* Committee on Medicare Payment Methodology for Clinical Laboratory Services, Division of Health Care Services; 2000. Available at: http://www.nap.edu/catalog/9997.html (accessed August 28, 2007).
2. Ramsey SD, Veenstra DL, Garrison LP, et al. Toward evidence-based assessment for coverage and reimbursement of laboratory-based diagnostic and genetic tests. Am J Manag Care 2006;12:197–202.
3. Streckfus CF, Bigler LR. Saliva as a diagnostic fluid. Oral Dis 2002;8:69–76.

4. Gustafson T. *Testimony before the Institute of Medicine Committee on Method-ology for Clinical Laboratory Services*, Washington, D.C., January 20, 2000.
5. The Lewin Group. *The Value of Diagnostics Innovation, Adoption and Dif-fusion into Health Care*. Report prepared for the Advanced Medical Tech-nology Association (AdvaMed), July 2005. Available at: http://www.advamed.org/publicdocs/thevalueofdiagnostics.pdf (accessed August 28, 2007).
6. Klipp J. *Lab Industry Strategic Outlook 2000: Market Trends and Analysis*. Washington, D.C.: Washington G-2 Reports; 2000.
7. Centers for Medicare & Medicaid Services. Clinical Laboratory Improve-ment Amendments (CLIA). Available at: http://www.cms.hhs.gov/clia/ (accessed September, 2007).
8. Young DS. Earning your keep: succeeding in laboratory reimbursement. Clin Chem 1998;44:1701–12.
9. Young DS. Reforming laboratory reimbursement: issues, impact and inno-vations. A summary of the clinical chemistry forum held on November 15, 2001. Clin Chem 2002;48:792–5.
10. Centers for Medicare & Medicaid Services. Glossary. http://www.cms.hhs.gov/glossary/ (accessed September, 2007).
11. Wolman DM, Kalfoglou AL, LeRoy L, eds. *Medicare Laboratory Payment Policy: Now and in the Future*. Washington, D.C.: The National Academies Press; 2000:17.
12. Garber AM. Cost-effectiveness and evidence evaluation as criteria for cov-erage policy. Health Aff 2004;W4:284–96.
13. Higashi MK, Veenstra DL. Managed care in the genomics era: assessing the cost-effectiveness of genetic tests. Am J Manag Care 2003;9:493–500.
14. Kaufman E, Lamster IB. The diagnostic applications of saliva—a review. Crit Rev Oral Biol Med 2002;12:197–212.
15. Bailey B, Klein J, Koren G. Noninvasive methods for drug measurement in pediatrics. Pediatr Clin North Am 1997;44:15–26.
16. Wong DT. Salivary diagnostics powered by nanotechnologies, proteomics and genomics. JADA 2006;137:313–21.
17. Huckle D. Point-of-care diagnostics: will the hurdles be overcome this time? Expert Rev Med Devices 2006 3:421–6.

Saliva diagnostics in the dentist's and physician's office

Chakwan Siew and Milton V. Marshall

SALIVARY GLAND ANATOMY AND PHYSIOLOGY

The salivary glands are mucus-producing glands primarily regulated by the parasympathetic nervous system that provide physiological functions within the gastrointestinal tract[1] (also see Chapters 1 and 2). Stimulation of saliva production occurs following sight and smell of food, taste, or tactile stimulation in the oral cavity. Compared with plasma constituents, saliva components vary in concentration, and some electrolytes and proteins found in saliva are not present in plasma; salivary components are typically found at lower concentrations than in plasma. Using saliva has advantages over venipuncture for obtaining plasma/serum, including ease of collection, reduced risk of percutaneous injuries, and lower collection cost. Noninvasive procedures can reduce anxiety and discomfort and simplify repetitive sample collection.

DIAGNOSTIC TESTS WITH SALIVA

In developing diagnostic tests within the oral cavity, it is important to consider which moieties provide useful information. Typically, small molecules such as drugs and hormones (and their metabolites) are easily isolated, assayed, and quantified. Additional information can also be obtained from analysis of nucleic acids and proteins present in saliva.

SALIVARY DIAGNOSTIC APPLICATIONS

Oral diseases

Salivary diagnostic applications fall into several broad categories (Table 25.1). One obvious application is detection of disease. Identification of pathogenic organisms in the oral cavity is important for diagnosis and treatment. Infectious agents in saliva are typically identified by isolation, culture, and differential identification, which is time-consuming and labor-intensive. A more rapid means of identification of microorganisms present in saliva is by

Table 25.1   Salivary diagnostic applications.

- Infectious agents
- Disease
    Local
    Systemic
- Hormone levels
- Therapeutic drug monitoring
- Drugs of abuse
- Forensic applications

amplification using polymerase chain reaction (PCR). However, this methodology cannot differentiate between living and dead organisms. Salivary biomarkers of inflammation, matrix metalloproteinase-8 (MMP-8) and interleukin-18,[2] have been identified. Disease detection from saliva analysis can reflect local or systemic changes related to a disease.

It is logical to assume that local disease factors would be present in saliva; moreover, biomarkers for cancer of the oral cavity have been identified.[3–5] MMP-8 has been implicated as a potential cofactor of systemic diseases.[6,7]

Systemic diseases

Systemic diseases, including infectious diseases such as human immunodeficiency virus (HIV), hepatitis A virus (HAV), hepatitis B virus (HBV), hepatitis C virus (HCV), and autoimmune diseases, endocrine disorders, Alzheimer's disease, and cancer frequently have circulating biomarkers[8–10] that can be monitored to determine treatment strategy and efficacy. For example, salivary c-*erb*B-2, a breast cancer biomarker,[11] may be useful in monitoring for disease recurrence following therapy.

Steroid hormone levels in saliva represent free, rather than protein-bound, hormones that are predominantly found in blood. Small unbound steroid molecules that are lipophilic and nonionized within the pH range of saliva readily diffuse into saliva. Circulating levels of predominantly protein-bound hormones do not correlate well with salivary hormone levels because the high molecular weight precludes transport into salivary glands and then into saliva. Elevated salivary cortisol levels are associated with episodic stress[12] and free salivary cortisol levels can identify persons with Cushing's syndrome.[13] Free levels of therapeutic drugs in saliva can also be monitored. Drugs of abuse can be identified in saliva, and a good correlation exists between serum and salivary levels.[14]

DENTISTS AND ORAL DISEASE DETECTION AND DIAGNOSES FROM SALIVA

Dental healthcare providers spend the majority of time monitoring the oral health of their patients, and the dental community is the first line of defense in early disease detection. Including generalists and specialists, there are over 140,000 dentists in the United States, and each one sees approximately 15 patients per day. According to the American Dental Association, over 60% of the US population sees a dentist every year. Disease monitoring of the existing patient population can yield many opportunities to catch potential oral and systemic diseases early in order to facilitate prevention or treatment. Historically, oral health professionals were pioneers in studying anticariogenic, remineralization, and antibacterial properties of saliva.[15] They are currently taking major initiatives in developing biosensor technologies to detect biomarkers in saliva, such as DNA, RNA, peptides, carbohydrates, and fatty acids that could signal potential disease conditions.

Detection technology has been developed and applied to identify individuals susceptible to developing caries, oral or systemic cancer, infectious diseases, and other systemic diseases. Several saliva-based tests are already approved by the Food and Drug Administration (FDA) for marketing. These are used to measure drugs of abuse and antigens/antibodies. Point-of-care (POC) salivary diagnostics is the first step in initiating the process of evaluating local and systemic patient health.[16] The ultimate goal of POC diagnostics is to accelerate the clinical decision-making process, which will in the long term reduce the overall cost of healthcare. As part of a general health-screening program, salivary diagnostic tests can be used to monitor overall health status, disease onset, disease progression, and treatment efficacy. Early detection is key to successfully treating patients and, simultaneously, to reducing the skyrocketing healthcare costs. For an effective reduction in mortality and morbidity associated with diseases outside the oral cavity, salivary diagnostic results must be shared with the person's physician.

Some types of tests, such as mass spectroscopy[17] or microarray analysis, do not work well in a clinical setting because of expensive instrumentation and training requirements. However, information from these diagnostic tests has been successfully translated to clinical use with the design of compact, handheld devices that could eventually be used for routine screening[18,19] in dental clinics.

For example, a saliva-based caries assessment and risk evaluation test has been developed.[20] Dental caries is an infectious disease, and colonization of tooth surfaces by acid-producing oral bacteria is initiated by an interaction between microbial surface lectins and saliva glycoproteins that form the pellicle on tooth surfaces. Amounts of specific glycoproteins produced in the saliva are genetically determined and, in turn, determine whether an individual will be caries-prone. A test for caries or caries potential evolved from quantitating more than 50 different lectin affinities from the saliva of individuals with varying caries histories. When applied to children, this test can be used to predict future caries development. This test outcome can then be used to provide specific preventive recommendations (see Chapter 14).

Other researchers have made major advances in the development of nanotechnology/microtechnology to detect salivary proteins and genomic biomarkers for POC applications for oral cancers and periodontal diseases. A salivary diagnostic instrument, the Oral Fluid NanoSensor Test (OFNASET), is a hand-held, automated system for rapid detection of multiple salivary proteins and nucleic acids[3,18]; another product is a microchip electrophoretic immunoassay (μCEI).[8] The μCEI relies on molecular sieving gels and electrophoresis to enrich samples and subsequently resolve a fluorescent antigen–antibody complex. Salivary MMP-8 levels have been measured with this instrument (see Chapter 15).

Salivary antibodies to tumor-suppressor protein p53 can be measured with ELISA to identify individuals with oral cancer. Tumors with high levels of p53 elicit an immune response with production of IgG and/or IgA antibodies to p53.[21]

MEDICAL/CLINICAL APPLICATIONS

Salivary diagnostics should prove useful in medical practice to rapidly identify drugs of abuse, monitor therapy, and identify predictive markers of systemic and infectious diseases.[22] Detection of antipertussis toxin in children with a salivary ELISA test would be especially advantageous when screening infants or young children in whom it is difficult to obtain blood samples.[23]

Oral fluid testing has evolved to the point that it is generally equivalent in accuracy and performance to urine testing for certain drugs of abuse.[24] The accuracy of urine testing has been eroded by adultering or substituting urine samples to circumvent drug screening tests. Saliva is readily accessible, and testing saliva avoids the privacy issues inherent in urine testing because saliva can be collected noninvasively under direct observation.

The potential also exists for personalizing medicine by identifying genetic polymorphisms from saliva to develop individual treatment regimens. Soluble HLA antigens in saliva can be used to identify persons with autoimmune diseases.[25] C-reactive protein (CRP) is an acute-phase reactant that is a general indicator of inflammation that bridges the dental and medical fields. Elevated blood levels of high sensitivity CRP (hs-CRP) are correlated with an increased risk for heart attack, restenosis of coronary arteries after angioplasty, stroke, and peripheral vascular disease.[26] Measurement of hs-CRP from saliva[27] has increased sensitivity compared with serum ELISA. The ELISA assay for hs-CRP is not as sensitive as the microchip assay, which can detect as little as 10 pg/mL saliva. Because antibody or antigen levels are lower in saliva compared with that in blood, higher sensitivity assays are required, and this sensitivity can be obtained with microfluidic assays.[8,19]

Detection of HIV in saliva is as sensitive as detection in serum. Venipuncture poses the risk of infection to healthcare workers through percutaneous injuries. Saliva offers a much safer alternative to blood testing and thus reduces the potential for contracting this blood-borne pathogen.

Salivary levels of antidengue IgM and IgG can be used to distinguish between primary and secondary infection with the dengue fever virus.[10] This differential diagnosis is important in managing complications such as dengue hemorrhagic fever and dengue shock syndrome.

MARKETING A DIAGNOSTIC DEVICE

Diagnostic tests must undergo FDA review of safety and efficacy before they can be marketed in the United States. Diagnostic tests must initially be characterized by risk associated with use. For economic feasibility, a diagnostic test must have a Current Procedural Terminology code for third-party reimbursement.

CONCLUSIONS

Salivary diagnostic testing has been used for a number of years, but with the explosion of knowledge in human genetics and major advancements in nanotechnology and miniaturization, salivary diagnostic tests are becoming available for routine screening. One major advantage of screening with saliva, compared with circulating blood, is the reduction in percutaneous injury risk and thus the reduction in the risk of transmission of pathogens from patients to healthcare workers. These tests will eventually be miniaturized and validated so that they can be used for routine screening in dental and medical offices. These diagnostic tests will not be limited to detection of local disease, but can be used to identify systemic disease. Effective use of salivary diagnostics requires a willingness by patients to share salivary diagnostic test results with their physicians.

REFERENCES

1. Whelton H. *Introduction: The Anatomy and Physiology of Salivary Glands*, 2nd edn. WM Edgar (ed.) London: British Dental Journal Publishing; 1996.
2. Orozco A, Gemmell E, Bickel N, Seymour GJ. Interleukin 18 and periodontal disease—critical reviews in oral biology & medicine. J Dent Res 2007;86(7):586–93.
3. Li Y, St John MA, Zhou X, et al. Salivary transcriptome diagnostics for oral cancer detection. Clin Cancer Res 2004;10(24):8442–50.
4. Mager DL, Haffajee AD, Devlin PM, Norris CM, Posner MR, Goodson JM. The salivary microbiota as a diagnostic indicator of oral cancer: a descriptive, non-randomized study of cancer-free and oral squamous cell carcinoma subjects. J Transl Med 2005;3(1):27.
5. Giusti L, Baldini C, Bazzichi L, et al. Proteome analysis of whole saliva: a new tool for rheumatic diseases—the example of Sjogren's syndrome. Proteomics 2007;7(10):1634–43.
6. Beck JD, Offenbacher S. Systemic effects of periodontitis: epidemiology of periodontal disease. J Periodont 2005;76:2089–2100.
7. Al-Zahrani MS, Kayal RA, Bissada NF. Periodontitis and cardiovascular disease: a review of shared risk factors and new findings supporting a causality hypothesis. Quintessence Int 2006;37:11–18.

8. Herr AE, Hatch AV, Throckmorton DJ, et al. Microfluidic immunoassays as rapid saliva-based clinical diagnostics. Proc Natl Acad Sci U S A 2007;104(13):5268–73.

9. Abrams WR, McCann K, Barber CA, et al. Development of a microfluidic device for detection of pathogens in oral samples using upconverting phosphor techonology (UPT), Ann NY Acad Sci 2007;1098:375–88.

10. Kaufman E, Lamster IB. The diagnostic applications of saliva—a review. Crit Rev Oral Biol Med 2002;13(2):197–212.

11. Streckfus C, Bigler L. The use of soluble, salivary c-erbB-2 for the detection and post-operative follow-up of breast cancer in women: the results of a five-year translational research study. Adv Dent Res 2005;18(1):17–24.

12. Hubert W, de Jong-Meyer R. Emotional stress and the saliva cortisol response. J Clin Chem Clin Biochem 1989;27:235–7.

13. Castro M, Elias PCL, Martinelli CE, Antonini SR, Santiago L, Moreira AC. Salivary cortisol as a tool for physiological studies and diagnostic strategies. Braz J Med Biol Res 2000;33:1171–75.

14. Toennes SW, Steinmeyer S, Maurer HJ, Moeller MR, Kauert GF. Screening for drugs of abuse in oral fluid—correlation of analysis results with serum in forensic cases. J Anal Toxicol 2005;29(1):22–7.

15. Mandel E. A contemporary view of salivary research. Crit Rev Oral Biol Med 1993;4(3–4):599–603.

16. Tabak LA. Point-of-care diagnostics enter the mouth. Ann N Y Acad Sci 2007;1098:7–14.

17. Schipper R, Loof A, de Groot J, Harthoorn L, van Heerde W, Dransfield E. Salivary protein/peptide profiling with SELDI-TOF-MS. Ann N Y Acad Sci 2007;1098:498–503.

18. Li Y, Zhou X, St John MA, Wong DT. RNA profiling of cell-free saliva using microarray technology. J Dent Res 2004;83(3):199–203.

19. Wong DT. Salivary diagnostics powered by nanotechnologies, proteomics and genomics. J Am Dent Assoc (1939) 2006;137(3):313–21.

20. Denny PC, Penny PA, Takeshimer J, et al. A novel caries risk test. Ann N Y Acad Sci 2007; 1098:204–15.

21. Liao PH, Chang Y, Huang M, Tai KW, Chou MY. Mutations of p53 gene codon 63 in saliva as a molecular marker for oral squamous cell carcinomas. Oral Oncol 2000;36:272–6.

22. Forde MD, Koka, S, Eckert S, Carr AB, Wong DT. Systemic assessments utilizing saliva: Part 1. General considerations and current assessments. Int J Prosthodont 2006;19:43–52.

23. Litt DJ, Samuel D, Duncan J, Harnden A, George RC, Harrison TG. Detection of anti-pertussis toxin IgG in oral fluids for use in diagnosis and surveillance of Bordetella pertussis infection in children and young adults. J Med Microbiol 2006;55(Pt 9):1223–8.

24. Cone EJ, Presley L, Lehrer M, et al. Oral fluid testing for drugs of abuse: positive prevalence rates by Intercept immunoassay screening and GC-MS-MS confirmation and suggested cutoff concentrations. J Anal Toxicol 2002;26(8):541–6.

25. Adamashvili I, Pressly T, Gebel H, et al. Soluble HLA in saliva of patients with autoimmune rheumatic diseases. Rheumatol Int 2002;22(2):71–6.

26. Rifai N, Ridker PM. Population distributions of C-reactive protein in apparently healthy men and women in the United States: implication for clinical interpretation. Clin Chem 2003;49(4):666–9.
27. Christodoulides N, Mohanty S, Miller CS, et al. Application of microchip assay system for the measurement of C-reactive protein in human saliva. Lab Chip 2005;5(3):261–9.

26

Salivary hormones in research and diagnostics

Douglas A. Granger, Christine K. Fortunato, and Leah C. Hibel

INTRODUCTION

More than 50 years of interdisciplinary study reveals that hormones influence, and are affected by, behavior. These reciprocal effects are highly dependent on social context.[1] Hormones have been used as markers of status and change in various physiological systems. Contemporary behavioral endocrinology research is focused on linking individual differences in the status and change in these systems with a variety of issues related to health, development, and psychosocial adjustment.

Monitoring hormones noninvasively has advanced this agenda by enabling the study of variation in endocrine function in the context of everyday life. The attention saliva has received as a research specimen is due to the perception that sample collection is quick, uncomplicated, and minimally invasive and salivary assays are reliable and accurate. In many circumstances, however, specialized issues threaten the measurement validity of salivary hormones. This chapter highlights several of these special issues in an effort to inform the most recent movement to develop diagnostic applications for oral fluids.

SALIVA COLLECTION IS CHALLENGING FOR THE YOUNG AND OLD

Saliva collection from preterm newborns, infants in neonatal intensive care units, and healthy infants less than 3 months of age, is especially challenging.[2] After repeated and sustained effort, the result is often insufficient (<25 μL) specimen volume for immunoassay.[3] Collecting saliva from older infants (5–10 months) is frequently not possible (or permitted) owing to their irregular sleep–wake cycles.[4] Moreover, infants' consumption of breast milk, formula, and diary-related products can contaminate specimens by cross-reacting with detection antibodies used in immunoassays.[5] Later in early childhood (12–18 months), saliva collection becomes complicated by stranger anxiety and noncompliance with collection procedures.[4]

On the other hand, collecting saliva from the oldest-old can be time-consuming and have a high failure rate. In a study of the oldest-old (73% older than 85 years), one-third of attempts failed to provide valid saliva samples. Xerostomia (dry mouth) affected more than half of the study's participants. Use of medications with direct, or iatrogenic, diuretic effects was high for those who had difficulty donating specimens.[6]

Using saliva, as opposed to urine or blood, enables sample collection in special populations and circumstances. However, investigators must be aware that this perception does not match reality in some unique person-by-situation circumstances. Specimen collection failure yields missing data, and these findings highlight that "missingness" may be related to age, physiological states (xerostomia), ethnic and poverty status,[4] as well as medications. For diagnostic applications, inadequate sample test volumes obviously negate many of the advantages of monitoring hormones in oral fluids and translate directly into missed opportunity, wasted time and resources.

EFFECTS OF SALIVA COLLECTION TECHNIQUES ON SALIVARY HORMONES

Historically, saliva collection devices involve cotton-absorbent materials (e.g., Sarstedt, Numbresht, Germany) placed under the tongue (2–3 min), cotton saturates with saliva. Then saliva is expressed into collection vials by centrifugation or compression. Most of the time, this approach is convenient, simple, and time efficient. However, when the absorbent capacity is large and sample volume small, the specimen absorbed can be diffusely distributed and recovery becomes problematic. Recoveries for the Salivette (Sarstedt, Numbresht, Germany) cotton pledget are only 38, 59, 74, and 83%, and for braided cotton rope (Richmond Dental, Charlotte, NC) only 15, 31, 64, and 74% when initial sample volumes were 0.25, 0.50, 1.0, and 1.5 mL. Poor saliva volume recovery has been associated with artificially low hormone estimates.[7] The process of absorbing saliva with cotton also interferes with immunoassay performance for testosterone, SIgA, dehydroepiandrosterone (DHEA), estradiol, progesterone, 17-OH Progesterone, and androstenedione.[8] Thus, the use of cotton-based material to collect salivary hormone data for research or diagnostic applications raises unique concerns.

Early literature on salivary hormones addressed low specimen volumes by "simply" stimulating saliva flow by chewing (gums, dental wax) or tasting (sugar crystals, powdered drink mixes, citric acid drops), or smelling a variety of substances (e.g., orange oil). When used more than minimally and/or inconsistently, some of these methods affect immunoassay performance. Saliva is poorly buffered and oral substances containing acids easily lower salivary pH. As pH declines, antibody–antigen binding is compromised and artificially high salivary hormone estimates may result.[9] Stimulants also influence measurement of the levels of analytes that are dependent on saliva flow rate. To minimize this validity threat, the immunodiagnostic industry has reduced saliva test volume requirements from >200 μL (prior to 1998) to <25 μL, and diluents now normalize sample pH or flag samples with pH problems. The need to stimulate saliva is obsolete. The risks of doing so for oral diagnostics far outweigh the benefit.

Behavioral science champions measurement of multiple endocrine markers in contemporary biosocial models of individual differences. To "multiplex" from a single sample, collection must minimize interference across different assay protocols. To achieve this aim, we ask participants to imagine they are chewing their favorite food, slowly move their jaws as if chewing, and to let saliva pool in their mouth without swallowing. Specimen is gently forced through a short drinking straw into a storage vial. The procedure's advantages include the following: (1) a large sample (1–5 mL) volume can be collected within 5 min; (2) sample can be assayed for multiple markers; and (3) samples can be archived for use in future assays. The disadvantage is that the procedure requires a competent, aware (and awake), and compliant sample donor. In situations that lack this type of donor, it is essential to have a material to absorb saliva from the mouth.

Collecting saliva on filter paper may be a viable option.[10] Dombrowski and colleagues[10] sampled newborns by placing filter paper on the anterior portion of the tongue and holding it in place until "sufficient" saliva was obtained. Despite standardizing the time of exposure in the mouth, there is considerable range in the volume of saliva collected between individuals, and saliva collected using filter paper returned at least fivefold higher cortisol estimates than passive drool.[11] More recently, Neu and colleagues[12] describe a filter paper collection procedure that has acceptable recovery and linearity. They report that saliva collection was very efficient, and only 2% of the samples from newborns were lost due to inadequate test volumes. When it is not possible to gather samples by other means, filter paper may be viable for some salivary hormones.

Granger and colleagues[11] evaluated hydrocellulose microsponge devices (BD Opthlamatic, Walton, MA) as an alternative saliva collection technique. Microsponges are used during ocular surgery to collect very small volumes of liquid (tears). The BD microsponge reaches its maximum capacity (∼300 μL saliva) within 60 s. The test volume for most salivary assays (25–50 μL) was obtained within 20–30 s.[11] Sample recovery under conditions designed to represent very small volume availability is also adequate. Percent recovery from the microsponge device was superior to cotton-based materials especially when sample volumes were below 100 μL. The small size also allows collection of sample from sleeping infants without waking them. For infants (5–18 months of age), a 1-min collection period and the use of two sponges per collection maximized success of collecting sufficient volume.[4] The microsponge is appropriate for use with samples to be assayed for cortisol, cotinine, and salivary alpha-amylase but is not appropriate for dehydroepiandrosterone (DHEA) or testosterone.[11]

In summary, each saliva collection approach is associated with a unique set of benefits and risks that prevent universal application. Specifying the manner that samples are collected, stored, and prepared for each analyte will be critical to ensure the future of oral diagnostics.

BLOOD "CONTAMINATION" AND SALIVARY HORMONES

Blood can leak into oral fluids due to injury (burns, abrasions, or cuts to the cheek, tongue, or gums). Blood in oral fluid is more prevalent for individuals suffering from poor oral health (i.e., open sores, periodontal disease, gingivitis), during the course of certain infectious diseases (e.g., HIV), and for those who routinely engage in behavior known to influence oral health negatively (e.g., tobacco use). Epidemiologic studies are equivocal that poor oral health is most prevalent among minority, lower socioeconomic status, rural, and third world populations. Blood leakage into saliva is more likely during teething and when shedding teeth.

To meaningfully index endocrine function, quantitative estimates of hormone levels in saliva must be highly correlated with the levels measured in serum. This correlation depends on consistency in the processes[13] that move circulating hormones into oral fluids. When the integrity of this process is compromised, the level of the serological marker (hormone) in saliva should be affected. The impact of this phenomenon for oral diagnostics has received only scant empirical attention.

Utilizing salivary transferrin as a surrogate marker of blood contamination,[14] we studied the degree of contamination needed to affect salivary hormone levels and whether the effects are long- (30–45 min) or short-lived (10–15 min). We found that the effects depend on which hormone is assessed.[14,15] Transferrin levels in saliva are positively associated with salivary DHEA, cortisol, and testosterone, but explain less than 5% of the variance,[16] and less than 0.1% of statistical outliers (+2.5 SDs) in salivary hormone distributions are due to blood contamination. Field studies also show that even in children at high risk for oral health problems, blood contamination in saliva is very infrequent. Finally, the findings demonstrate that blood contamination is a characteristic of individual specimens rather than of individual donors.

The presence of blood in oral fluids has the potential, albeit small, to introduce error variance in the levels of hormones measured in saliva. Sample donors should be screened for events in their recent history that could cause blood leakage into saliva by asking questions related to oral health, teething, shedding teeth, open sores, and injury. Sampling saliva for diagnostic use within 45 min of microinjury to the oral cavity should be avoided. Samples should be systematically inspected at the collection point and if visibly contaminated with blood,[15] excluded from analyses.

MEDICATION USE AND SALIVARY HORMONES

Using saliva as a specimen enables measurement of individual differences and intra-individual change in endocrine function in the context of everyday life. Advances in modern medicine have made over-the-counter and prescription medication use a common feature of most social worlds, and highly salient for those suffering from physical or mental illness. Knowing whether medications influence the measurement of salivary hormone levels seems imperative. Medications that dehydrate and reduce salivary flow (as noted earlier) and, simultaneously, have the potential to act directly on the function of endocrine tissues are of obvious concern (e.g., contraceptives, glucocorticoid containing medicines). Medications that alter subjective psychological experiences (e.g., antidepressants, narcotics) may indirectly influence salivary hormones by changing the impact of environmental events (e.g., stress) on endocrine activity. Other medications may affect movement of small molecules into oral fluids (e.g., blood thinners, vasoconstrictors), or leave residue that interferes with salivary assay function (e.g., teething gels). Finally, the most prevalent medications require examination, just in case.

In three recent studies, we have addressed some of these possibilities. The effects of exogenous glucocorticoid use on salivary cortisol measurements were dependent on both the type and amount of inhaled/nasal steroid used.[17] Compared to infants not taking any medications, stress-related cortisol reactivity was less pronounced for those taking acetaminophen.[18] Also, cortisol levels were higher for mothers taking oral or transdermal contraceptives and acetylsalicylic acid (e.g., Aspirin®) but lower for mothers taking pure agonist opioids (e.g., Oxycontin®) compared with mothers not taking medications.[18] Relative to a no-medication comparison group, children taking (1) antipsychotic medications had higher DHEA levels and flat cortisol diurnal rhythms, (2) Ritalin® or Adderall® had flat testosterone diurnal rhythms, (3) Concerta® had higher testosterone levels, (4) antidepressants had flat DHEA diurnal rhythms, and (5) hypotensives had flat cortisol and DHEA diurnal rhythms and higher testosterone levels.[19]

A variety of medications are capable of introducing variance in salivary hormones. Medication use must be considered when interpreting the meaning of individual differences in salivary hormones in any research, screening, or diagnostic application.

BACTERIA AND SALIVARY HORMONES

Saliva specimens are often gathered in conditions that restrict how they can be handled and stored. Typically, once specimens are collected, samples are kept cold or frozen to maintain sample integrity. Refrigeration prevents degradation of some salivary hormones, restricts activity of proteolytic enzymes and growth of bacteria. For large-scale national surveys, investigators working in remote areas, or patients collecting samples at home, freezing and shipping samples can be cost-prohibitive. In the past, to preserve a sample when refrigeration is not possible, sodium azide (NaN_3) has been added. Disappointingly, NaN_3 interferes with the activity of horseradish peroxidase in enzyme-based saliva immunoassays.

The impact of bacteria-related issues on the measurement of salivary hormones by immunoassay has recently been explored. There are significant declines in the levels of some salivary hormones when samples are stored at RT or 4°C in comparison to −60°C after 96 h.[20] Attempts to minimize this phenomenon by filter-sterilization[21] were largely unsuccessful because passing saliva through 0.22-µm pores was impractical. Subsequently, we treated saliva with penicillin/streptomycin (Pen-Strep, Hyclone, SV30010) to inhibit bacteria growth. Samples were treated either a priori (immediately after collection and then left at RT) or post hoc (samples were collected and then stored at RT prior to treatment). Within 48 h at RT, salivary alpha-amylase (sAA) and salivary cortisol levels had declined by 34 and 5%, respectively. The negative effect of RT storage on sAA and cortisol was minimized by a priori, but not post hoc, treatment with Pen-Strep.

There are considerable individual differences in the quality of saliva that may interact with how samples are handled, stored, and transported after collection. When these potential sources of error variance remain unaccounted for, researchers, medical professionals, and patients should question specimen integrity and any conclusions drawn from the measurement of salivary hormones.

CONCLUDING COMMENTS

More than 25 years of research involving the measurement of hormones in saliva reveal that (1) there are wide-ranging individual differences between individuals and within individuals over time in the levels of most salivary hormones; (2) cross-study consistency in findings linking salivary hormones to social forces, specific behaviors, developmental trajectories, or health status and outcomes are the exception rather than the rule; and (3) even our most elegant theoretical and measurement models account for only a small portion of the variation in individual differences or intra-individual change.

This chapter has highlighted many subtle and special characteristics of oral fluid as a biological specimen that may threaten measurement validity. We suspect that these issues have reduced the ability to detect hormone–behavior associations in previous studies, or contributed to cross-study inconsistency in findings involving salivary hormones, or both. To the extent that either of these possibilities is true, the ability to refine and advance biosocial models of health and human development, to understand stress-related vulnerabilities and resilience, and to extend the knowledge of how individual differences and intra-individual change in salivary hormones relate to adverse physical, mental health, and cognitive outcomes has been compromised.

We expect drawing attention to these issues will increase the probability that salivary hormones will be more successfully integrated into the next generation of biobehavioral research and, in doing so, set a more solid foundation for the eventual translation of the basic findings into clinical investigation and diagnostics.

REFERENCES

1. Nelson RJ. *An Introduction to Behavioral Endocrinology*, 2nd edn. Sunderland, MA: Sinauer; 2000.

2. Bettendorf M, Albers N, Bauer J, Heinrich UE, Linderkamp O, Maser-Gluth C. Longitudinal evaluation of salivary cortisol levels in full-term and preterm neonates. Horm Res 1998;50(6):303–308.

3. Herrington CJ, Olomu IN, Geller SM. Salivary cortisol as indicators of pain in preterm infants: a pilot study. Clin Nurs Res 2004;13(1):53–68.

4. Fortunato CK, Kivlighan KT, Davis L, Granger DA, Investigators TFLP. Trials and tribulations of collecting saliva samples from infants: prevalence and impact on salivary alpha-amylase and cortisol. Poster presented at the Biennial Meeting of the Society for Research on Child Development, Boston, MA; 2007.

5. Magnano CL, Diamond EJ, Gardner JM. Use of salivary cortisol measurements in young infants: a note of caution. Child Dev 1989;60(5):1099–1101.

6. Hodgson N, Freedman VA, Granger DA, Erno A. Biobehavioral correlates of relocation in the frail elderly: salivary cortisol, affect, and cognitive function. J Am Geriatr Soc 2004;52(11):1856–62.

7. Harmon AG, Hibel LC, Rumyansteva O, Granger DA. Measuring salivary cortisol in studies of child development: watch out—what goes in may not come out of saliva collection devices. Dev Psychobiol 2007;49(5):495–500.

8. Shirtcliff EA, Granger DA, Schwartz E, Curran MJ. Use of salivary biomarkers in biobehavioral research: cotton-based sample collection methods can interfere with salivary immunoassay results. Psychoneuroendocrinology 2001;26(2):165–73.

9. Schwartz EB, Granger DA, Susman EJ, Gunnar MR, Laird B. Assessing salivary cortisol in studies of child development. Child Dev 1998;69(6):1503–13.

10. Dombrowski MAS, Huang M, Wood C, Anderson GC. A successful and non-stressful method of collecting saliva from pre-term infants in the neonatal intensive care unit. Poster presented at the Biennial meeting of the Society for Research on Child Development, Tampa Bay, FL; 2001.

11. Granger DA, Kivlighan KT, Fortunato C, et al. Integration of salivary biomarkers into developmental and behaviorally-oriented research: problems and solutions for collecting specimens. Physiol Behav 2007;92(4):583–90.

12. Neu M, Goldstein M, Gao D, Laudenslager ML. Salivary cortisol in preterm infants: validation of a simple method for collecting saliva for cortisol determination. Early Hum Dev 2007;83(1):47–54.

13. Malamud D, Tabak, L. Saliva as a diagnostic fluid. Ann N Y Acad Sci 1993;694.

14. Schwartz EB, Granger DA. Transferrin enzyme immunoassay for quantitative monitoring of blood contamination in saliva. Clin Chem 2004;50(3):654–6.

15. Kivlighan KT, Granger DA, Schwartz EB, Nelson V, Curran M, Shirtcliff EA. Quantifying blood leakage into the oral mucosa and its effects on the measurement of cortisol, dehydroepiandrosterone, and testosterone in saliva. Horm Behav 2004;46(1):39–46.

16. Granger DA, Cicchetti D, Rogosch FA, Hibel LC, Teisl M, Flores E. Blood contamination in children's saliva: prevalence, stability, and impact on the measurement of salivary cortisol, testosterone, and dehydroepiandrosterone. Psychoneuroendocrinology 2007;32(6):724–33.

17. Masharani U, Shiboski S, Eisner MD, et al. Impact of exogenous glucocorticoid use on salivary cortisol measurements among adults with asthma and rhinitis. Psychoneuroendocrinology 2005;30(8):744–52.
18. Hibel LC, Granger DA, Kivlighan KT, Blair C, Investigators TFLP. Individual differences in salivary cortisol: associations with common over-the-counter and prescription medication status in infants and their mothers. Horm Behav 2006;50(2):293–300.
19. Hibel LC, Granger DA, Cicchetti D, Rogosch F. Salivary biomarker levels and diurnal variation: associations with medications prescribed to control children's problem behavior. Child Dev 2007;78(3):927–37.
20. Schwartz EB, Eppihimer L, Nelson VJ, Granger DA. Effects of sample storage temperature on the measurement of salivary analytes: degradation of testosterone, estradiol, and progesterone. Clin Chem 2005;51:A48–A49.
21. Whembolua GL, Granger DA, Singer S, Kivlighan KT, Marguin JA. Bacteria in the oral mucosa and its effects on the measurement of cortisol, dehydroepiandrosterone, and testosterone in saliva. Horm Behav 2006;49:478–83.

27

Crossroads between saliva diagnostics and salivary gland gene therapy

Bruce J. Baum, Ana P. Cotrim, Corinne M. Goldsmith, Fumi Mineshiba, Senrong Qi, Gabor Z. Racz, Yuval Samuni, Takayuki Sugito, Antonis Voutetakis, and Changyu Zheng

INTRODUCTION

Diagnostic accuracy obviously enhances therapy. Advances in biomedical research, while increasing our understanding of fundamental physiological processes and pathological events, facilitate the broader societal goals of developing more precise clinical diagnostic tests and, consequently, more effective therapies. There are numerous examples of such progress, including many now-commonplace, "simple" procedures, for example, monitoring of blood glucose level to enable convenient, patient-centered insulin therapy and the determination of bacterial sensitivities to allow specific antibiotic treatments for potentially virulent infections.

Particularly rapid advances in the detection of HIV, and in understanding lentivirus biology, have led to the development of novel antiviral regimens that have practically turned an AIDS "death sentence" of 1990 into a "life sentence" with a chronic disease in 2007. Similarly, as the etiology of many systemic single protein deficiency disorders became clear, improved diagnosis and therapy quickly followed, for example, a molecular understanding of hematopoiesis resulted in the availability of recombinant erythropoietin for treating anemias associated with chronic renal failure. Perhaps, some of the best examples of a symbiotic relationship between biomedical scientific advances, molecular diagnostics, and novel therapies are found in oncology. Thus, novel biologicals are being developed to target key molecules in a tumor-specific manner, for example, VEGF[1] and the epidermal growth factor receptor type 2 (HER2)[2] in breast cancer.

Gene transfer to salivary glands, so-called salivary gland gene therapy, has been shown to be feasible in numerous small and large animal studies.[3–9] Potential clinical applications of this therapeutic approach include treatments to repair salivary glands damaged either as a result of irradiation during the treatment of head and neck cancers or from the autoimmune exocrinopathy

Sjögren's syndrome (SS).[10–13] In addition, salivary gland gene transfer could prove useful in helping to manage various oral and upper gastrointestinal tract disorders, for example, irradiation- or chemotherapy-induced mucositis[14] as well as certain systemic single-protein deficiency disorders, such as a deficiency of growth hormone.[6,15] With all these conditions, improvements in salivary diagnostics will facilitate realization of the full clinical potential of salivary gland gene therapy. It is the purpose of this chapter to review briefly the status of such potential applications of salivary gland gene therapy and to speculate as to how advances in saliva diagnostics could lead to enhanced clinical benefits.

GENE TRANSFER TO SALIVARY GLANDS

The general approach used for transferring genes to salivary glands is comparable to that used for taking contrast x-rays (sialographs) of salivary glands. The orifices of a major salivary gland can be readily cannulated intraorally, but instead of infusing a contrast medium within the gland and taking a radiograph, a solution containing a vector that encodes the gene or genes of interest is infused.[3]

The vectors used for salivary gland gene transfer can be viral or nonviral. Viral vectors, for example, those derived from serotype 5 adenovirus (Ad5) or serotype 2 adeno-associated virus (AAV2), have the advantage of mediating highly efficient gene transfer to a salivary target cell in vivo. This process of viral vector-mediated gene transfer is known as transduction. Nonviral vectors, for example, plasmid DNA mixed with cationic liposomes, while currently unable to mediate efficient gene transfer to salivary cells in vivo, provide a much safer means of gene transfer than viral vectors. The process of nonviral gene transfer is known as transfection.

Successful gene transfer to salivary glands has been demonstrated in several animal model species, including mice ($\sim$20 g), rats ($\sim$300 g), miniature pigs ($\sim$25–30 kg), and nonhuman primates (rhesus macaques; $\sim$5 kg). In virtually all these studies, gene transfer has been accomplished using viral vectors. In rodents, the submandibular glands (SMGs) typically have been targeted for gene transfer, as cannulation is relatively easier than with parotid glands. In addition, the SMGs are modestly encapsulated, limiting undesirable vector spread.[4–6] In miniature pigs and rhesus macaques, gene transfer has targeted the parotid glands,[7–9] which are fairly easy to cannulate and well encapsulated. In all these animal studies, anesthesia was used only for restraint. For each animal species studied, there is an optimal volume of solution in which to infuse vectors. With murine SMGs, 50 µL is optimal, while for rat SMGs 200 µL is best. In miniature pigs and rhesus macaques, the optimal infusion volumes for parotid glands are 4,000 µL and 500 µL, respectively.

At present, one salivary gland gene transfer clinical protocol has been approved at all regulatory levels (http://www.clinicaltrials.gov/ct/show/NCT00372320?order=1). This is a phase I study (i.e., primarily monitoring safety, though with some efficacy measures) that uses an Ad5 vector (termed AdhAQP1) to transfer the cDNA encoding the human water channel protein aquaporin-1 to repair irradiation-damaged parotid glands. Preclinical studies in irradiated rats and miniature pigs showed that this strategy could return salivary flow to near normal levels, albeit transiently.[10,11]

STUDIES OF GENE TRANSFER IN ANIMAL MODELS OF SJÖGREN'S SYNDROME

The overall strategy in gene transfer studies related to SS is to deliver genes encoding immunomodulatory proteins locally to SMGs in a murine model of SS, the NOD mouse.[16] Similar to human SS, this mouse model develops an age- and gender-related (female) chronic sialadenitis with focal inflammatory infiltrates in the SMGs and marked reductions in salivary flow.[16] For these SS-model studies, AAV2 vectors have been used, primarily because, compared to Ad5 vectors, they are only mildly immunogenic and mediate transgene expression for more extended periods (>1 year in mice). Two genes, encoding human interleukin-10 (hIL10) and vasoactive intestinal peptide (hVIP), appear to be useful in this SS model (see Table 27.1). Both genes are thought to blunt proinflammatory and enhance antiinflammatory signaling. Administration of AAV2hIL10 to NOD mice before they developed frank SS-like disease, that is, a prevention strategy, prolonged normal salivary secretion and diminished the presence of focal glandular inflammatory infiltrates.[12] AAV2hIL10 also had some beneficial effects when administered to NOD mice after SS-like disease had developed,[12] that is, as a treatment strategy. AAV2hVIP was tested in mice prior to disease onset. This vector had no effect on the presence of inflammatory infiltrates in SMGs, but it was able to prolong predisease salivary secretion levels.[13]

While these initial studies provide proof of concept that local immunomodulatory gene transfer can be effective in managing autoimmune sialadenitis, these studies are a long way from clinical applications. The major problem in developing an effective gene or conventional therapy for SS is that currently

Table 27.1   Effectiveness of transgenes in preserving salivary flow and reducing inflammatory infiltrates in the NOD mouse model of Sjögren's syndrome.[a]

	8 weeks	16 weeks	20 weeks	FS (20 weeks)
Control	100%	~30%	~15%	~3
hIL10 pre	100%	~95%	~65%	~1.5
hIL10 post	100%	ND	~50%	~1.5
hVIP pre	100%	100%	ND	NC

[a]Percentages show salivary flow results that are normalized to predisease levels at 8 weeks. "Pre" means animals administered vectors (AAV2hIL10 or AAV2hVIP) at 8 weeks. "Post" means animals administered vector (AAV2hIL10) after disease onset, at 16 weeks. hIL10, human interleukin 10; hVIP, human vasoactive intestinal peptide; FS, focus score of inflammatory infiltrates; ND, not done; NC, no change from control. For details of these studies, see references 12 and 13.

there is no mechanistic understanding of the pathogenesis of SS. Since we do not understand how SS disease develops, we essentially are guessing at possible therapeutic strategies and, as indicated earlier, employing genes that are generally immunosuppressive rather than specific for a particular event or process.

The SS disease paradigm thus presents an excellent example of how improved salivary diagnostics could potentially greatly influence a field. At present, most patients diagnosed with SS have had the disease for a long while. There are no useful early markers of disease activity, which might not only facilitate earlier and likely better patient care but also might shed light on early pathways to target for therapy. The animal models available, the NOD mouse and others, while useful, are neither perfect models of the human disease nor free from problems.[17] That makes patient samples especially valuable. Typically, from each patient a minor salivary gland biopsy, salivary fluid, and serum are obtained: all rich resources available for diagnostic study. This disease is a diagnostic black box that would greatly benefit from intensive investigations using available sensitive molecular tools.

STUDIES OF GENE TRANSFER IN ANIMAL MODELS RELATED TO TREATING SYSTEMIC SINGLE-PROTEIN DEFICIENCIES

One ubiquitous application of gene transfer, with potential utility to many tissues, is gene therapeutics, the use of a gene as a drug.[18] In this application, genes can be employed in much the same way as recombinant proteins (e.g., insulin, growth hormone, erythropoietin), by following classical pharmacotherapeutic principles. However, instead of injecting a recombinant protein frequently, a gene can be transferred and theoretically will provide stable and regulated transgenic therapeutic proteins for extended periods. While many tissues have been examined for their utility with this application of gene transfer (e.g., most commonly muscle, liver, and lung), salivary glands present some distinct advantages. Salivary glands are (i) easily accessible, (ii) a secretory organ by nature and thus designed to produce and secrete copious amounts of protein, (iii) readily transduced in a fairly noninvasive manner, and (iv) not critical for life in case of the occurrence of a severe adverse event.

In our studies, we have often employed human erythropoietin (hEpo) as a model transgene. Physiologically, hEpo is produced in kidney epithelial cells and secreted by the constitutive secretory pathway. Constitutive pathway proteins are secreted from cells at the same rate as they are synthesized and in a nonpolarized manner, that is, they can cross the plasma membrane and exit the cell in any direction. Since most of the plasma membrane in salivary epithelial cells faces the interstitium (i.e., the basolateral membrane) we have sought to take advantage of hEpo's secretion via this pathway to deliver this therapeutic protein into the bloodstream.

A good example of our studies, as well as of the problems necessary to address for this potential clinical application, can be found in studies using an AAV2 vector encoding Epo (AAV2Epo) to transfer the Epo cDNA

Table 27.2 Secretion of erythropoietin (Epo) from male murine and macaque salivary glands after transduction with AAV2Epo.[a]

	Serum	Saliva	Ratio
Balb/c mice	~80	~0.5	160:1
Rhesus macaque	~1,000	~140	7:1

[a]Data shown are the average amounts of total Epo secreted into saliva or serum. In murine experiments, whole saliva was collected after transduction of submandibular glands. For rhesus macaques, whole saliva was collected after transduction of parotid glands. For mice, 10^9 AAV2hEpo particle units (pu)/gland were administered in 50 μL, that is, a multiplicity of infection (MOI) = 2 × 10^7 pu/μL. For macaques, 10^{10} pu/gland of a similar vector, but encoding Rhesus Epo were delivered in 500 μL, that is, a MOI = 2 × 10^7 pu/μL. Data based on references 4 and 9.

into murine and rhesus macaque salivary glands.[4,5,9] As summarized in Table 27.2, hEpo is secreted from SMGs of male mice almost entirely into the bloodstream, approximately 160:1 by total amount measured (serum: saliva; ~10:1 by concentration, not shown). These findings are consistent with what is known about secretion of constitutive pathway proteins from in vitro cell culture studies.[19] However, when the rhesus Epo transgene is expressed in male rhesus macaque parotid glands very different results are seen. When assessed by the concentration of Epo present, it seems more Epo is secreted into macaque parotid saliva than into serum (~4:1, not shown). However, when the total amount detected is considered (i.e., concentration × volume), it is clear that most Epo is found in macaque serum (~7:1). This distribution is significantly different from that seen in mice.

Since rhesus macaques are phylogenetically much closer to humans than mice, we would speculate that secretion of hEpo from a human salivary gland would most likely be more similar to what was seen in rhesus macaques.

One important component to any eventual clinical application of hEpo gene transfer to salivary glands involves the convenient and specific detection of hEpo levels in saliva for ease of monitoring. For example, it would be very useful if the relationship between salivary and serum levels could be defined, something which would allow hEpo levels to be monitored by patients frequently and easily. Excessive hEpo levels would be dangerous to patients (e.g., could lead to stroke), somewhat analogous to the situation of excessive insulin levels being dangerous for patients with insulin-dependent diabetes mellitus. Advances in the diagnosis and measurement of salivary components clearly would be helpful to this goal.

An important problem in using salivary glands for systemic gene therapeutic applications is that many therapeutic proteins are not normally secreted by the constitutive pathway, but rather by the regulated secretory pathway, for example, human growth hormone (hGH). After synthesis, regulated pathway proteins are sequestered into dense-core granules, where they remain within the cell until an external stimulus signals the cell to secrete. Following the stimulus, these granules fuse with the plasma membrane and release their contents.

Regulated pathway secretion is also highly polarized, occurring in a specific direction unlike constitutive pathway secretion.

Physiologically, hGH is secreted from somatotrophs in the anterior pituitary gland by the regulated pathway, which in this tissue leads directly to the bloodstream. In salivary gland epithelial cells, the regulated pathway leads to secretion into saliva, which for hGH would be biologically wasteful. Indeed, in studies with an AAV2 vector encoding hGH, most (~5:1) hGH was secreted into murine saliva.[5] If this hGH distribution is the same after gene transfer to salivary glands of nonhuman primates, then it will be necessary to develop strategies to redirect hGH secretion into the bloodstream.[6] Whatever the distribution of transgenic hGH between serum and saliva will be in humans, as mentioned earlier for hEpo, it will be helpful if hGH levels in saliva could be monitored in a convenient, sensitive, and specific manner.

STUDIES OF GENE TRANSFER IN ANIMAL MODELS RELEVANT TO THERAPIES FOR OROPHARYNGEAL DISEASE

This application of gene transfer to salivary glands is the most obvious, that is, getting the salivary glands to secrete a new protein into saliva that would provide therapeutic benefits in the mouth and upper GI tract. The principles are the same as for systemic gene therapeutics, only the disease targets and direction of secretion are different. Our original studies addressed the problem of azole-resistant mucosal Candidiasis, which approximately 15 years ago was a significant problem in severely immunosuppressed patients, for example, AIDS.[20] While azole-resistant Candidiasis is less of a clinical concern now, our initial goal and approach, that is, providing saliva with an antimicrobial protein that would be effective against a drug-resistant microorganism, is still valid.[21] In addition, considering this strategy is informative about the kind of problems that would likely benefit from improved salivary diagnostic methods.

Normally, human major salivary glands secrete a group of potent anti-Candidal peptides called histatins.[22] These small proteins are found only in humans and Old World primates and, in addition to their anti-Candidal activity, the histatins also possess antibacterial activities.[22] We posited that increasing the levels of histatins in the saliva of AIDS patients would be effective in reducing the azole-resistant Candidal species present orally. For this proof of concept study, we constructed an Ad5 vector encoding histatin-3, Ad-CMVH3. Normally, histatin-3 is secreted via the regulated secretory pathway into saliva. As indicated earlier, regulated pathway secretory proteins are efficiently secreted in the saliva of mice and rats.[5,6,14] Indeed, the vector-encoded histatin-3 was secreted into rat saliva at levels that could be useful clinically, and the transgenic histatin-3 also was capable of killing azole-resistant Candida species (Table 27.3).[20]

The significant problem encountered in this study was the lack of a convenient assay for monitoring histatin-3 levels. Histatin-3 is a highly cationic protein and, because of that characteristic, technically difficult to assay. Advances in salivary diagnostic methods doubtless would prove beneficial for this

Table 27.3 Production and activity of human histatin-3 (H3) from male rat submandibular glands after transduction with AdCMVH3.[a]

	AdCMVH3	Control
H3 mRNA	+	−
H3 Protein	+	−
Saliva H3 concentration (mean, µg/mL)	302	0
Activity vs *Candida albicans*		
FLC-sensitive	>90%	0
FLC-resistant	>90%	0

[a]AdCMVH3 (4 to 5 × 10^9 plaque-forming units/gland) was administered to submandibular glands. Glands and saliva were obtained and the indicated parameters measured. Control samples were either transduced with an irrelevant Ad5 vector or nontransduced. Protein production was demonstrated on cationic gels or by HPLC. *Candida albicans* species were either sensitive or resistant to fluconazole (FLC). Results shown are taken from reference 20.

particular problem. More generally, many transgenic therapeutic proteins secreted into saliva might be difficult to monitor with conventional assays because of degradation, aggregation with other salivary proteins, adherence to mucosal or dental surfaces, or complicating structural characteristics. Advances in the general field of salivary diagnostics (i.e., sample handling, methodologies) also will contribute to the solution of such difficulties.

In addition to the application described earlier, there are other potential uses of salivary gene transfer for augmenting saliva. One example of interest to us has been for patients who receive either chemotherapy or head and neck irradiation during cancer treatment. These individuals commonly develop a severe oral mucositis.[23] This painful condition, which affects all normal oral functions (e.g., alimentation, speech), can provide oral microbes with a systemic entry point and serve as a dose-limiting toxicity for the therapy. Currently, there are no fully effective treatments for oral mucositis. Theoretically, a transgenic protein, which could promote mucosal wound healing and could be secreted in saliva so that it could continually bathe the damaged tissue, would be beneficial, for example, keratinocyte growth factor (KGF) or interleukin-11.[24,25] Recently, and consistent with this notion, transfer of the murine KGF gene was shown to be useful for ameliorating acute hypoxic lung injury and enhancing survival in mice.[26] If a similar approach using salivary gland gene transfer proved useful, then having convenient tools for the measurement of salivary KGF levels would allow a simple way to follow transgene expression levels in conjunction with clinical assessments of efficacy.

CONCLUSIONS

Based on studies published for more than a decade, it is clear that gene transfer to salivary glands is feasible in many small and large animal models and is potentially of use for multiple clinical applications. These studies have been valuable for demonstrating proof of concept and for showing that the procedure of gene transfer to salivary glands with the approach described herein is safe and reasonably efficacious.

However, all the studies published thus far have used first-generation viral vectors that are not ideal. For example, these vectors can elicit host immune responses.[27,28] In addition, for almost all studies cited, the vectors used directed transgene expression continuously, versus a more idealized controlled expression.[29] In the future better vectors will be available, and these vectors, consequently, will minimize host toxic responses and permit stable and controlled transgene expression. Advances in salivary diagnostics will facilitate the development of salivary gland gene transfer by providing additional insights on pathological conditions, as well as more sensitive and convenient monitoring of the produced transgenic proteins.

Acknowledgment

The research on which this chapter is based is supported by the Division of Intramural Research, National Institute of Dental and Craniofacial Research, NIH.

REFERENCES

1. Schneider BP, Sledge GW Jr. Drug insight: VEGF as a therapeutic target for breast cancer. Nat Clin Pract Oncol 2007;4:181–9.
2. Geyer CE, Forster J, Lindquist D, et al. Lapatinib plus capecitabine for HER2-positive advanced breast cancer. New Engl J Med 2006;355:2733–43.
3. Baum BJ, Wellner RB, Zheng C. Gene transfer to salivary glands. Int Rev Cytol 2002;213:93–146.
4. Voutetakis A, Kok MR, Zheng C, et al. Re-engineered salivary glands are stable endogenous bioreactors for systemic gene therapeutics. Proc Natl Acad Sci U S A 2004;101:3053–8.
5. Voutetakis A, Bossis I, Kok MR, et al. Salivary glands as a potential gene transfer target for gene therapeutics of some monogenetic endocrine disorders. J Endocrinol 2005;185:363–72.
6. Hoque ATMS, Baccaglini L, Baum BJ. Hydroxychloroquine enhances the endocrine secretion of adenovirus-directed growth hormone from rat submandibular gland in vivo. Hum Gene Ther 2001;12:1333–41.
7. Li J, Zheng C, Zhang X, et al. Developing a convenient large animal model for gene transfer to salivary glands in vivo. J Gene Med 2004;6:55–63.
8. O'Connell AC, Baccaglini L, Fox PC, et al. Safety and efficacy of adenovirus-mediated transfer of the human aquaporin-1 cDNA to irradiated parotid glands of non-human primates. Cancer Gene Ther 1999;6:505–13.
9. Voutetakis A, Zheng C, Mineshiba F, et al. Adeno-associated virus serotype 2-mediated gene transfer to the parotid glands of non-human primates. Hum Gene Ther 2007;18:142–50.

10. Delporte C, O'Connell BC, He X, et al. Increased fluid secretion after adenoviral-mediated transfer of the aquaporin-1 cDNA to irradiated rat salivary glands. Proc Natl Acad Sci U S A 1997;94:3268–73.

11. Shan Z, Li J, Zheng C, Liu X, et al. Increased fluid secretion after adenoviral-mediated transfer of the human aquaporin-1 cDNA to irradiated miniature pig parotid glands. Mol Ther 2005;11:444–51.

12. Kok MR, Yamano S, Lodde BM, et al. Local adeno-associated virus-mediated interleukin 10 gene transfer has disease-modifying effects in a murine model of Sjögren's syndrome. Hum Gene Ther 2003;14:1605–18.

13. Lodde BM, Mineshiba F, Wang J, et al. Effect of human vasoactive intestinal peptide gene transfer in a murine model of Sjögren's syndrome. Ann Rheum Dis 2006;65:195–200.

14. Wang J, Voutetakis A, Zheng C, et al. Rapamycin control of exocrine protein levels in saliva after adenoviral vector-mediated gene transfer. Gene Ther 2004;11:729–33.

15. Kagami H, O'Connell BC, Baum BJ. Evidence for the systemic delivery of a transgene product from salivary gland. Hum Gene Ther 1996;7:2177–84.

16. Yamano S, Atkinson JC, Baum BJ, Fox PC. Salivary gland cytokine expression in NOD and normal BALB/C mice. Clin Immunol 1999;92:265–75.

17. Lodde BM, Mineshiba F, Kok MR, et al. NOD mouse model for Sjögren's syndrome: lack of longitudinal stability. Oral Dis 2006;12:566–72.

18. Felgner PL, Rhodes G. Gene therapeutics. Nature 1991;349:351–2.

19. Burgess T, Kelly RB. Constitutive and regulated secretion of protein. Annu Rev Cell Biol 1987;3:243–93.

20. O'Connell BC, Xu T, Walsh TJ, et al. Transfer of a gene encoding the anticandidal protein histatin 3 to salivary glands. Hum Gene Ther 1996;7:2255–61.

21. Martin JM, Green M, Barbadora KA, Wald FR. Erythromycin-resistant group A streptococci in schoolchildren in Pittsburgh. New Engl J Med 2002;364:1200–6.

22. Van Nieuw Amerongen A, Veerman EC. Saliva—the defender of the oral cavity. Oral Dis 2002;8:12–22.

23. Sonis ST, Peterson DE, McGuire DB, Williams DA. Prevention of mucositis in cancer patients. J Natl Cancer Inst Monogr 2001;29:1–2.

24. Dorr W, Noack R, Spekl K, Farrell CL. Modification of oral mucositis by keratinocyte growth factor: single radiation exposure. Int J Radiat Biol 2001;77:341–7.

25. Sonis ST, Peterson RL, Edwards LJ, et al. Defining the mechanisms of action of interleukin-11 on the progression of radiation-induced oral mucositis in hamsters. Oral Oncol 2000;36:373–81.

26. Baba Y, Yazawa T, Kanegae Y, et al. Keratinocyte growth factor gene transduction ameliorates acute lung injury and mortality in mice. Hum Gene Ther 2007;18:130–41.

27. Adesanya MR, Redman RS, Baum BJ, O'Connell BC. Immediate inflammatory responses to adenovirus-mediated gene transfer in rat salivary glands. Hum Gene Ther 1996;7:1085–93.

28. Kok MR, Voutetakis A, Yamano S, et al. Immune responses following salivary gland administration of recombinant adeno-associated virus serotype 2 vectors. J Gene Med 2005;7:432–41.
29. Wang J, Voutetakis A, Papa M, et al. Rapamycin control of transgene expression from a single AAV vector in mouse salivary glands. Gene Ther 2006;13:187–90.

28

Saliva diagnostics—a new industry

Stuart R. Smith, David T. Wong, and R. Michael Buch

INTRODUCTION

This chapter will consider the various challenges faced by researchers and industry in establishing saliva diagnostics as a routine part of health screening and disease diagnosis.

For many years, saliva has been viewed as having the potential to be a very important diagnostic fluid following pioneering work in the late 1960s indicating that salivary calcium is elevated in cystic fibrosis.[1] The number of diagnostic tests available today (Table 28.1) underscores the growth of diagnostic opportunities that capitalize on the attributes of saliva as a diagnostic fluid.

ADVANTAGES OF SALIVA AS A DIAGNOSTIC FLUID

Although the field is referred to as saliva diagnostics, pure saliva is rarely tested. Typically, resting or stimulated whole saliva, which will also include a variety of other constituents such as bacteria, gingival crevicular fluid, and cell debris is collected. There are many advantages associated with the use of whole saliva as a diagnostic fluid, and these have been a major factor in increasing the uptake of saliva testing. Advantages include easy noninvasive collection, avoidance of needlestick injuries, no need for a phlebotomist, and acceptability to those with needle phobias. The range of analytes that can be evaluated in saliva is also rapidly increasing.[2–4]

Key challenges that saliva diagnostics have had to overcome include familiarizing people with the process of saliva collection, measuring analytes present in low concentrations, and the development of methods to stabilize markers in the sample to avoid degradation after collection. The potential advantage of a saliva sample compared with a blood sample has been demonstrated by one of the authors since, at least in the case of oral cancer detection, salivary markers appear to be more robust than the corresponding serum markers.[5,6]

An appreciation of the potential value of saliva diagnostics has also been reflected in the increasing number of research publications in the area, and greater levels of funding and commitment from organizations such as the National Institute of Dental and Craniofacial Research (NIDCR).[7] In light of such

Table 28.1 Oral fluid diagnostics commercially available in the United States.

Purpose	Product	Markers	Supplier
General saliva collection	Omni-SAL	N/A	Saliva Diagnostic Systems
General saliva collection	Saliva Sampler	N/A	Saliva Diagnostic Systems
General saliva collection	Saliva Filter	N/A	Saliva Diagnostic Systems
General saliva collection	Saliva Sampler™	N/A	StatSure Diagnostic Systems, Inc.
Substance abuse	Intercept®	"NIDA 5" blood panel + barbiturates, methamphetamines, benzodiazepines, methadone	Orasure Technologies, Inc.
Blood alcohol	Q.E.D.® Saliva Alcohol Test	Ethanol	Orasure Technologies, Inc.
HIV	OraQuick ADVANCE® Rapid HIV-1/2 Antibody Test	HIV antibodies	Orasure Technologies, Inc.
HIV	Orasure® HIV1 Western Blot	HIV antibodies (Confirmatory Test)	Orasure Technologies, Inc.
Insurance and toxicology assays	MICRO-PLATE EIA	Cocaine metabolite, cotinine, cannabinoids, opiates, phencylidine	Orasure Technologies, Inc.
Hormones	ZRT Saliva Test	Estradiol, progesterone, testosterone, DHEA, cortisol	ZRT Laboratory
Substance abuse	SALIVASCREEN™ 5 Professional	"NIDA 5" blood panel	Craig Medical Distribution, Inc.

developments, saliva is taking on a more prominent role as a diagnostic fluid with a promise of even greater importance in the future.

APPLICATIONS

Saliva diagnostic tests have the potential to be used within a broad spectrum of applications encompassing population-based screening programs, confirmatory diagnosis as part of a battery of special tests, and monitoring the state of previously diagnosed disease. Each approach raises different challenges particularly with regards to the accuracy of the test.

Screening the entire population for disease to enable early diagnosis and intervention would appear, on initial inspection, to have significant appeal. However, this approach has not been successful owing to the lack of sufficient predictive values of the tests. The results of diagnostic tests only represent a snapshot in time, so the appropriate frequency of repeat testing also needs to be established. Sadly, it is often the people most at risk of a disease who are least likely to be tested. Programs based on screening the entire population are, therefore, not universally undertaken because they are simply not cost-effective.

No diagnostic test is perfect, and the current level of accuracy of tests means that inevitably some people with the disease will be missed (false-negative), and that some healthy people will be identified as having the disease (false-positive). The implications of false-positive and false-negative results are extremely important. When screening for a life-threatening disease, a false-negative will often lead to delayed diagnosis. This may result in a poorer prognosis and treatment that will be more complex and more expensive. A false-positive result will lead to considerable patient anxiety and a requirement for further tests, usually under the care of a specialist, to exclude the disease. These additional tests may be invasive, expensive, and expose the patient to an increased risk related to the test procedures.[8]

However, screening becomes much more effective when it is possible to target a smaller sample of the population at greater risk of having the disease in question (see Tables 28.2 and 28.3).[9] Hence for prostate cancer, the predictive value of a prostate-specific antigen test is much greater if the population sample tested is men over 50 and results are combined with those of a digital rectal examination.[10–13]

UTILITY OF DIAGNOSTIC TESTS

When considering the development of a new diagnostic test, its utility will be influenced by accuracy, cost-effectiveness, and ease of administration (convenience and acceptability).

Clearly, a diagnostic test needs to be accurate, but no test is 100% accurate. The ability of a diagnostic test to correctly detect positive and negative results is generally reported as its sensitivity and specificity. To evaluate a test's predictive value, it is very important to understand how many false-positive results and how many false-negative results are likely to occur. Even for very accurate tests, the predictive value is heavily influenced by the prevalence of the condition in the sample of the population that receives it. The ability to target a high-risk group (such as long-term heavy smokers in the case of lung cancer) can improve the predictive value of a test dramatically.

The impact of specificity, sensitivity, and the selection of a targeted patient population on the predictive value of a test is illustrated using a hypothetical example in Table 28.2.

Table 28.2 Impact of sensitivity, specificity, and low prevalence on predictive value.

	Disease +ve	Disease −ve		
Test +ve	9,990 (TP)	990 (FP)	All with +ve test (TP + FP) 10,980	+ve Predictive value (TP/TP + FP) 91%
Test −ve	10 (FN)	989,010 (TN)	All with −ve test (FN + TN) 998,020	−ve Predictive value (TN/FN + TN) 99.1%
	All with disease 1,000	All without disease 999,000	Everyone TP + FP + FN + TN	
	Sensitivity 99.9%	Specificity 99.9%	Pretest probability 0.1%	

Let us assume that a new saliva diagnostic has been developed for testing disease X, and that the method has a very high sensitivity of 99.9% and a specificity of 99.9%. If this test were applied to 1 million people where 1% (10,000 people) of the population has the disease, the following situation would exist. Since the test is 99.9% sensitive, it will correctly detect 9,990 cases of the disease out of the total of 10,000 (true positives: TP) and miss 10 (false negatives: FP). Considering the 990,000 people who do not have the disease (out of the original sample of 1 million persons), the test (with 99.9% specificity) will indicate that 989,010 are free of the disease (true negatives: TN). However, 990 individuals who do not have the disease are found to be positive (false positives: FP). This means that 10 people with the disease would have been missed and 990 people would have been informed that they had a positive test result when they did not have the disease. This gives a positive predictive value of 91% and a negative predictive value of 99.1%

If we target a sample of the population known to be at higher risk through simple criteria (e.g., age-related), we may be able to increase the proportion of the sample with the disease from 1% to, say, 10%. This means that many fewer people in the population would be tested, and of a total sample of 1 million people within the risk group, 100,000 people would have the disease and 900,000 would not. Our saliva test would find 99,900 true positives and 100 false negatives. Of the 900,000 without the disease, the saliva test would show 899,100 to be negative (TN) and misdiagnose 900 as positive (FP). Clearly, the sensitivity and specificity of the test has not changed, but even for a test with very high sensitivity and specificity (99.9%), the predictive value of the test has increased (positive predictive value 99%, negative predictive value 99.99%) as a result of more targeted testing (Table 28.3). The predictive values that are necessary for any test to be adopted would need to be determined on an individual basis.

The need to consider the cost-effectiveness of any new treatment is an important consideration. Generally, the greater the cost of a treatment or diagnostic test, the greater the expected outcome benefit.

Table 28.3   Impact of sensitivity, specificity, and high prevalence on predictive value.

	Disease +ve	Disease −ve		
Test +ve	99,900 (TP)	900 (FP)	All with +ve test (TP + FP) 100,800	+ve Predictive value (TP/TP + FP) 99%
Test −ve	100 (FN)	899,100 (TN)	All with −ve test (FN + TN) 899,200	−ve Predictive value (TN/FN + TN 99.99%
	All with disease 100,000	All without disease 900,000	Everyone TP + FP + FN + TN	
	Sensitivity 99.9%	Specificity 99.9%	Pretest probability 10%	

Saliva tests can offer a number of cost advantages because whole saliva collection is relatively straightforward and does not necessarily require specialist healthcare professionals, expensive equipment, or dedicated facilities. These same advantages make saliva a suitable fluid for self-collection.

The health economic argument in favor of a screening test becomes stronger if the test targets an important life-threatening disease, where early diagnosis using existing methods is difficult but where early treatment leads to much-improved prognosis and risk groups can be identified.

A test that is easy to administer has an advantage in enabling more rapid and widespread acceptance by health care professionals and patients. Uptake of a test that is used as part of a diagnostic panel to investigate signs or symptoms under hospital conditions is unlikely to be significantly affected by patients' attitudes. However, in most situations, where screening is involved and attendance is voluntary, tests that are invasive, painful, or embarrassing are likely to have a lower uptake than a convenient noninvasive test. Saliva diagnostics are ideally suited to address these issues. Saliva is particularly useful when observation of the sample collection is required, as is the case for illicit drug testing.

In addition to convenience for the patient, the burden on the healthcare provider should also be considered. The test needs to be appropriate for the chosen setting. For example, if the test is to be used in a doctor's office, the equipment should ideally be easy to store and simple to use with results available quickly. The analysis of the sample should be automated and the results clearly displayed. In the United States, the device would require a Clinical Laboratory Improvement Amendments waiver.

RECENT DEVELOPMENTS AND CONSIDERATIONS

There have been major advances in genomic and proteomic research and the application of this science to diagnostics. For example, the Tag-It device is a

DNA-based test to detect cystic fibrosis from a patient's blood or saliva. The TRUGENE HIV-1 genotyping test determines if a patient has a drug-resistant form of the virus. The AmpliChip P450 Genotyping Test is a DNA test that measures how quickly particular drugs are cleared from the body so that medication levels can be customized for individual patients.[14] Further developments in molecular-based saliva diagnostic tests will enable earlier and more precise diagnosis. An additional advantage of these techniques is that they can be miniaturized and put on small chips that can analyze very small volumes of fluid. It is also possible to amplify the signal to measure the relatively low levels of analytes in saliva.

For any new diagnostic to gain acceptance by the healthcare professionals who are expected to use it, there should also be an extensive data package of publications supporting the science.

THE FUTURE

A test that would enable patients at risk of a fatal disease to be screened frequently and easily would not only save lives but also have a dramatic effect on morbidity. There is currently considerable interest in a saliva diagnostic test for Oral Squamous Cell Carcinoma, and this has been discussed in other chapters of this book (Chapters 11, 12, and 17). There are numerous other oral and systemic conditions that could equally benefit from early diagnosis and treatment.

Recent scientific advances and the priority that is currently being given to research into saliva diagnostics mean that this area of research will continue to grow. More products will be commercialized and will build on what has been achieved to date with existing tests such as those for HIV. Given the current rate of progress, saliva diagnostics may yet achieve a key role in routine health monitoring. This may enable the early diagnosis of oral and systemic disease at a stage when intervention can be much simpler and more effective. Thus, salivary diagnostics will not only help save lives but also preserve the quality of those lives that have been saved.

REFERENCES

1. Mandel ID, Kutscher A, Denning CR, Thompson RH Jr, Zegarelli EV. Salivary studies in cystic fibrosis. Am J Dis Child (1960) 1967;113(4):431–8.
2. Hodinka RL, Nagashunmugam T, Malamud D. Detection of human immunodeficiency virus antibodies in oral fluids. Clin Diagn Lab Immunol 1998;5(4):419–26.
3. Kaufman E, Lamster IB. The diagnostic applications of saliva—a review. Crit Rev Oral Biol Med 2002;13(2):197–212.
4. Wong DT. Salivary diagnostics powered by nanotechnologies, proteomics and genomics. J Am Dent Assoc (1939) 2006;137(3):313–21.
5. Li Y, Elashoff D, Oh M, et al. Serum circulating human mRNA profiling and its utility for oral cancer detection. J Clin Oncol 2006;24(11):1754–60.

6. Li Y, St John MA, Zhou X, et al. Salivary transcriptome diagnostics for oral cancer detection. Clin Cancer Res 2004;10(24):8442–50.
7. Dove A. The hunt for cancer biomarkers. Drug Discov Devel 2007;10(8):16–20.
8. Marcus PM, Bergstralh EJ, Fagerstrom RM, et al. Lung cancer mortality in the Mayo Lung Project: impact of extended follow-up. J Natl Cancer Inst 2000;92(16):1308–16.
9. Wagner H, Ruckdeschel JC. *Lung Cancer*. In: Reintgen DS, Clark RA, eds, *Cancer Screening*. St. Louis, MO: Mosby; 1996:118–49.
10. Bretton PR. Prostate-specific antigen and digital rectal examination in screening for prostate cancer: a community-based study. South Med J 1994;87(7):720–3.
11. Catalona WJ, Richie JP, Ahmann FR, et al. Comparison of digital rectal examination and serum prostate specific antigen in the early detection of prostate cancer: results of a multicenter clinical trial of 6,630 men. J Urol 1994;151(5):1283–90.
12. Muschenheim F, Omarbasha B, Kardjian PM, Mondou EN. Screening for carcinoma of the prostate with prostate specific antigen. Ann Clin Lab Sci 1991;21(6):371–80.
13. Richie JP, Catalona WJ, Ahmann FR, et al. Effect of patient age on early detection of prostate cancer with serum prostate-specific antigen and digital rectal examination. Urology 1993;42(4):365–74.
14. Rados C. Genomics and medical devices: a new paradigm for health care. FDA Consumer 2005;39(6):34–9.

Index

Persistent or intermittent major salivary gland
enlargement, 190
PGE2, 161–2
Phenycyclidine (PCP), 177
Phlebotomy, 94
Phospholipase C (PLC)/inositol trisphosphate
(IP3)-dependent pathway, 15
Phosphoproteins, 85
Phosphoserine, 86
Pipette, 52
Plasma membrane-associated proteins, 22
POC testing, 136
Point-of-care (POC) diagnostics, 136
salivary testing, 261
Point-of-care (POC) salivary diagnostics, 265
Polyacrylamide gel electrophoresis (PAGE),
122
Polyethylene tubing, 48–9
Polymerase chain reaction/reverse
transcriptase-polymerase chain reaction
(PCR/RT-PCR) system, 112
Polypeptide peaks, 96
Poor saliva volume recovery, 271
Portable point-of-care medical diagnostic
systems, 111–2
Positivity rate of drugs in saliva and blood,
174
Posttranslationally modified proteins, 85
Potassium channels, molecular identity, 20
Predicate product, 248
Premarket approval application (PMA), 248–9
Primary acute infection with HIV, 145
Primary biliary cirrhosis (PBC), 201
Primary SS, 66, 191
Prostaglandins, 161
Protein components, proteome-wide study,
233
Protein expression, proteomics-based
approach for monitoring changes, 122
Proteomics databases, 235
Pyridinoline cross-linked carboxyterminal
telopeptide of type I collagen (ICTP),
164

Rapid point-of-care (POC) oral diagnostics,
165
RDx reader from AvagoTech Inc., 252, 252f
Reagent storage cartridge (RSC), 117
Real-time quantitative PCR (qPCR)
technology, 230
Receiver operating characteristic (ROC) curve
analysis, 115–6, 116f
Reference protein sequence database, 237–8
Reliability
collecting saliva from the minor salivary
glands, 53–5
flow rate data of PAR saliva, 44

flow rate data of whole saliva, 41–3
SM/SL saliva, flow rate data of, 51
RNA viruses, 143
RNAprotect Saliva, 70

Salimetrics, 246
Saliva collection
from older infants, 270
from the oldest-old, 271
imitations, 37
noninvasive nature, 71
techniques on salivary hormones, 271–2
Saliva diagnostics, 111
advantages, 288–9
applications, 289–90
challenges in testing, 119–20
Saliva pH, 169
Saliva stains, 226
microarray data on gene expression, 229
Saliva-based cardiac diagnostic tests, 115–6
Saliva-based caries assessment and risk
evaluation test, 265
Saliva-based diagnostics, technologies for, 114f
Saliva
antimicrobial mechanism, 33
as an alternative medicine in Africa, 106–7
correlaton with urine and blood, 173–5
as a diagnostic fluid, 98–101
detection of HIV, 266
digestive functions, 27–9
disease protein biomarkers, 126
functional value of, 109
global cultural views, 104–7
Greek traditions, 106
protective systems, 32–3
psychological aspects, 107–9
rheological (viscoelastic) properties of, 70–1
secretion, proteomic analysis, 21–3
steroid hormone levels, 264
treatment with penicillin/streptomycin, 275
viral infections, 73
Salivary carcinoembryonic antigen (CEA), 185
Salivary cortisol levels, 72
Salivary diagnostic applications, 263–4
systemic diseases, 264
Salivary diagnostic tests, 255–61, 289–90.
See also Oral fluid testing.
(FDA) review of safety and efficacy, 267
cost advantages, 292
utility of, 290–2
Salivary diagnostics, 259–60
barriers to wide-scale implementation, 260
HNSCC, approaches and applications, 181–2
medical/clinical applications, 266
microfiber array technology, 87
optical fiber array methodology, 87
Sjögren's syndrome (SS), 192–3